HAZEN AND SAWYER
Environmental Engineers & Scientists

Disinfection Alternatives for Safe Drinking Water

Principal Authors:
Edward A. Bryant
George P. Fulton
George C. Budd

VNR VAN NOSTRAND REINHOLD
New York

Library of Congress Catalog Card Number 91-45497
ISBN 0-442-31841-3

Manufactured in the United States of America

Published by Van Nostrand Reinhold
115 Fifth Avenue
New York, New York 10003

Chapman and Hall
2–6 Boundary Row
London, SE1 8HN, England

Thomas Nelson Australia
102 Dodds Street
South Melbourne 3205
Victoria, Australia

Nelson Canada
1120 Birchmount Road
Scarborough, Ontario M1K 5G4, Canada

16 15 14 13 12 11 10 9 8 7 6 5 4 3 2 1

Library of Congress Cataloging-in-Publication Data

Bryant, Edward A., 1931–
Disinfection alternatives for safe drinking water / Edward A. Bryant, George P. Fulton, George C. Budd.
p. cm.
Includes bibliographical references and index.
ISBN 0-442-31841-3
1. Drinking water—Purification. 2. Disinfection and disinfectants. 3. Water—Purification—filtration. I. Fulton, George P. II. Budd, George C. III. Title.
TD459.B78 1992
628.1′662—dc20 91-45497
CIP

Contents

Preface

This book addresses the current and emerging practices of disinfection as related to the comprehensive aspects of water treatment design and operation. Previously published references have concentrated on the use of individual disinfectants, on families of disinfectants, or on interpretation of the regulations.

The primary purpose of this book is to compile relevant information to assist the practicing engineer in understanding the significant disinfection issues that should influence the planning and design of new or modified disinfection facilities for both new and existing water treatment plants. Such facilities would provide efficient disinfection action while minimizing unwanted side effects.

The book informs the reader of current trends and regulations and describes the status of knowledge regarding the mechanisms of disinfection and the techniques for determining which chemicals are toxic and the relative accuracy of these techniques. Included are detailed descriptions of the ramifications of the use of disinfection and related processes, including chlorine, chloramination, chlorine dioxide, ozonation, potassium permanganate, ultraviolet radiation systems, membrane processes, air stripping, and activated carbon adsorption.

Under the new Surface Water Treatment Rule, microorganism inactivation by disinfection is now considered to be a part of an overall treatment process that may also include filtration. This book considers the role of filtration as a baseline treatment that can reduce both the extent of microorganism inactivation required and the formation of unwanted by-products. Two chapters are devoted to improving design and operation of existing filtration plants to achieve these objectives and include new design recommendations. The final chapter details the studies necessary to arrive at effective and economical water treatment plant designs for varying conditions of treatment needs, along with an emphasis on the need for sufficient flexibility in design to adjust to revised regulation requirements as more is learned in the future.

Acknowledgments

The following people contributed to this book:

James P. Black and Dennis O. Rester, American Norit Co., Inc.—Activated Carbon
Kenneth J. Ficek and Arnold H. Reidies, Carus Chemical Co.—Potassium Permanganate
Robert E. Fergen, Hazen and Sawyer—Air Stripping
Francis A. DiGiano, Professor, University of North Carolina—Activated Carbon
W. J. Masschelein, Brussels, Belgium—Chlorine Dioxide
A. David Nickols, Hazen and Sawyer—Ozonation and Granular Activated Carbon
François van Hoof, Antwerp Water Supply, Belgium—Genotoxic Evaluations
Alex J. Varas, Hazen and Sawyer—Chlorination, Chlorine Dioxide, and Ozonation
Ian C. Watson, Rostek Services, Inc.—Membrane Processes

The following people reviewed the book or portions of the book:

Barry Schwartz, Director, Water Quality Control and Treatment, Hackensack Water Company—entire book
Richard J. Bull, Professor, College of Pharmacy, Washington State University—Chapter 3
M. Robin Collins, Associate Professor, University of New Hampshire—Chapter 2 and Biodegradation Methods

Brian A. Dempsey, Associate Professor, The Pennsylvania State University—Chapter 11
Robert M. Gore, Hazen and Sawyer—Chapter 7
Raymond W. McIndoe, Consultant—Chapters 11, 12, and 13
Rip G. Rice, Consultant—Chapter 7

Some of the text in Chapters 11 and 12 is courtesy of *Public Works Magazine*. We would like to thank them for their kind permission to use this material.

Jillian Williams, Hazen and Sawyer, illustrated this book.

Disinfection Alternatives for Safe Drinking Water

1

Introduction

TRENDS IN DISINFECTION PRACTICE

In the past, the primary emphasis of disinfection was to control waterborne diseases through the control of associated bacterial indicator organisms such as coliforms. Two findings made in the 1970s have resulted in significant reevaluation of this long established disinfection practice. The first finding was that disinfection byproducts, formed in the reaction of disinfectants and certain source water organic matter, may be harmful to human health. The second finding was the discovery of newly recognized waterborne disease-causing organisms that could not be effectively controlled by the then accepted disinfection procedures. This latter finding made it apparent that use of discrete indicator organisms was not sufficient to provide proof of inactivation of a broad range of pathogenic microorganisms.

These new concerns require a high level of understanding of what disinfection is and how it can be accomplished with minimal side effects. In many instances, design studies will have to be carried out to result in treatment plants that will not only meet current regulations, but also be flexible enough to adjust to new regulations as more is learned.

Past Practices

Past success of disinfection of drinking water in the control of waterborne disease has been well established. With the use of disinfectants, epidemic outbreaks of diseases such as cholera and typhoid have been virtually unknown for decades. This almost complete elimination of these serious diseases, once a major cause of mortality, has represented a significant public health achievement.

Historically, chlorine has been the primary disinfectant employed by most water utilities in the United States. Chlorine disinfection has produced and continues to produce excellent results in terms of *kill* or inactivation of pathogenic microorganisms. Chlorine, a strong oxidant, has provided many additional water treatment benefits such as the removal of iron, manganese, and color. Under certain source water quality conditions, chlorination has also been effective in reducing tastes and odors. In treatment plant operation, the practice of prechlorination has provided major benefits in reducing algae blooms in open settling basins and in controlling biological growths in water plant filter media. In addition, where the natural organic content might inhibit or interfere with coagulation, prechlorination has often been effective in enhancing the coagulation process.

Disinfection Byproducts

Products or byproducts of disinfection occur as a result of reactions between a disinfecting chemical and naturally occurring background constituents or synthetic compounds found in many source waters. These constituents and compounds are more commonly known as *precursors*. Initial concerns about byproducts were mainly related to the possible carcinogenic potential of trihalomethanes (THMs) formed in chlorine reactions. Improved analysis techniques have since detected additional disinfection byproducts, and there are now concerns for health effects other than cancer.

Waterborne Disease

The newly recognized waterborne diseases include those associated with viruses and protozoan organisms. Others include more resistant forms of bacteria. Some of the new waterborne disease outbreaks have occurred in water systems designed and operated in accordance with the prevailing treatment regulations of the time. Investigations ultimately indicated that water treatment plant designs and operating protocols, established in accordance with the prevailing criteria, were sometimes inadequate for control of the new disease organisms. In other instances the outbreaks occurred in systems where clearly identified treatment facility and operation defects existed that did not meet those previous regulations.

Apparent Contradiction

In many ways, the remedies for resolving the waterborne disease and disinfection byproduct concerns appear to be in opposition. While reduced use of disinfectants is encouraged in order to limit byproduct formation, the concern about more resistant waterborne diseases discourages such reductions. Because disinfection is such an essential water treatment process, either these concerns need to be reconciled under revised disinfection approaches, or additional technologies need to be employed to achieve control over development and removal of disinfection byproducts.

DISINFECTION AND BYPRODUCT FORMATION

Definitions

Strictly speaking, disinfection may be defined as the inactivation of (pathogenic) microorganisms. The major and first disinfection step normally employed in the treatment of drinking water is *primary disinfection*. In essence, primary disinfection is intended to completely kill pathogens present in the source water, thereby preventing the introduction of such pathogens into the water distribution network.

A supplemental disinfection effect may also be accomplished by the separation and removal of pathogens in the filtration of drinking water. This is reflected in the latest regulations, which provide credit for the removal of these pathogens; credit varies according to the type of filtration employed and, more importantly, according to the diligence of operation. No matter what facilities might be provided, the potential for effective pathogen removal can be realized only in well-operated treatment plants. In the new concept, the filtration system, which often includes coagulation and preliminary solids removal, provides *baseline treatment*. Disinfection protocols are usually integrated into this baseline process train.

Usually a secondary or final disinfection step is added to the treatment train to maintain a disinfectant residual concentration throughout the water distribution system. The role of this disinfectant residual is to provide protection against subsequent microbial intrusion or regrowth following treatment. Sufficient disinfectant is added to the flow leaving the treatment facilities to ensure that some residual is available throughout a distribution system. The level of disinfectant addition must take into account the residence time in conveyance and storage elements of the distribution network as well as the possibility of disinfectant loss by degradation.

Principal Disinfectants/Byproducts

The more common disinfecting chemicals include chlorine, chloramines (chlorine/ammonia), chlorine dioxide, and ozone. Not only do these chemicals cause the inactivation of the pathogens in different ways, but each disinfectant reacts differently under various water quality conditions such as pH, temperature, disinfectant concentration, and the presence of other chemicals. Depending on the particular disinfectant, the basic mechanisms for inactivation include alterations in the permeability of the pathogen cell wall, interference with its cell enzymes or other key cell components, and oxidative attack.

Although chemical reactivity is a desirable trait for achieving disinfection, such reactivity makes disinfectants susceptible to other chemical reactions, some of which can form undesirable byproducts. Chemical precursors that react with disinfectants to form disinfection byproducts (DBPs) can come from several sources. In most cases, naturally occurring organic matter (NOM) is the predominant source of a diverse group of precursors. Originally, precursors for THMs were observed to be humic substances in the source water supply that occur as a consequence of natural plant matter decay processes. However, hydrophilic acids and amino compounds may also produce THMs in reactions with chlorine. Algal precursors—both the material contained within the original algal cell and the extracellular material that may be excreted—have also been identified as precursor candidates. Another source of precursors is the discharge of waste materials into the environment. Such wastes can include a wide range of synthetic organics.

As analytical methods have been developed and improved, an increasing number of byproducts (other than THMs) have been identified. In spite of such analytical improvement, limitations still exist. Although new byproducts continue to be detected, evidence suggests that potentially significant groups of byproducts still remain to be identified. In addition, areas of uncertainty still exist with respect to evaluation of health effects of already identified byproducts. As health effect evaluation methodologies improve, it is possible that the level of scientific concern for byproducts may change. Such changes may result in either an increase or a decrease of currently established maximum contaminant levels (MCLs) of various DBPs. As a result, there is a significant opportunity for change in scientific views of these issues over time.

Role of Chlorine

Because much of the original concern was for chlorinated byproducts rather than the byproducts of other disinfectants, chlorine first appeared to be the least attractive disinfection alternative. As knowledge of other disinfectant byproducts develops, however, it is possible that additional, potentially harmful constituents may be disclosed. Therefore, some flexibility is appropriate in planning for water system disinfection and the management of disinfection byproducts to allow for possible changes in understanding of the byproducts of all disinfectants.

As previously mentioned, most treatment plants must achieve two disinfection goals: disinfection to remove source-related pathogens (primary disinfection) and provision of a disinfection residual in the distribution system to prevent subsequent regrowth of harmful microbes (secondary disinfection). Among the available disinfecting agents, only chlorine is widely proven for achieving both primary and secondary disinfecting goals. If it becomes necessary to use alternative disinfecting agents to control the formation of undesired byproducts, it is possible that the overall disinfection process may become significantly more complex, requiring separate disinfecting agents to meet specific primary and secondary disinfection goals.

NEW REGULATORY APPROACH

Development

Under the Surface Water Treatment Rule (SWTR), the EPA has published disinfection regulations for treatment of surface water sources. The basic presumption in this rule is that the specific combination of disinfectant concentration and contact time (CT) will result in a certain degree of inactivation of the target pathogen groups. Many of these target pathogen groups are more difficult to control than the more traditional coliform indicator groups, which is the principal reason for the new disinfection requirements. In addition, a new approach is specified in the regulations that emphasizes the use of baseline water treatment techniques as part of a disinfection program. As a result of recognition of the importance of filtration in the removal of pathogens, requirements for turbidity removal are being implemented. Credit for removal of certain target pathogens is given to various particulate removal processes, depending on the particular mode of filtration. As a result, less primary disinfection may be required for treatment facilities that meet established particulate removal goals than for facilities with little or no particulate removal capability. The regulations also emphasize proper and careful operation of filters through adequate maintenance of filter media and operating procedures to limit filter breakthrough.

Before promulgation of the Surface Water Treatment Rule, the principal regulatory requirement for drinking water disinfection was maintenance of a minimum residual of chlorine and limitations on coliform count in the product drinking water. Some state standards also stipulated a minimum detention period between the time of chlorine application and the time the water enters the distribution system or the time the water reaches the first customer. These regulations were based on the ability to detect coliform bacteria, which served as an index or surrogate for the principal pathogens of concern at the time. Simple and inexpensive tests are available for the detection of coliform bacteria. Although coliform tests are still applicable for assessing some aspects of microbial quality, such tests are not indicators of the possible presence of viruses or protozoa pathogens such as *Giardia lamblia* cysts. Tests to monitor the presence of cysts and viruses are not only expensive, but are also difficult to use in water plant water quality–monitoring laboratory routines—hence, the development of the new treatment-based criteria stipulating CT and type of filtration.

Surface Water Treatment Rule

The EPA Surface Water Treatment Rule of June 1989 is the first regulation to adopt the new approach to disinfection. This SWTR is applicable to all water treatment systems that use surface water. The regulations are based on the assumption that all water systems that use surface water sources may be at risk, at least to some degree, from contamination by protozoan cysts like *Giardia lamblia*, as well as enteric viruses and other forms of microbial contamination like *Legionella*. Surface water is defined as all water sources open to atmosphere, such as rivers, streams, lakes, reservoirs, and other impoundments. Springs, infiltration galleries, wells, or other collectors that are directly influenced by surface water are also subject to these regulations.

"Directly influenced by surface water" means that the source is subject to pathogenic contamination from surface waters. The determination of such direct influence is to be made on a site-specific or case-by-case basis. Where primacy has been granted by the EPA, the state is responsible to determine which systems are subject to such influence and, therefore, are subject to the requirements of the SWTR.

A regulation regarding disinfection of groundwater sources not influenced by surface water contamination will be promulgated in the future. Deviations from the SWTR disinfection requirements may be expected for these sources. For instance, *Giardia lamblia* may not be considered to be a pathogenic contaminant of concern for groundwater systems. Viral inactivation would, most likely, be of concern in future groundwater treatment regulations.

With the elimination of requirements for removal of *Giardia* from groundwater sources, other treatment technologies not effective for *Giardia* removal may become applicable. Such other treatment methods may include ultraviolet radiation and the high pH of lime softening, both of which may be effective for virus inactivation. Potassium permanganate is another oxidant that may receive consideration as a disinfecting agent for some groundwaters.

Microorganisms and Other Criteria to Be Regulated

The intent of the SWTR is to control *Giardia lamblia*, viruses, heterotrophic plate count, and *Legionella* in addition to the turbidity of the treated drinking water. Turbidity requirements, significant in this rule, are discussed below. While the maximum contaminant level goal (MCLG) for microorganisms should be zero, EPA's intent is to approach the MCLG by requiring specific treatment technologies (disinfection and filtration) for surface water.

Appropriate Baseline Treatment

Table 1–1 is a list of potential baseline filtration processes along with tested water turbidity goals that must be achieved as part of the overall

TABLE 1–1. Baseline Filtration—Disinfection Credits

Filter Process	Maximum Turbidity[b] (NTU)	*Giardia lamblia* Removals		Virus Removals	
		(log)	(%)	(log)	(%)
Conventional: coagulation, flocculation, sedimentation, rapid rate (granular) filtration	0.50	2.5	99.3	2.0	99.0
Direct filtration: coagulation, rapid rate (granular) filtration	0.50	2.0	99.0	1.0	90.0
Slow sand filtration	1.0	2.0	99.0	2.0	99.9
Diatomaceous earth filtration	1.0	2.0	99.0	1.0	90.0
Total (including disinfection)[a]	—	3.0	99.9	4.0	99.99

[a] If the presence of *Giardia* cysts is estimated to exceed 1/100 l, greater inactivation is required.

[b] Maximum turbidity limits must be achieved in at least 95 percent of the measurements made. Turbidity of drinking water must never exceed 5 NTU.

Source: Adapted from Ref. 1.

microorganism removal process. Comparison of the removal credits indicates that EPA considers conventional treatment with coagulation, flocculation, sedimentation, and rapid rate (granular media) filtration to offer the highest level of pathogen removal. Conventional treatment with sedimentation provides an additional barrier of protection in pretreatment compared to the other modes of filtration, where particulate solids are removed only in the filter units. The variations in baseline treatment credits are related to removals of *Giardia lamblia* and enteric viruses. Each baseline treatment system must be supplemented with a specified level of disinfection to achieve the total CT shown in Table 1–1. Those baseline processes rated at lower removal effectiveness than conventional filtration must, therefore, be provided with disinfection facilities that are rated at higher microorganism inactivation levels.

Minimum Disinfection Requirements

Table 1–2 lists the relative CT values for various disinfectants required to achieve 1 log inactivation of *Giardia lamblia*. This table illustrates how the requirements for such inactivation vary according to the particular disinfectant and the pertinent water temperature. In addition, chlorination effectiveness varies with pH of the water. In actual practice, credit for baseline treatment removals would first be assigned. Disinfection needs would then be determined based on the difference remaining when such credits are subtracted from the overall removal requirements.

Table 1–3 shows CT values for achieving 3 log inactivation of viruses using various disinfectants. Detailed tables showing CT values for varying

TABLE 1–2. CT Values for Achieving 1 Log Inactivation[a] of *Giardia lamblia*

		Temperature				
Disinfectant	pH	0.5°C	5°C	10°C	15°C	20°C
Free chlorine[b]	6	49	35	26	18	13
	7	70	50	37	25	19
	8	101	72	54	36	27
	9	146	104	78	52	39
Ozone		0.97	0.63	0.48	0.32	0.24
Chlorine dioxide		21	8.7	7.7	6.3	5
Chloramines		1,270	735	615	500	370

[a] 0.5 log inactivation can be achieved with one-half the values.

[b] CT for chlorine varies somewhat with chlorine residuals. Values shown are based upon 1 mg/l residual.

Source: Adapted from Ref. 1.

TABLE 1–3. CT Values for Achieving 3 Log Inactivation of Viruses

Free chlorine:	2–9, depending upon temperature (20–0°C, respectively)
Ozone:	0.4–1.4, depending upon temperature (20–0°C, respectively)
Chlorine dioxide:	6.4–25.6, depending upon temperature (20–0°C, respectively)
Chloramines:	534 to 2,063, depending upon temperature (20–0°C, respectively)
UV:	36

Source: Adapted from Ref. 1.

removal requirements for the respective disinfectants may be found in Appendix E of the 1989 EPA *Guidance Manual for Compliance with the Filtration and Disinfection Requirements for Public Water Systems Using Surface Water Sources*. It is obvious that significant differences exist in the pathogen inactivation capabilities of the alternative disinfectants.

Disinfectant Byproducts

Table 1–4 shows the general classifications of disinfectant byproducts included in the 1991 Drinking Water Priority List by the EPA for future consideration. Existing regulations have established maximum contaminant levels (MCLs) only for THMs. Total concentration of these compounds has been regulated at 100 μg/l.

Investigations on the toxicity of readily identifiable byproduct compounds are being conducted on an ongoing basis. In addition to chlorine, these include studies of the byproducts of ozone, chloramines and chlo-

TABLE 1–4. Disinfectants and Disinfectant Byproducts on the U.S. Environmental Protection Agency 1991 Drinking Water Priority List

Disinfectants: Chlorine, hypochlorite ion, chlorine dioxide, chlorite ion, chlorate ion, chloramine

Four trihalomethanes: Chloroform, bromoform, dibromochloromethane, dichlorobromomethane

Chlorination/Chloramination byproducts (misc.): haloacetic acids, haloketones, chloral hydrate, MX-2 (3-chloro-4-(dichloromethyl)-5-hydroxy-2(5H)-furanone), *N*-organochloramines

Ozone byproducts: aldehydes, epoxides, peroxides, nitrosamines, bromate, iodate

Haloacetonitriles: bromochloroacetonitrile, dichloroacetonitrile, dibromoacetonitrile, trichloroacetonitrile

Other: chloropicrin (trichloronitromethane), cyanogen chloride

Source: Adapted from Ref. 2.

rine dioxide. It is important that flexibility to accommodate future modifications be a part of any planning.

While MCLs have been established only for THMs, tests to date indicate potential health effects associated with a number of other byproducts. (These are discussed in the chapters that follow.) In the design of disinfection systems it is important to be aware of the potential for adverse health effects of byproducts that may be identified in the future.

OTHER BENEFITS OF DISINFECTING AGENTS

Most disinfectants are highly reactive and have chemical properties that provide benefits in addition to the ability to inactivate pathogens. In water treatment, disinfecting chemicals can often be effective in the removal of color and unpleasant taste and odor. Disinfectants can also oxidize certain dissolved inorganic constituents to produce precipitates, which then are more readily removed in the filtration process. This latter oxidation property can be especially important for the removal of iron and manganese, which are of an esthetic concern and have secondary standards of 0.3 and 0.05 mg/l, respectively.

Other benefits in the use of disinfectants include enhancement of the performance of coagulation and filtration processes and the control of operating problems that may result from the growth of biological slimes or algae in both raw water pipelines and certain water treatment units. These ancillary roles for disinfecting chemicals are often important considerations in the development of a comprehensive approach to disinfection. In many cases, the extent to which these ancillary benefits are available can influence the selection of the disinfection agents.

It should be emphasized that the response of a water to disinfecting chemicals can be site specific. For example, in some treatment situations, certain disinfectants may improve taste and odor conditions. These same disinfectants, however, may increase taste and odors under other treatment conditions. Site-specific considerations can also influence the oxidation of inorganic constituents. It is, therefore, necessary to exercise care in the selection of disinfectant or disinfectants for treatment of a particular source water.

BIOLOGICAL STABILITY

In recent years, microbial growth or regrowth has been observed in water distribution systems where biologically assimilable substances have been available. While it is true that regrowth is inhibited where disinfectant residuals are maintained, the presence of biodegradable organic matter can increase the potential for regrowth in some parts of a distribution system where residuals may be depleted. This condition can be difficult to control by secondary disinfection strategies due to the inevitable reduction of disinfecting residuals in some locations of water distribution systems as well as in customer service lines. As a result, the use of biological processes has been proposed as a method for removing or reducing the biodegradable matter at the treatment plant.

Biological stability can be altered by disinfecting agents that react with naturally occurring source water organic matter to make it more biodegradable. Tests have shown that ozonation of certain source waters can generate a significant increase in biodegradable (or assimilable) organic content. Other disinfectants will also generate an increase in the biodegradable content, but to a lesser extent than ozone.

DISINFECTION BYPRODUCT STRATEGIES

Evolving regulatory concerns for disinfection byproducts have resulted in consideration of several alternative water treatment approaches. These strategies fall into one of the following categories:

- Use of alternative disinfectants that minimize the formation of regulated byproducts. Alternatives to free chlorine include chlorine dioxide, ozone, chloramines, potassium permanganate, and ultraviolet radiation.
- Removal of organic precursors prior to addition of disinfecting agents. Varying degrees of removal are possible with processes that employ coagulation, activated carbon, and oxidation with chemical agents. Membrane and biological processes also can provide effective removals in some treatment situations.
- Processes such as activated carbon and air stripping to remove byproducts once they are formed.

Locations of the disinfectant feed, special precursor removal technologies, and methods to limit contact times with disinfectant should all be considered to minimize byproduct formation. Reducing precursors and disinfectant demand prior to the disinfectant feed could be an important method for meeting otherwise difficult concentration goals for disinfection byproducts.

Among the general approaches, removal of disinfection byproducts following their formation is often the most expensive approach and normally would be used only if all other techniques prove to be inadequate. If the best combination of alternative disinfection and precursor removal techniques fails to keep the byproduct level within EPA requirements, it may be necessary to include some form of byproduct removal such as granular activated carbon contact with provision for regeneration or replacement. Air stripping might be considered if a large portion of the byproducts is highly volatile. However, this may not prove to be the case for products other than THMs, and this approach may not be adequate for removing the full range of disinfection byproducts being considered for future regulation.

DISINFECTION FACILITY DESIGN AND IMPROVEMENT PROGRAMS

The principal elements that may be involved in the conception, planning, evaluation, and design of disinfection facilities or other facility improvements are shown in Table 1–5. The actual background data and procedures employed will depend upon the particular evaluation and design situation. For new water treatment plant designs, all of the elements in the table might be included. In special situations, alternatives other than those shown might be included. Some operating plants may require simple evaluations to show that minor adjustments in chemical feed would achieve the disinfection objectives, while others may require more involved evaluations and treatment modification.

The requirements of the SWTR apply to treatment of all water from surface sources. Under this rule variances may be granted to exempt the filtration requirement for certain surface supplies that meet applicable surface water quality criteria. Apparent groundwater sources may be classified as actual surface water supplies as defined by identification criteria included in the SWTR. The first step in many treatment and design evaluation programs, therefore, would be to identify how a supply should be classified and, in some cases, whether filtration should be included in the water treatment process.

In the evaluation of the treatment performance of operating water plants, it is essential that the potential and actual efficiency of such operation be determined first. Many existing plants do not perform well simply because of inadequately maintained treatment facilities or because of unsuitable operating procedures. Such inadequacies must be corrected and optimum performances established before the appropriate design improvements can be selected.

The development of a disinfection program for either new or existing plants should include three basic objectives:

1. Adequate disinfection
2. Minimizing the formation of unwanted disinfection byproducts
3. Consideration of the full oxidation benefits within a treatment plant

TABLE 1–5. Elements of Disinfection Design and Improvement Programs

Element	Principal Features and Objectives
Source water quality	Basic water quality features such as turbidity, pH, organics (TOC, THMFP), coliforms, alkalinity, hardness, iron, manganese, color, taste and odors, temperature, and total dissolved solids.
Established federal and state standards	Surface Water Treatment Rule—turbidity MCL, CT requirements for filtration (conventional and direct filtration with granular media, slow sand filtration, diatomaceous earth filtration), disinfection byproducts–disinfectant residual (distribution system). Systems that do not filter—turbidity, coliform rule, CT for overall *Giardia* and virus inactivation, disinfection byproducts—disinfectant residual. All systems—miscellaneous constituents, MCLs, and other requirements of the primacy (state) agencies.
Baseline treatment	Capabilities and requirements of alternative methods of filtration and the appropriate methods to achieve particulate and dissolved solids reduction and other non–microorganism-associated drinking water quality objectives.
Disinfection alternatives	Disinfection byproduct formation and other properties of alternatives to be used as: *Primary disinfectants*—chlorine, ozone, and chlorine dioxide. *Secondary disinfectants*—(residual)—chlorine, chlorine dioxide, chloramines. *Nondisinfection oxidation*—chlorine, ozone, chlorine dioxide, and potassium permanganate.
Disinfection byproduct treatment alternatives	Changes in sequence of disinfectant addition to baseline treatment; changes in disinfectants; supplementary treatment additions to baseline treatment to achieve reductions in byproduct precursors or reduction in formed by products.
Bench tests, pilot, and full-scale tests	To demonstrate the effectiveness of individual process steps or treatment trains to produce drinking water quality meeting the established standards.

The last feature can be important to the relative cost of certain disinfection improvements. For example, ozonation would perhaps be the most costly disinfection alternative for many treatment situations. Proper application of the strong oxidation properties of ozonation, however, might make it possible to significantly reduce coagulant requirements or to eliminate the need for supplemental treatment facilities. Such savings in materials and facilities might reduce the overall cost of treatment sufficiently to make the use of ozone the least costly alternative. Moreover, at this time, known byproducts of ozone seem to be of less concern. This situation could, however, change with the development of more background knowledge.

Each water treatment requirement and disinfection situation will be different. When disinfection design alternatives are considered, final water quality goals must be paramount. In most instances, however, more than one disinfection arrangement will be able to achieve the established quality goals. Economic as well as functional evaluations should determine which alternative is the most advantageous for the particular application.

References

1. *Guidance manual for compliance with the filtration and disinfection requirements for public water systems using surface water sources.* October 1989. EPA 68-01-6989. Washington, DC: U.S. Environmental Protection Agency, Office of Drinking Water.
2. 1991. *Fed. Reg.* 54(9): 1470–74.

2

Disinfection

ROLE OF DISINFECTION

Until the turn of the century, waterborne disease was a serious, ubiquitous health problem. It continues to be a problem today in many parts of the world where proper water treatment is not available. The more prominent diseases that have long been associated with a waterborne route of transmission include those principally of bacterial origin: cholera, typhoid, salmonellosis, shigellosis. While these bacterial pathogens have largely been controlled by modern water treatment practice, other waterborne diseases can also be transmitted through the water supply route, including those of viral and protozoan origin. Long established examples of diseases caused by these other groups include hepatitis, a disease due to a viral pathogen, and amoebic dysentery, a disease due to a class of protozoan pathogens. While these two particular types of diseases have been recognized for some time, other virus- and protozoa-related diseases have been more recently recognized, as well as some additional bacteria-related diseases. Many of these newly recognized organisms have proven to be more resistant to water treatment practices than the more familiar waterborne diseases listed above. In addition, while bacteria may require hundreds or thousands of viable organisms to achieve infection, viruses and protozoan pathogens can be infective at doses as low as 1 to 100 organisms (1).

Some of the recently recognized waterborne pathogens have been associated with animal carriers, including the bacteria *Campylobacter* (2) and *Yersinia* (3) and the protozoa *Giardia*. Therefore, use of watersheds protected from human contamination may not provide complete protec-

TABLE 2–1. Major Microbial Disease-Causing Agents Identified in Water and Wastewater

Organism	Major Diseases
Enteric viruses (typical size range: 0.025–0.100 μm diameter):	
Enteroviruses	
Polioviruses	Poliomyelitis
Coxsackievirus A viruses	Aseptic meningitis
Coxsackievirus B viruses	Aseptic meningitis
Echoviruses	Aseptic meningitis
Other enteroviruses	Acute hemorrhagic conjunctivitis
Hepatitis A virus	Infectious hepatitis
Adenoviruses	Upper respiratory illness and gastroenteritis
Reoviruses	Mild upper respiratory illness and gastroenteritis
Rotaviruses	Gastroenteritis
Norwalk-type viruses	Gastroenteritis
Enteric bacteria (typical size range: 0.5–2.0 μm diameter):	
Salmonella	
S. typhi	Typhoid fever
S. paratyphi	Paratyphoid fever
Other Salmonella	Gastroenteritis
Shigella sp.	Bacillary dysentery
Escherichia coli (enteropathogenic)	Gastroenteritis
Campylobacter jejuni	Gastroenteritis
Yersinia enterocolitica	Gastroenteritis
Vibrio sp.	Cholera, gastroenteritis
Leptospira sp.	Fever, jaundice, meningitis, rash
Legionella sp.	Pneumonia
Mycobacteria sp.	Tuberculosis, respiratory illness, granulomas
Protozoans (typical size range: 2–50 μm diameter):	
Entamoeba histolytica	Amoebic dysentery
Giardia lamblia	Giardiasis
Balantidium coli	Dysentery
Cryptosporidium sp.	Gastroenteritis
Acanthamoeba sp.	Meningoencephalitis
Helminths (worms) (typical size range: 50 μm diameter):	
Nematodes (roundworms)	
Ascaris lumbricoides	Pneumonitis, gastroenteritis
Trichuris trichiura	Chronic gastroenteritis
Dracunculus medinensis	Dracontiasis

TABLE 2–1. (*Continued*)

Organism	Major Diseases
Hookworms	
Ancylostoma duodenale	Chronic anemia
Necator americanus	Chronic anemia
Strongyloides stercoralis	Chronic gastroenteritis
Cestodes (tapeworms)	
Taenia saginata	Variable symptoms
Taenia solium	Chronic illness
Hymenolepis nana	Gastroenteritis
Trematodes (flukes)	
Schistosoma sp.	Schistosomiasis

Source: Ref. 4, with permission.

tion against these diseases. Beavers have widely been cited as carriers of *Giardia*. However, dogs, sheep, elk, muskrats, and other animals have also been found to have the capability to transmit this disease.

Table 2–1 summarizes waterborne pathogens that have been identified in both water and wastewater, along with the associated effects. Of these organisms, the major concerns are for viruses, bacteria, and protozoa. Helminths (worms) can be effectively removed by water filtration and have not been considered to be a significant problem except in less developed areas where overall sanitation is a problem (4). However, one study reported the occurrence of nematodes in filtered water in some locations in the United States (29).

The significance of disinfection as it is related to the inactivation of organisms is discussed in this chapter. Depending on the specific disinfectant used, reactions with certain source water constituents can generate unwanted byproducts. (This byproduct aspect of disinfection is discussed in Chapter 3.)

Significant Pathogens in Treatment

Giardia in particular has become important for determining baseline water supply disinfection and filtration needs for two essential reasons. First, it has become a prominent waterborne disease that must be controlled. Second, out of the full range of known waterborne pathogens, *Giardia* is among the most resistant to disinfection, thereby making it difficult to inactivate. When steps are taken to assure *Giardia* removal, a more complete level of control is thought to be achieved over the full range of waterborne pathogens.

Giardia has proven to require highly effective water treatment for its removal. Unlike lower forms of microbes, such as viruses and bacteria, *Giardia* is a protozoa that undergoes changes throughout a life cycle. It typically occurs in water as a dormant cyst that is more protected from disinfection than the lower forms of microbial pathogens. To be controlled, these cysts must either be physically removed by filtration and associated coagulation/sedimentation processes or be inactivated by disinfection. If this dormant form is not inactivated or removed, it can transform to the active or trophozoite form upon ingestion.

Concern for *Giardia* and other pathogens requiring similar levels of control has resulted in the application of new, more stringent criteria or standards for disinfection and filtration. As a result, measures required for the effective reduction of *Giardia* can become a major determining feature in the design and operation of disinfection systems where this pathogen is considered to be a risk. However, it should be noted that, under certain conditions, other pathogens may require more stringent control criteria. For example, enteric viruses can be difficult to disinfect with chloramines and may have a higher disinfection requirement than *Giardia* in some cases. Therefore, the base pathogen group to consider when assessing chloramine disinfection is likely to be enteric viruses when this pathogen group is a possible risk. Criteria for enteric viruses can also affect ozone disinfection needs under some conditions.

Significantly, it has not been possible to identify the causative organism in many waterborne disease outbreaks. It is also probable that many such outbreaks have gone unreported and are unknown. Therefore, further refinements in criteria for control of waterborne disease are likely to occur in the future as more becomes known about causative organisms. This has been illustrated by recent outbreaks associated with another protozoan pathogen, *Cryptosporidium,* which is under evaluation by the EPA for future regulations. Like *Giardia, Cryptosporidium* is more difficult to control than most of the other known pathogens and has the potential for requiring further modification to established disinfection practices.

Proliferation in Distribution Systems

Most of the organisms shown in Table 2–1 are associated with human and animal feces and are initially discharged from these external sources to subsequently reside in raw water. A number of bacteria, however, can subsequently proliferate in water distribution systems under proper conditions. These include *Legionella* and *Mycobacterium,* as well as several others. In addition, several fungi have also been found to grow in distribution systems. Some of these naturally occurring organisms that can become established within distribution system piping can also act as opportunistic pathogens in humans. In other words, when ingested, these organisms can convert to pathogens when the opportunity presents itself. In the case of *Legionella,* the route of transmission is thought to be by water droplets (aerosols) that are formed by water heaters, certain types of air conditioning systems, and showers. Although the most severe form of this disease, sometimes known as Legionnaires' disease, is often fatal, milder forms of *Legionella* known as Pontiac fever also exist. The former form occurs less frequently, whereas the milder form is much more widespread (15, 16).

The potential for growth of naturally occurring pathogens in distribution system piping has resulted in additional criteria for disinfection beyond those necessary for simply achieving pathogen removal at water treatment plants. As a consequence, overall disinfection strategies must also consider the capability for effectively limiting the subsequent growth and regrowth of these naturally occurring organisms. This has led to the development of two categories of disinfection: primary and secondary. Primary disinfection criteria are intended to provide for the removal and/or inactivation of raw water source–related pathogens at the water treatment plant, whereas secondary disinfection criteria are intended to provide a disinfecting residual in the distribution system that will prevent subsequent growth of naturally occurring, opportunistic pathogens.

CHEMICAL PROPERTIES OF DISINFECTANTS

Chlorine

Chlorine can occur in several different chemical forms. As an example, chlorine gas, which is in the form of molecular chlorine, $Cl_2(g)$, rapidly reacts in water to form hypochlorous acid, HOCl, and chloride, Cl^-:

$$Cl_2(g) + H_2O = HOCl + Cl^- + H^+ \qquad (2\text{–}1)$$

In normal practice, the initial Cl_2 form of chlorine is not present except for the brief period of time required for this reaction. Reaction products such as HOCl and Cl^- are, therefore, the most prominent forms remaining. In the case of the reaction shown above, the portion of chlorine that is transformed to Cl^- is relatively inert and does not significantly contribute to disinfection or to further chemical reaction. Instead, the active portion of chlorine is the portion that is transformed to HOCl. This form of chlorine can be further transformed by other reactions so that the overall disinfecting effectiveness and reactivity of chlorine may actually result from a composite effect of several different forms. As an example, HOCl can form the hypochlorite ion OCl^- by the following reaction:

$$HOCl = H^+ + OCl^- \quad (2\text{–}2)$$

The reaction is driven to the right with increasing pH and reaches a point at which OCl^- becomes the dominant chlorine form at pH > 8. At pH < 7, HOCl is the dominant form; a transition region occurs between pH 7 and 8. This phenomenon has a significant impact both on disinfection in particular and chemical reactivity in general, since OCl^- is much less effective than HOCl as a disinfectant and is less reactive. Because of this, it is important to consider the pH influence when evaluating chlorine disinfection processes.

Chlorine gas represents just one of several alternative chlorine sources from which HOCl and OCl^- may be formed and ultimately become the active disinfecting agents. Other examples include sodium hypochlorite, NaOCl, which is also used as household bleach, and calcium hypochlorite, $Ca(OCl)_2$. Reactions of these chemicals with water are as follows:

$$NaOCl + H_2O = HOCl + Na^+ + OH^- \quad (2\text{–}3)$$

$$Ca(OCl)_2 + 2H_2O = 2HOCl + Ca^{2+} + 2OH^- \quad (2\text{–}4)$$

In both instances, HOCl and OCl^- become the active end products as in the case of gaseous chlorine. Therefore, disinfection and chemical reaction characteristics of these approaches are generally similar to those of gaseous chlorine systems in spite of differences in the original form of chlorine. The distribution of HOCl and OCl^- is determined by pH just as for gaseous chlorine. Some difference in pH control, however, may be required since gaseous chlorine reacts as an acid, whereas hypochlorite solutions tend to be slightly alkaline.

A common characteristic of HOCl and OCl^- is that chlorine exists within both of these chemical forms in a +1 oxidation state:

$$(H^{+1}O^{-2}Cl^{+1})$$

$$(O^{-2}Cl^{+1})^{-1}$$

Chloramines

In chloramination, ammonia (NH_3) is added and its reaction with HOCl is as follows:

$$NH_3 + HOCl = NH_2Cl + H^+ + OH^- \quad (2\text{–}5)$$

The result is the formation of monochloramine, NH_2Cl, a compound in which the reactivity and disinfecting capability of chlorine differs from HOCl and OCl^-, even though chlorine remains in the +1 oxidation state.

Chloramines formed by reactions such as these are frequently used in water treatment in situations where lower reactivity provides advantages such as reduced formation of unwanted byproducts and increased disinfectant life due to slower degradation and reaction rates. Although monochloramine is the predominant form of chloramine in most water treatment applications, two other forms exist: dichloramine ($NHCl_2$) and nitrogen trichloride (NCl_3). The chlorine associated with chloramines is distinguished from that available in free chlorine and is termed *combined chlorine*. Total chlorine is the sum of free and combined chlorine.

Unlike HOCl, none of the chloramine forms readily undergo dissociation with change in pH. Therefore, pH does not have the same effect on the chemical reactivity of chloramines, although reactivity of other chemicals in a solution and the susceptibility of certain organisms to disinfection may still be affected in varying degrees. Indirect pH effects are, therefore, still possible.

Chlorine Dioxide

Chlorine dioxide is another disinfecting chemical that contains chlorine. However, unlike HOCl, OCl^-, and chloramines, where chlorine is in the +1 oxidation state, a +4 oxidation state of chlorine is present in chlorine dioxide, and significant differences occur in its chemistry. For example, this form of chlorine does not substitute into ammonia and can take part in different types of chemical reactions. It also is a somewhat stronger disinfectant for the inactivation of most organisms than other forms of chlorine.

Ozone

Another disinfecting chemical, ozone (O_3), is a highly reactive and relatively unstable form of oxygen that is derived from the more common O_2 or diatomic (two atoms in one oxygen molecule) form. The actual formation can be envisioned as occurring in two steps:

$$O_2 + \text{energy} = 2O^{\cdot} \quad (2\text{–}6)$$

$$2O^{\cdot} + 2O_2 = 2O_3 \quad (2\text{–}7)$$

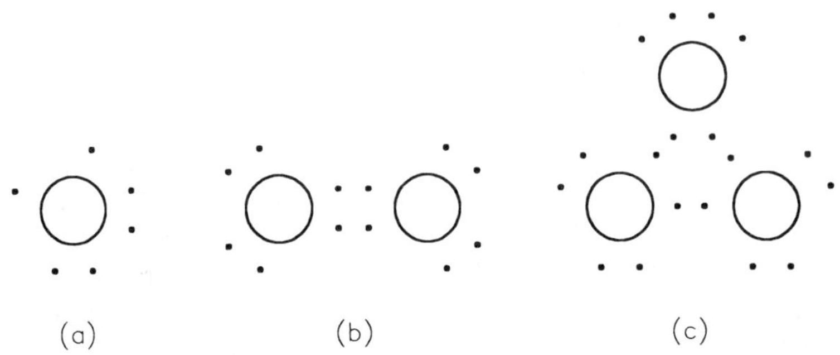

FIGURE 2–1. Forms of the oxygen atom and molecule: (a) oxygen atom (oxygen free radical); (b) oxygen molecule (diatomic); (c) ozone molecule (triatomic).

The first step in the reaction cleaves two pairs of electrons that are shared between the two oxygen atoms in O_2, leaving two unpaired electrons in the outer shell of the individual atoms, as shown in Figure 2–1. This is an unstable condition since outer shell configurations tend to be stabilized by maintaining four paired sets of electrons to achieve a full complement of eight electrons for each atom. In the single atom configuration, each atom provides only six electrons, two of which are unshared, resulting in a very unstable condition. The unpaired electron configuration is termed a free radical in chemical terminology. The dot in $O^{\cdot}$ represents this unpaired electron phenomenon and is used to represent free radical compounds.

The introduction of free radical chemistry into ozonation can have a significant effect on its overall chemistry. For example, ozone can form uncharged hydroxyl radicals ($OH^{\cdot}$), which are even more reactive than ozone itself. Formation of these radicals tends to be encouraged as pH is increased and leads to a more rapid rate of ozone degradation because of the higher reactivity. Therefore, pH has a significant effect on the capability for maintaining an ozone residual over a specified period of time.

MECHANISMS OF DISINFECTION

Although the general effects of disinfectants on bacteria and other organisms are known, the precise mechanisms are not as firmly established. Even the mechanisms by which chlorine kills microorganisms are not firmly understood in spite of its widespread use as a disinfectant since the early 1900s (5). A review in 1980 by the Safe Drinking Water Committee of the National Academy of Science (6) indicated that HOCl can affect bacteria by altering the permeability of the cell wall in a manner that disrupts cell function. However, a subsequent study indicated that gross damage to the cell wall may not occur except at extremely high dosages, although damage to an inner cytoplasmic membrane may take place (25). Some studies (6, 7) have noted that chlorine may act through interference with certain enzymes such as those with sulfhydryl groups (—SH). Damage to cell DNA has been reported as yet another mechanism. A recent evaluation indicates that chlorine is very reactive with a wide range of nucleic acids such as DNA and amino acids similar to those found in proteins that are responsible for enzyme function and cell structure. It is, therefore, apparent that a number of potential chlorine disinfection pathways exist.

Less information is available about the inactivation of bacteria with chloramines. A review of this information by the Safe Drinking Water Committee in 1980 suggested that chloramine inactivation of bacteria may be due to reactions with enzymes, although effects on nucleic acids such as DNA were also thought to be possible (6). Subsequent study by Jacangelo et al. (7, 25), indicates that chloramines do not readily react with nucleic acids and DNA. Instead, they are more likely to participate in reactions such as those with sulfhydryl groups found in enzymes, although other factors may be involved (25). Significantly, some chloramine reactions with sulfhydryl groups may be reversible unless an adequate chloramine dose is provided, thereby raising the possibility of regrowth in situations where the residual is lost. Moreover, bacteria can contain a large number of sulfhydryl groups thereby requiring multiple reactions before a cell can be fully inactivated (6). All of these factors may contribute to a lower chloramine disinfecting capability for many organisms.

Chlorine dioxide is also thought to be capable of affecting bacterial enzyme functions, more specifically those associated with synthesis of proteins. Ozone, on the other hand, is thought to exert its strong oxidizing capability to achieve disinfection by disrupting the function of the bacterial cell membrane (6), although enzyme and other internal cell interactions are also possible (24). In general, both ozone and chlorine dioxide have been observed to be very strong disinfectants.

The effect of disinfectants on viruses is less well understood than the disinfection of bacteria. Viruses are lower forms of organisms that are generally comprised of a protective protein coating that surrounds a strand of nucleic acid (i.e., DNA or RNA). Essentially, viruses are parasites that rely on a host organism for the synthesis reactions needed to form new viral particles. Unlike bacteria, viruses do not appear as susceptible to inactivation through pathways such as those involving sulfhydryl groups. The lack of this disinfection pathway may be responsible for the relative ineffectiveness of chloramines for disinfecting viruses (7). In contrast, free chlorine has a greater array of disinfection pathways, some of which are effective for disinfecting viruses. Because of these conditions, the use of coliforms and other bacterial indicator organisms, which are effectively disinfected by both chlorine and chloramine, must be applied with some caution when assessing disinfection of viruses.

With respect to viral disinfection by other agents, ozone is thought to achieve viral disinfection through oxidative attack of the protective protein coating (6); possible interactions with DNA or RNA may be a factor as well (24). Little information is available on the specific mechanisms for disinfection by chlorine dioxide (6), although it has been observed to be an effective viricide.

Protozoan pathogens are a higher order of microorganism that can take on different forms in different stages throughout a life cycle. These may include a dormant cyst stage that can excystate and form an active pathogen when it encounters the proper condition in the host animal. Although the active stage may be susceptible to disinfection, the cyst stage, which is often the initial infective agent, may not be readily disinfected. This has proved to be the case for both *Giardia* and *Cryptosporidium,* two protozoan species that have become of concern as waterborne pathogens. The cyst stages of both of these protozoan pathogens have proved to be less susceptible to inactivation by free chlorine than other pathogen categories. Also, coliform bacteria have proved to be poor indicators of disinfection of these cysts, and disease outbreaks have occurred in cases where coliform criteria have been met.

DISINFECTION KINETICS

The rate of disinfection determines the reduction in the quantity of pathogenic organisms that occurs in a given time of contact. Relationships that define these rates form the basis for selecting disinfection dose and contact time. The following empirical relationship, commonly referred to as Chick's law, has proven to be a convenient method for characterizing the decay patterns of organisms during disinfection.

$$dN/dt = -kN \qquad (2\text{–}8)$$

In this expression, N is the number of viable organisms that remain after exposure to a disinfectant for a time of contact, t. The negative sign is an indication of a decrease in the number of organisms over time. For a given organism, the rate coefficient, k, can vary with water quality factors. This coefficient defines the rate of organism inactivation over time.

Under a defined set of conditions that result in a constant value for k, integration of the above equation yields the following relationship:

$$\ln N/N_0 = -kt \qquad (2\text{–}9)$$

where N_0 is the initial number of viable organisms. The rate coefficient k can be redefined to incorporate the effect of a specified disinfectant concentration, C.

$$k = k'C^n \tag{2–10}$$

In this expression, n is a constant exponent term and k' is a revised coefficient. Using this modification, Chick's law can be rewritten as follows:

$$\ln N/N_0 = -k'C^n t \tag{2–11}$$

or

$$\log N/N_0 = \frac{-k'C^n t}{2.3} \tag{2–12}$$

These expressions can be further rearranged to calculate the level of $C^n t$ required to achieve the objective for N/N_0:

$$C^n t = \frac{-1}{k'} \ln N/N_0 = \frac{-2.3}{k'} \log N/N_0 \tag{2–13}$$

Based on this modified relationship, variations in log N/N_0 can be related to variations in $C^n t$. It is this relationship that forms the basis for CT disinfection criteria that have been developed by the EPA for regulation of disinfection practices in drinking water. (The EPA has chosen to use T for time in spite of the traditional scientific use of t to denote time and T to denote temperature.)

The coefficient n can have a significant influence on the characteristics of the decay relationship. The simplest relationship occurs when $n = 1$. In this case, the logarithm of the decay ratio N/N_0 is proportional only to CT, and it is not necessary to specify individual values for C and T. For cases where n is not equal to 1, C and T must be specified individually in order to fully define the relationship. Where n is greater than 1, disinfectant concentration strongly influences the decay rate and the disinfection effectiveness tends to be significantly reduced at lower disinfectant levels. Conversely, if n is less than 1, reaction time becomes the more important factor for pathogen inactivation (5).

It should be noted that the rate coefficient, k', is specific to a given organism and can vary as a result of changes in temperature and water quality factors such as pH. In fact, pH can affect both the chemistry of the disinfecting agent as well as the survival rate of an organism. Typically, when the pH is less than 6 or greater than 8, enteric pathogens exhibit an increased rate of die-off (1). Therefore, these and other effects of significance must be taken into account. Decay rates can also be affected by interfering factors such as the presence of particulate matter that might protect organisms from exposure to the disinfectant. As such, solids removal can become a consideration for achieving a desired decay rate.

Although the Chick's law CT relationships presented here are the most recognized approach for characterizing disinfection rates, several other modeling approaches are available. In some cases these may be more appropriate than Chick's law (8). For example, CT relationships may not characterize the multiple reactions that appear to be required for inactivation when monochloramine is applied for disinfection of bacteria (7). Hoff (9) acknowledges some of the difficulties in applying CT relationships under Chick's law for extrapolation to regulatory criteria. As a consequence of the uncertainties, he indicates that a cautious and conservative approach is appropriate for setting CT criteria.

EFFECT OF PARTICULATE REMOVAL PROCESSES

Although not specifically designed for the purpose, conventional coagulation/filtration and other particulate removal processes can have an important role in removing pathogens. These processes can play important roles in either supplementing or assisting the disinfection process as a result of the following phenomena and can be particularly important for providing an overall strategy for control of pathogens that are somewhat resistant to disinfecting agents:

- Removal of particulate matter that may provide a degree of protection for pathogens against disinfectants.
- Removal of aggregates of microbes that may be protected to a greater degree than a single microbe.
- Supplemental removal of pathogenic organisms, thereby reducing the level of removal required in the disinfection step.

While these roles have not always been widely acknowledged, conventional particulate removal processes have long been established as important in the control of waterborne disease. In the early 1890s, water filtration was observed to markedly reduce the incidence of typhoid fever (10). Much of this reduction occurred prior to the widespread use of chlorine, which achieved an additional level of control over the proliferation of waterborne disease in general. Even though the practice of chlorination continued, eventually to become the primary focus of disinfection, there have been suggestions of the importance of particulate removal processes. For example, in 1962, Hudson presented data that suggested a correlation between effective turbidity removal and reduction in virus-related diseases (11). His observations indicated that low virus disease rates occurred in cities where operation was oriented towards the highest possible turbidity removal as opposed to just meeting regulatory criteria for such removals.

Recently, waterborne outbreaks caused by pathogens such as *Giardia* and *Cryptosporidium* have underscored the importance of proper filtration. These pathogens are more resistant to the action of disinfectants, placing an increased emphasis on the need for particulate removal processes as a supplement to disinfection. Research has indicated that *Giardia* cysts can be effectively reduced in number by filtration processes (12, 13). Filtration also appears to be capable of reducing the levels of *Cryptosporidium,* but less is known about its adequacy for effective control of this disease (17).

PRIMARY DISINFECTION

The goal of the primary disinfection process is to destroy or inactivate pathogenic organisms found in the source water. Primary disinfecting agents are summarized in Table 2–2 based on a review prepared in 1980 by the Safe Drinking Water Committee of the National Academy of Science. As a result of this review, free chlorine, chlorine dioxide, and ozone are regarded as having the greatest potential for primary disinfecting agents. Because of its widespread use, chloramines were also evaluated in detail. Chloramines were found, however, to have weak disinfecting properties for *Giardia* and were thought to be particularly ineffective for inactivating enteric viruses. Their chief value was thought to be as a secondary disinfecting agent to inhibit aftergrowth of *Legionella* and other microbes that might grow in the distribution system.

Other disinfecting agents were also reviewed, but less information was available at that time. As more becomes known about some of the other disinfecting agents, there may be greater acceptance of their role for primary disinfectants under certain conditions. For example, recent work has been done on the disinfecting capability of potassium permanganate (see Chapter 8). Design of ultraviolet (UV) radiation equipment has improved, and more operating experience has been obtained since the 1980 review. The UV technique, while not currently considered adequate for disinfection of certain protozoan pathogens such as *Giardia*, may be ap-

TABLE 2–2. 1980 Evaluation of Primary Disinfecting Capabilities by the Safe Drinking Water Committee of the National Research Council

Disinfection Agent	Suitability as Inactivating Agent	Limitations	Suitability for Primary Disinfection[a]
Chlorine	Yes	Efficacy decreases with increasing pH; affected by ammonia or organic nitrogen	Yes
Ozone	Yes	On-site generation required; no residual; other disinfectant needed for residual	Yes
Chlorine dioxide	Yes	On-site generation required; interim MCL 1.0 mg/l	Yes
Iodine	Yes	Biocidal activity sensitive to pH	No
Bromine	Yes	Lack of technological experience; activity may be pH sensitive	No
Chloramines	No	Mediocre bactericide; poor virucide	No[b]
Ferrate	Yes	Moderate bactericide; good virucide; residual unstable; lack of technological experience	No
High pH conditions	No	Poor biocide	No
Hydrogen peroxide	No	Poor biocide	No
Ionizing radiation	Yes	Lack of technological experience	No
Potassium permanganate	No	Poor biocide	No
Silver	No	Poor biocide; MCL 0.05 mg/l	No
UV light	Yes	Adequate biocide; no residual; use limited by equipment maintenance considerations	No

[a] This evaluation relates solely to the suitability for controlling infectious disease transmission.

[b] Chloramines may have use as a secondary disinfectant in the distribution system in view of their persistence.

Source: Reprinted from "Drinking Water and Public Health," 1980, with permission from the National Academy Press, Washington, DC.

propriate under conditions where *Giardia* is not thought to represent a risk, and it has been found to be effective for control of enteric viruses under appropriate conditions (12).

The EPA is engaged in setting disinfecting criteria for two separate categories of water supply: surface waters and groundwaters. Under the Suface Water Treatment Rule, criteria have been developed using *Giardia* and enteric viruses as the most restrictive pathogen categories. These pathogens were selected because they tend to be more resistant to disinfection than most other pathogens encountered in these water sources.

The Groundwater Treatment Rule has not been developed. A major decision in establishing this rule will be the selection of pathogen categories to be included. The particular pathogen categories selected will control the disinfection methods permitted. For example, if *Giardia* is not thought to be a concern in groundwater, alternative disinfecting agents such as UV radiation may prove to be effective for primary disinfection for the remaining pathogen categories. This alternative could be of particular value for certain groundwater systems that would otherwise exert a high demand for chlorine, chlorine dioxide, and ozone, thereby resulting in a high cost of disinfection. An indication of its effectiveness for removal of enteric viruses is provided in the EPA *Guidance Manual for Compliance with the Filtration and Disinfection Requirements for Public Water Systems Using Surface Water Sources* (12).

CT Criteria for Primary Disinfection

Using Chick's law (Equations 2–8 through 2–13) as a basis, the EPA has developed CT criteria for the Surface Treatment Rule. Table 2–3 shows criteria for 99.9 percent *Giardia* removal. Several water quality factors influence disinfection effectiveness, as reflected in this table. Temperature has an effect on disinfection rates; for most microorganisms, disinfection occurs at higher rates (i.e., lower CT) as water temperature is increased. With free chlorine, an increase in the required CT for *Giardia* inactivation occurs as pH is increased. This corresponds to increases in the dissociation of the more effective hypochlorous acid, HOCl, to form the less effective hypochlorite ion, OCl^-, as described by Equation 2–2.

It should be emphasized that CT values shown in Table 2–3 for free chlorine are for a residual concentration of 2.0 mg/l. In the case of chlorine, CT criteria also vary with chlorine concentration, indicating that the

TABLE 2–3. CT Values for Achieving 99.9 Percent Inactivation of *Giardia lamblia*[a]

		Temperature			
	pH	0.5°C	5°C	10°C	15°C
Free chlorine[b]	6	165	116	87	58
	7	236	165	124	83
	8	346	243	182	122
	9	500	353	265	177
Ozone	6–9	2.9	1.9	1.43	0.95
Chlorine dioxide	6–9	63	26	23	19
Chloramines	6–9	3,800	2,200	1,850	1,500

[a] Criteria for enteric virus disinfection are somewhat less restrictive. Also, credit is given to filtration processes for different degrees of removal of *Giardia* and viruses. In these cases, disinfecting agents are required to achieve an adjusted CT.

[b] CT levels will vary depending on concentration of free chlorine. Levels indicated are for 2.0 mg/l free chlorine. CT levels for different free chlorine concentrations are specified in tables in the proposed rule.

Source: Adapted from Ref. 12.

value of the exponent, n, in the Chick's law relationship shown in Equation 2–13 deviates significantly from 1. Therefore, appropriate adjustments are necessary for different concentrations. Additional information is available on specific requirements in the U.S. EPA *Guidance Manual for Compliance with the Filtration and Disinfection Requirements for Public Water Systems Using Surface Water Sources* (12).

Evaluation of Contact Time

An important factor for establishing compliance with CT criteria is the actual distribution of contact times within a system. For pipelines, where flow is somewhat confined and the potential for short-circuiting is limited, time of contact can reasonably be computed based on flow rate and pipe volume. Long-term experience has shown, however, that for many treatment structures and storage tanks, short-circuiting of portions of the flow can occur. To account for these effects, EPA has developed criteria based on tracer tests for evaluating contact time distributions under procedures prescribed in the *Guidance Manual for Compliance with the Filtration and Disinfection Requirements for Public Water Systems Using Surface Water Sources* (12). The recommended basis for determining allowable contact time under these criteria corresponds to a time of retention that can be achieved by 90 percent of the flow. This is sometimes referred to as

T_{10}, since a 10 percent portion of the flow will pass through the structure or short circuit in less time. A summary of the prescribed test is included in Chapter 13.

Note that the prescribed EPA basis of evaluation is substantially more conservative than the use of calculated contact times. Basin configuration is extremely important; considerable variation can occur with different basin arrangements. This is illustrated by the fact that unbaffled basins are estimated to have a T_{10} of only 10 percent of the calculated contact time, whereas this ratio varies upwards with the degree of baffling provided in other structures. For example, baffled basins with an element of plug flow are estimated to have T_{10} values of 30 to 70 percent of the calculated hydraulic retention times (HRT) (12).

Approaches to consider for improving disinfection time of contact include providing characteristics that increase the tendency towards plug flow and decrease the tendency for short-circuiting. In many cases, it is appropriate to take steps to improve flow patterns by providing baffles in tankage in order to minimize short-circuiting. Basin and tankage inlet and outlet conditions also are important considerations to attain the desired flow patterns.

Storage tanks and clear wells often require the capability for an extreme degree of drawdown in order to function in the intended manner. Storage provides the fill and draw capability to reduce pumping variations. This tends to minimize the volume that can be reliably made available for contact times. As a consequence, it may be better to add other structures, not subject to fill and draw cycling, to expand contact time. This relative efficiency of structures for achieving contact should be considered when comparing alternative methods for providing additional contacting volume. Other aspects, such as site considerations and the capability for achieving multiple goals within an added structure or expansion, should also be evaluated.

Multiple Pathogen Removal Steps

For most water treatment plants, several pathogen removal steps can be employed that use both disinfection and nondisinfection processes. In these instances, it may be necessary to establish an aggregate CT for the process combinations. An example might be a situation where nondisinfection pathogen removal is achieved by physical removal of pathogens with filtration, and ozone is used as a primary disinfectant followed by the addition of chlorine or chloramine applied later in the water treatment process to provide a disinfecting residual in the distribution system.

Where such multiple steps are applied in sequence, the total inactivation is an aggregate of the effect of each of the individual pathogen removal or inactivating steps. The CT available for each disinfection step would be equal to the credited travel time during peak hourly flow through that segment of the plant multiplied by the residual disinfectant concentration maintained (measured during peak hourly flow). Where pH and temperature effects are a consideration, the inactivation achieved should be based on the worst-case conditions for pH and temperature in the respective segments of the plant.

The following formula can be used to determine overall percent inactivation achieved by sequential pathogen removal steps:

$$G_{t,n} = G_{t,n-1} + \frac{G_n(100 - G_{t,n-1})}{100} \tag{2–14}$$

where

n = number of points of pathogen removal

G_n = the percent inactivation achieved by the nth pathogen removal step

$G_{t,n}$ = the total percent inactivation achieved by the n pathogen removal steps

$G_{t,n-1}$ = the total percent inactivation achieved by the $n - 1$ pathogen removal steps

To illustrate the use of this equation, assume that a 99.9 percent removal (sometimes termed 3 log removal since the logarithm of the fraction remaining, 0.001, is equal to −3) of *Giardia* cysts is required for the example plant. Assume that this plant employs rapid sand filtration for turbidity removal, ozone for primary disinfection, and chlorine for secondary disinfection. In this example, assume that criteria provide for a rapid sand filter credit of 99 percent *Giardia* removal and that the CT conditions achieved in secondary disinfection with chlorine provide a supplemental primary disinfection credit equal to a 50 percent removal of the *Giardia*. The following relationship can be written for the aggregate inactivation provided by the filtration and chlorination steps, $G_{t,n}$, by assigning 99 percent for removal by the filtration step, designated as $G_{t,n-1}$ for purpose of this calculation, and 50 percent removal to the chlorination step, designated G_n.

$$G_{t,n} = 99 + \frac{50(100 - 99)}{100}$$

$$= 99.5\% \tag{2–15}$$

To now determine ozonation requirements, Equation 2–14 is again applied to compute the required percent ozone inactivation, designated as G_n. The value of $G_{t,n-1}$ for the other inactivation steps is 99.5 percent, computed in the preceding calculation, and the total required percent inactivation of 99.9 percent is set equal to $G_{t,n}$:

$$99.9 = 99.5 + \frac{G_n(100 - 99.5)}{100} \tag{2–16}$$

Solving this expression yields:

$$G_n = \text{Required Ozone Inactivation} = 80\%$$

Because CT criteria specified for ozone in Table 2–3 are based on a 99.9 percent inactivation by ozone, an adjustment in criteria is needed to produce the criterion for 80 percent inactivation. The relationship for development of the multiplier is a logarithmic expression:

$$\frac{\log(1 - \text{removal A})}{\log(1 - \text{removal B})} = \frac{(\text{CT})_\text{A}}{(\text{CT})_\text{B}} \tag{2–17}$$

Based on this relationship, the required CT for ozone would be equal to the CT required for 99.9 percent removal multiplied by 0.23 [i.e., log (1.0 − 0.8) divided by log (1.0 − 0.999)] to arrive at the CT required for 80 percent removal.

Role of Testing for Determining CT Criteria

It should be noted that the EPA CT criteria represent a general basis for attaining credit for required removals of 99.9 percent for *Giardia* cysts and 99.99 percent for enteric viruses, respectively. These criteria are intended for use in the absence of site-specific information on disinfection effectiveness. However, the regulations allow development of site-specific criteria as an option. This might allow a less costly approach to primary disinfection to be justified. Development of site-specific criteria could also be used to demonstrate the primary disinfecting capability of an alternative primary disinfecting agent, such as chloramines, that might not otherwise meet published criteria. Another test consideration might be for assessing capabilities of modified disinfection methods such as peroxone and photozone (see Chapter 7) where reliance on measured residuals may not give an accurate indication of the actual disinfection effectiveness of these modifications to ozonation.

SECONDARY DISINFECTION

The principal goals of secondary disinfection are to inhibit regrowth of organisms in distribution systems and to protect against microbial contamination due to cross-connection. Although cross-connections might ostensibly be prohibited and controlled by proper plumbing procedures, a degree of protection against the potential for this type of occurrence is still considered prudent by many regulatory agencies.

The problem of microbial regrowth is related to the fact that a number of bacteria and other microbes can colonize in water distribution systems. Some of these bacteria can subsequently become opportunistic human pathogens under the proper conditions of exposure. The more significant bacteria included in this category are *Legionella, Pseudomonas, Mycobacterium, Aeromonas* (13), *Bacillus subtilis,* and *Flavobacterium* (17).

Although not investigated as extensively as bacteria, fungi have also been isolated in water distribution systems. Possible effects from fungi include those of human health (allergenic, pathogenic, or toxigenic species), interference with capability for maintaining chlorine residual, contamination of foodstuffs, deterioration of gaskets and joint materials, and generation of tastes and odors. Although most fungi have been observed to be successfully disinfected by chlorine levels of 1 to 2 mg/l in raw water, some species have proved to be resistant, even at levels greater than 3 mg/l (14).

Thus far, the greatest regulatory concern for regrowth organisms has been associated with *Legionella* bacteria. *Legionella* is responsible for respiratory disease, creating a significant clinical problem estimated to cause up to 50,000 cases per year, most of which occur in a milder form that is not fatal (15). These bacteria can be transported by waterborne aerosols that emanate from sources such as water coolers, showers, and air conditioning systems that use cooling towers. In its most severe form, Legionnaires' disease is of particular risk to individuals in a generally weakened physical condition, where it can be fatal. Control of this disease in hospital environments has become an important consideration because of the presence of a significant population of people in poor health. Less severe forms are usually experienced by individuals in normal health as a result of exposure in office environments and in the home.

Because of its established significance, *Legionella* is being regulated as one of the pathogenic contaminants listed in the 1986 Amendments to the Safe Drinking Water Act. However, other types of pathogens have also been identified. These include fungi such as *Aspergillus niger* (14), *Aspergillus fumigatus* (14), and *Petriellidium boydii* (26), as well as the bacteria that have been previously discussed. The extent of these and other building services–related illnesses is not well characterized. Further research in this area will probably be required to determine the possible need for additional controls regarding these pathogens. However, significant changes may not occur since many of the control strategies applicable for *Legionella* are likely to be adequate for these pathogens as well (17).

Legionella bacteria can colonize within the distribution system and in plumbing systems, especially in areas where scale and sediment accumulate. This accumulation provides a media for a general biological growth that produce byproducts on which *Legionella* can subsequently grow. *Legionella* can be found in hot water tanks in spite of the fact that high temperatures are not favorable for its growth. Temperature strata can occur in these tanks, and favorable conditions can exist in the cooler portions of tanks, especially if high temperature settings are not used. At temperature settings greater than 140°F, *Legionella* growth tends to be limited (15).

Secondary Disinfection Approaches

Secondary disinfection, as traditionally practiced, has typically involved provision of a protective disinfecting residual with the goal of inhibiting biological regrowth phenomena. The most commonly used disinfecting agents have been chlorine and chloramines, although chlorine dioxide has also been used, but predominantly in European applications.

While disinfecting agents can represent an important component of a secondary disinfection strategy, other factors exert a significant influence over regrowth phenomena. For example, dead-end or low velocity conditions in distribution systems have long been recognized as critical areas where disinfecting residuals can be dissipated, thereby increasing the potential for regrowth. To the extent possible, these conditions should be minimized or corrected.

Flushing of low velocity areas has been regarded as one method for improving conditions by removing sediment material that can offer a place for bacteria to grow. While this may be helpful, difficulties have also been reported in some cases in which bacterial counts appeared to elevate following flushing as a result of detachment and suspension of accumulated biogrowths. In some cases, this might be corrected by flushing for a longer time or at higher flushing velocities. Flushing has also been reported to offer only short-term improvement when other conditions conducive to biogrowth (e.g., depleted disinfectant residuals and presence of adequate nutrients) were not entirely eliminated (18).

Corrosion-related tuberculation is one condition that is not corrected by flushing. Tubercles can offer an excellent media on which or in which biogrowth can take place. In addition, tubercles can partially protect such growth from disinfecting residuals in the bulk liquid flowing through a pipe. Depletion of disinfecting residuals and elevated levels of bacteria can occur in tuberculated piping sections even in the absence of dead-end conditions that usually eliminate disinfecting residuals due to long retention times (19). Although free chlorine is a strong disinfectant, it can be readily consumed in transport into the tubercles, thereby reducing its effectiveness under these conditions. In spite of a lower disinfection potential, chloramine is less reactive than free chloride and is more capable of penetrating the tubercles, sometimes resulting in better disinfection under these conditions. Tubercle penetration by free chlorine has been observed to improve with a slightly alkaline pH (18). This probably results from conversion from the highly reactive HOCl to the less reactive OCl^- (see Equation 2–2), thereby achieving a characteristic similar to chloramine. For other biofilm conditions, the relative effect of HOCl can vary compared to chloramine OCl^- (31).

Where pipeline corrosion is a problem, corrosion control can be an important adjunct to secondary disinfection strategies (18). This can be achieved by approaches such as the addition of corrosion inhibitors, elevated pH, or the use of lime-based strategies to form a protective scale. Adequate corrosion control will inhibit the generation of tubercles or sediments, which can provide protection for certain pathogens. In some circumstances, corrosion control will also inhibit the acidlike reactions of certain disinfectants with metal piping.

Although chloramines may provide some advantage for penetrating biofilms, other microbial problems can be encountered to confound such advantage. Some utilities have reported another type of bacterial regrowth phenomenon when converting to chloramination. These appear to result from biological nitrification, which appears to occur in response to the available ammonia used in forming chloramines (27, 28). Heterotrophic plate counts can increase during these events, possibly as a result of increased availability of biodegradable substrates from nitrifying bacteria. Several utilities have found it necessary to rigorously control the chloramine process and periodically switch from chloramination to free chlorine to "burn out" the system when these erratic trends occur.

Supplemental *Legionella* Control

While secondary disinfection considerations are important for achieving goals for limiting microbial growth in order to meet criteria such as those contained in EPA rules governing coliforms, heterotrophic plate counts, and disinfecting residuals, more specific strategies have evolved for control of *Legionella*. To control *Legionella,* the EPA intends for primary disinfection to be used as the major barrier to limit transport into the system, and secondary disinfection is intended to inhibit its subsequent growth in the distribution system (16). CT criteria adequate for primary disinfection of *Giardia* are considered to be adequate for preventing the introduction of *Legionella*. Of the available disinfection approaches for secondary disinfection, chlorine is a strong candidate for maintaining the necessary disinfecting residual. Chloramines represent another possible alternative, and in some cases chlorine dioxide might be appropriate. Restrictive limitations on allowable residuals for chlorine dioxide and its degradation products, chlorate and chlorite, however, may limit its application for providing a systemwide residual.

When established, *Legionella* colonies are somewhat resistant to chlorine and doses as high as 4 to 6 mg/l may be required for adequate control (15). Since these levels are not feasible on a systemwide basis, the main effect of a systemwide residual is to limit the extent to which these colonies can become initially established. Disinfection of susceptible home plumbing fittings such as shower heads and water taps is a consideration for dealing with contamination during installation. Heat treatment and shock chlorination are alternatives for subsequent control measures in building water systems (12).

Supplemental hypochlorination, which consists of the installation of a chlorinator in a building system, has sometimes been used to provide an elevated residual for continuous protection in office and institutional buildings. However, this approach is limited by difficulties in maintaining a chlorine residual in hot water systems and is not completely effective for these particular components of plumbing systems. In addition, undesirable levels of chlorine byproducts may be formed with higher levels of chlorine residual. Alternative approaches for localized control of *Legionella* include thermal inactivation by operating water heaters at sufficiently high temperatures and supplemental disinfection using ozone and UV radiation. Neither ozone nor UV radiation provides a disinfecting residual that can prevent regrowth, and while control may be achieved at specific points or locales in the piping, *Legionella* colonization can still occur at more remote points of the system (15).

Other methods of control include specially designed hot water tanks that more evenly distribute temperature throughout a tank and periodic maintenance by cleaning, disinfection, and monitoring of stagnant tanks. Some reports have also indicated that black rubber washers and gaskets used in pipe and tank fittings offer protection to *Legionella* from chlorine and heat. Replacement with Proteus 80 compound washers has been recommended as a possible remedy for limiting these potenital host locations (12).

Removal of Biodegradable Organic Matter as a Supplement to Secondary Disinfection

The application of secondary disinfecting agents is one approach for inhibiting microbial regrowth. Under some conditions, however, microbes can be protected from disinfecting residuals by distribution system characteristics such as accumulated sediment and tuberculation. Another factor affecting the capability to disinfect is the rate of depletion of the disinfectant in locations with long detention. These considerations have led some utilities to consider a supplemental approach that involves the removal of biodegradable organic matter as a means of limiting the food source for microbial growth (22, 30). Applicability of this type of approach may vary depending upon the specific distribution system characteristics.

The addition of strong oxidizing disinfectants such as ozone, chlorine, and chlorine dioxide can increase the level of biodegradable organic material. While these disinfectants are often necessary for primary disinfection, they appear to convert some of the natural organic content to lower molecular weight compounds that are more susceptible to biodegradation (13). An increase in production of biodegradable organic content can be especially significant with ozone disinfection. Where this creates enough of a problem, it can result in a need for processes to remove this organic content. The need for such removal is likely to depend on the initial dissolved organic carbon (DOC) content in raw water and the extent to which such DOC may be removed prior to ozonation. As a rule of thumb, these problems tend to become significant at DOC levels of greater than 3 mg/l. It will be necessary, however, to evaluate the requirement for biodegradable organic removals for each site.

Specific processes used for removing biodegradable organic material rely on biological treatment by microorganisms attached to a media such as sand or granular activated carbon (referred to as biological activated carbon or BAC). The basic concept is to encourage microbial growth within a confined treatment step in order to consume the food source that would otherwise be available at downstream locations within the distribution system. Some removals may also be obtained by nonbiological mechanisms in coagulation, sedimentation, and filtration processes.

Several measures of biodegradable matter have been developed to evaluate the relative availability of food source. Initially the more common methods were based on assimilable organic carbon (AOC) tests. These involve the use of certain strains of the bacteria. A strain of

Pseudomonas fluorescens, known as P-17, and a strain of *Spirillum,* referred to as NOX, have been used in the past. Pure strains of these bacteria are applied to a sample, and the extent of growth is determined. AOC is then estimated based on the observed level of cell growth and is expressed in terms of acetate equivalent growth levels, using a standard curve. Other cell enumeration methods have been developed, including a coliform growth rate method. Methods are also being developed that use biodegradable organic carbon (BDOC) as a measurement (32). All of these tests have some elements that are not fully resolved, and further refinements are likely.

Although these types of analyses are relatively recent, some preliminary criteria have been developed for levels at which biogrowth problems can become significant. One study indicated that bacterial growth tended to decline significantly at BDOC levels less than 0.3 mg/l based on work in France (20). Observations in the Netherlands (21) on the effect of AOC indicated that heterotrophic plate counts could be maintained at levels less than 100/100 ml if the AOC was less than 10 μg acetate equivalent carbon/l. This HPC criterion is more restrictive than the 500 counts/100 ml limit used in the United States. Therefore, this AOC level may be lower than necessary for many utilities. A study by one U.S. utility indicated that coliform growth can be limited with AOC levels less than 50 μg acetate equivalent carbon/l (31).

FUTURE TRENDS IN DISINFECTION

Although the need for treatment to control waterborne disease has long been recognized, methods for identifying and detecting pathogens are evolving and provide an improved understanding of water treatment needs. For example, it has been estimated that an average of two new enteric viruses per year have been associated with waterborne routes for the 15-year period that preceded 1984 (23). Similar discoveries for resistant protozoan species such as *Cryptosporidium* and *Giardia* have had significant ramifications in primary disinfection practice in recent years, and further changes are possible.

Understanding of microbial phenomena in distribution systems is also evolving. This involves an examination of secondary disinfection techniques and methods for removing biodegradable organic matter.

This evolving understanding of waterborne disease and associated effects has resulted in a potentially dynamic regulatory situation, which indicates a need for flexibility in disinfection to adapt to changing requirements. The principal process features that may be influenced by changing needs are filtration, the type of disinfectants employed in both the primary and secondary disinfection, the locations at which disinfectants are applied, and the level of supplemental treatment that may be required to reduce the extent of microbial regrowth in the distribution systems.

References

1. *Comparative health effects assessment of drinking water technologies: Report to Congress.* November 1988. EPA 68-03-3417. Washington, DC: U.S. Environmental Protection Agency, Office of Drinking Water.
2. Blaser, M. J. 1983. Occurrence and detection of *Campylobacter* in water. Paper presented at 11th Annual AWWA Water Quality Technology Conference, seminar on *Waterborne Pathogens: Their Detection and Occurrence,* 4–7 December, 1983, Norfolk, VA.
3. Schiemann, D. A. 1983. Occurrence and detection of *Yersinia enterocolitica* in water. Paper presented at 11th Annual AWWA Water Quality Technology Conference, seminar on *Waterborne Pathogens: Their Detection and Occurrence,* 4–7 December, 1983, Norfolk, VA.
4. Sobsey, M. D. 1988. Disinfection: Principles and applications relative to the new regulations. Paper presented at workshop on *Disinfection By-Products: Prevention and Control,* 10 March, 1988, at University of North Carolina, Chapel Hill, NC.
5. Gaudy, A. F., and E. T. Gaudy. 1980. *Microbiology for environmental scientists and engineers.* New York: McGraw-Hill Book Company.
6. National Academy of Science. 1980. The disinfection of drinking water. In *Drinking water and health,* Vol. 2. Washington, DC: National Academy Press.
7. Jacangelo, J. G., V. P. Oliveri, and K. Kawata. 1987. *Mechanism of inactivation of microorganisms by combined chlorine.* Denver: AWWA Research Foundation.
8. Severin, B. F., and C. C. K. Churn. 1987. Kinetics of microbial inactivation. Paper presented at AWWA Annual Conference, seminar on *Assurance of Adequate Disinfection, C-T or Not C-T,* June 1987, Kansas City, MO.
9. Hoff, J. C. 1987. Strengths and weaknesses of using C-T values to evaluate disinfection practice. Paper presented at AWWA Annual Conference, seminar on *Assurance of Adequate Disinfection, C-T or Not C-T,* June 1987, Kansas City, MO.
10. AWWA. 1971. *Water quality and treatment: Handbook of public water supplies.* New York: McGraw-Hill.
11. Hudson, H. E. 1962. High quality water production and viral disease. *JAWWA* 54(10): 1265–74.
12. *Guidance manual for compliance with the filtration and disinfection requirements for public water systems using surface water sources.* October 1989. EPA 68-01-6989. Washington, DC: U.S. Environmental Protection Agency, Office of Drinking Water.

13. AWWA Research Foundation. 1988. *The search for a surrogate*. Denver: AWWA.
14. Rosenzweig, W. D., H. Minnigh, and W. O. Pipes. 1986. Fungi in distribution systems. *JAWWA* 78(1): 53–55.
15. Muraca, P. W., V. L. Yu, and J. F. Stout. 1988. Environmental aspects of Legionnaires' disease. *JAWWA* 80(2): 78–86.
16. 1989. *Fed. Reg.* 54(124): 27486–541.
17. Galbraith, N. S., N. J. Barrett, and R. Stanwell-Smith. 1987. Water and disease after Croydon: A review of waterborne and water-associated disease in the United Kingdom, 1937–1986. Paper presented at IWES Summer Conference, 1987.
18. LeChevallier, M. W., C. D. Lowry, and R. G. Lee. 1990. Disinfecting biofilms in a model distribution system. *JAWWA* 82(7): 87–99.
19. LeChevallier, M. W., T. M. Babcock, and R. G. Lee. 1987. Examination of and characterization of distribution system biofilms. *Appl. Environ. Microbiol.* 53: 2714.
20. Levi, Y., J. C. Joret, and J. C. Block. 1990. Measurement of bioremovable dissolved organic carbon: Applications for the maintenance of water quality in networks. Presented at Annual Water Quality Technology Conference of AWWA, November 1990, San Diego, CA.
21. Van der Kooij, D. 1990. The definition of biological stability as a new quality criterion for drinking water. Presented at Annual Water Quality Technology Conference of AWWA, November 1990, San Diego, CA.
22. Schellart, J. A. 1986. Disinfection and bacterial regrowth: Some experiences of the Amsterdam water works before and after stopping the safety chlorination. *Water Supply* 4: 217–25.
23. Gerba, C. P. 1984. *Strategies for the control of viruses in drinking water: Report to the American Association for the Advancement of Science*. Washington, DC: Environmental Science and Engineering Program.
24. Bablon, G., et al. 1991. Practical application of ozone; principles and case studies. In *Ozone in water treatment: Application and engineering*. Langlais, B. et al., eds.; Chelsea, MI: Lewis Publishers.
25. Jacangelo, J. G., et al. 1991. Investigating the mechanism of inactivation of *Escherichia coli* B by monochloramine. *JAWWA* 83(5): 80–87.
26. Roesch, S. C., and L. Y. C. Leong. 1983. Isolation and identification of *Petriellidium boydii* from municipal water system. In Abstracts of Annual Meeting American Society for Microbiology, Washington, DC, p. 276.
27. Robinson, K., and R. Elefritz. 1990. Monitoring organic performance and disinfection of a surface water ozonation-softening facility in south Florida. *Proceedings AWWA WQTC*, San Diego, CA, pp. 877–99.
28. Wolfe, R. L., et al. 1989. Biological nitrification in covered reservoirs containing chlorinated water. *JAWWA* 80(9): 109–14.
29. Brazos, B. J., and J. T. O'Connor. 1990. Seasonal effects on the generation of particle-associated bacteria during distribution. *Proceedings AWWA WQTC*, San Diego, CA, pp. 1073–1101.

30. Rittman, B. E., and V. L. Snoeyink. 1984. Achieving biologically stable drinking water. *JAWWA* 76(10): 93–106.
31. Le Chevallier, M. W., B. H. Olson, and G. A. McFeters. 1990. Assessing and controlling bacterial regrowth in distribution systems. Report prepared for AWWA Research Foundation, Denver, CO, January 1990.
32. Servais, P., et al. 1987. Determination of biodegradable dissolved organic carbon in water. *Water Res.* 21: 445–50.

3

Identifying and Characterizing Effects of Disinfection Byproducts

with contributions by

François van Hoof
Antwerp Water Supply, Belgium
on *Genotoxic Evaluations*

EVOLUTION OF THE DISINFECTION BYPRODUCT ISSUE

Although waterborne disease and the need for disinfection to control this risk have long been recognized, awareness of possible health implications of disinfection byproducts has only recently emerged. Concern for these byproducts began to surface in the 1970s as newer analytical methods were applied for identifying constituents of drinking water. Two studies completed in 1974 identified chloroform, a potential carcinogen, as a byproduct formed in the chlorination of drinking water (1, 2). During this same year, Congress passed the Safe Drinking Water Act, which established authority through the EPA for Federal regulation of public water supplies throughout the country. Subsequent to passage of this act, the EPA performed the National Organics Reconnaissance Survey in 1975 (3) and the National Organic Monitoring Survey in 1976 and 1977 (4). These investigations confirmed the presence of chloroform in a number of water supplies throughout the country.

Studies have indicated that chloroform is a commonly generated byproduct of reactions between chlorine and portions of naturally occurring organic matter (NOM) that is widely found in raw water sources. The component of the organic material that can react to form chloroform and other disinfection byproducts is typically referred to as organic precursor material.

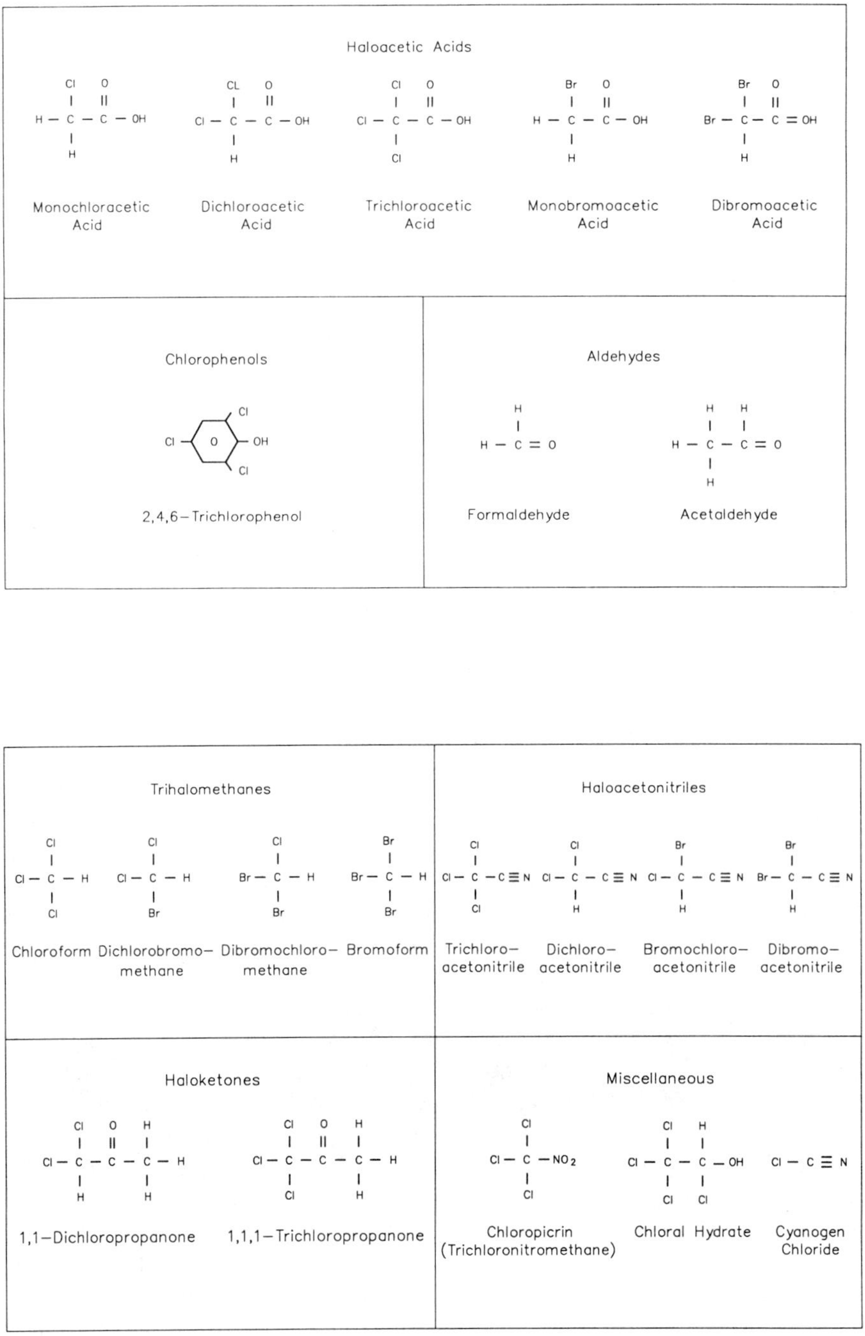

FIGURE 3–1. Structural formulas for disinfection byproducts. (Reprinted from *Journal American Water Works*, Vol. 81, No. 8 (August 1989), by permission. Copyright © 1989, American Water Works Association.)

Chloroform has a relatively simple organic structure, consisting of a methane molecule substituted with three chlorine atoms (Figure 3–1). Chlorine is a halogen, leading to the designation of chloroform as a halomethane compound. Because three halogen atoms in the form of chlorine are incorporated into chloroform, it is more specifically designated as a trihalomethane (THM).

Bromide, another form of halogen that is frequently present in raw waters, can be oxidized by chlorine and subsequently react with the background organic matter to form bromine and combined chlorine/bromine forms of trihalomethanes, also shown in Figure 3–1. Although other halogens exist that can potentially form additional trihalomethanes, the species shown in Figure 3–1 are those most frequently encountered in drinking water. The sum of these four chemical species has therefore been designated as the total trihalomethane (TTHM) content for regulatory purposes. In the past, TTHM content has been regulated under the Safe Drinking Water Act at a running average concentration of 0.10 mg/l or less for four consecutive quarters of sampling.

Although most of the attention on disinfection byproducts has focused on regulation of trihalomethanes, there has been a growing recognition that other disinfection byproducts may also be of significance. The Safe Drinking Water Committee of the National Academy of Science has, therefore, performed two reviews to compile information on the significance of other byproducts of chlorine, as well as byproducts of alternative disinfectants (5, 6). Specific regulatory intent for other disinfection byproducts was initially indicated in the first Drinking Water Priority List, published by the EPA in January 1988. A subsequent list, which indicates disinfection byproducts for possible future regulation, was developed in 1991 (Table 3–1). While these lists represent initial steps towards a more

TABLE 3–1. Disinfectants and Disinfectant Byproducts on the U.S. Environmental Protection Agency 1991 Drinking Water Priority List

Disinfectants: chlorine, hypochlorite ion, chlorine dioxide, chlorite ion, chlorate ion, chloramine
Four trihalomethanes: chloroform, bromoform, dibromochloromethane, dichlorobromomethane
Chlorination/Chloramination byproducts (misc.): haloacetic acids, haloketones, chloral hydrate, MX-2 (3-chloro-4-(dichloromethyl)-5-hydroxy-2(5H)-furanone), *N*-organochloramines
Ozone byproducts: aldehydes, epoxides, peroxides, nitrosamines, bromate, iodate
Haloacetonitriles: bromochloroacetonitrile, dichloroacetonitrile, dibromoacetonitrile, trichloroacetonitrile
Others: chloropicrin (trichloronitromethane), cyanogen chloride

Source: Adapted from *Fed. Reg.* 1991. 54(9): 1470–74.

comprehensive basis for regulating disinfection byproducts and will be subject to change upon further evaluation, they are significant because they have opened the range of possibilities beyond a confined focus on trihalomethanes.

GENERAL CHEMICAL REACTION CHARACTERISTICS OF DISINFECTANT CHEMICALS

Chlorine

As discussed in Chapter 2, HOCl and OCl^- are the predominant active forms of what is termed *free chlorine*. These are distinguished from *combined chlorine*, which refers to chlorine that has combined with other compounds such as those that result from reactions with ammonia to form chloramines.

The chemical reactivity of free chlorine varies significantly in the HOCl and OCl^- forms. These variations occur even though chlorine exists in the +1 oxidation state in both forms:

$$(H^{+1}O^{-2}Cl^{+1})^0$$

$$(O^{-2}Cl^{+1})^{-1}$$

In the case of HOCl, chlorine in the +1 oxidation state, designated hereafter as Cl(+1), is attached to an $H^{+1}O^{-2}$ component that has a net −1 charge. On the other hand, the Cl(+1) in OCl^- is attached to O^{-2} with a net −2 charge. This tends to create a much higher level of internal attraction for Cl(+1) in an OCl^- ion, a factor that would reduce its availability for external reaction. This explanation is somewhat simplified, and other factors can also influence strength of bonding and availability for chemical reaction. This discussion is illustrative for this particular case since OCl^- is a much less reactive form of Cl(+1) as indicated by this relatively simple concept.

Other factors that can affect the properties of HOCl/OCl^- are transport properties associated with ionic character. Ionic character can influence disinfection effectiveness and toxicity since neutrally charged molecules, such as HOCl, are more readily transported across cell membranes than the charged OCl^- ion. This may contribute to the effectiveness of HOCl as a disinfectant, although a number of other factors may also be involved. More important, it represents a major difference in the character of two separate species of chlorine, emphasizing the importance of distinguishing between the species for both toxicity and disinfection evaluations

When considering chlorine chemistry, it is important to understand the different types of reactions that can take place. For example, although chlorine is widely recognized as a strong oxidizing chemical, reactions of considerable significance can also occur in which chlorine remains in the Cl(+1) form and no oxidation occurs. These are reactions in which chlorine is added or substituted into the structure of another molecule in the form of Cl(+1). Reactions of this type are responsible for the formation of chloramines as well as the chlorinated organics that comprise many of the disinfection byproducts of concern. In contrast, oxidation reactions involving chlorine result in a modification of the oxidation state of chlorine to the relatively inert chloride form, Cl^-, and do not result in the formation of chlorinated compounds.

Two factors have focused attention on chlorinated disinfection byproducts that are formed by substitution-type reactions:

- A general concern about the health significance of chlorinated organics as a class of compounds.
- The availability of analytical methods for readily detecting certain types of chlorinated organics such as the trihalomethanes. This has allowed the presence of chlorinated byproducts to be more readily identified than other byproducts. In a sense we have become more concerned about chlorinated byproducts, because we are more aware of them.

Oxidation byproducts that do not contain chlorine may also be significant and are receiving increasing attention as understanding of such byproducts develops.

The complete oxidation of a simple organic compound by oxygen to produce relatively innocuous end products—carbon dioxide and water—illustrates the oxidation of organic compounds:

$$\underset{\text{Hydrocarbon}}{2CH_4} + 4O_2 = 4H_2O + 2CO_2 \tag{3–1}$$

For the most part, if this type of complete oxidation were to occur, there would be little or no concern for oxidation byproducts. However, intermediate organic products can also be formed prior to complete oxidation, which results in a sequence of oxidation illustrated by the progression of oxidation of relatively simple organic compounds (7):

$$\underset{\text{Hydrocarbon}}{CH_4} \longrightarrow \underset{\text{Alcohol}}{CH_3OH} \longrightarrow \underset{\text{Aldehyde}}{H_2C{=}O} \longrightarrow \underset{\text{Acid}}{HCOOH} \longrightarrow H_2O + CO_2 \tag{3–2}$$

Intermediate oxidation products such as those above and others can exist in most chlorine reaction circumstances since complete oxidation does not normally take place. In other words, the chlorine reaction may be arrested before complete oxidation can occur, a condition that leaves intermediate products. Molecular structures and other phenomena can have a significant influence on chemical reactions and pathways are not as simple or direct as shown in Equation 3–2.

In the case of reactions occurring along nonoxidation substitution pathways, several phenomena can also influence the type of chemical reaction. For example, the tendency for a reaction to occur can be affected by what may appear to be relatively small differences in molecular structures. This is illustrated in Figure 3–2 for reactions between HOCl and benzene-type compounds. Note that benzene itself does not readily react with HOCl. However, the inclusion of an electronegative group, such as the addition of OH to form phenol, has a *destabilizing* or activating effect on the benzene ring that allows chlorine substitution to occur at either the adjacent or the opposite carbon site (8). Further modification of the benzene ring by the introduction of OH groups on either side of a reaction site, such as is the case for resorcinol, activates the reaction site to such

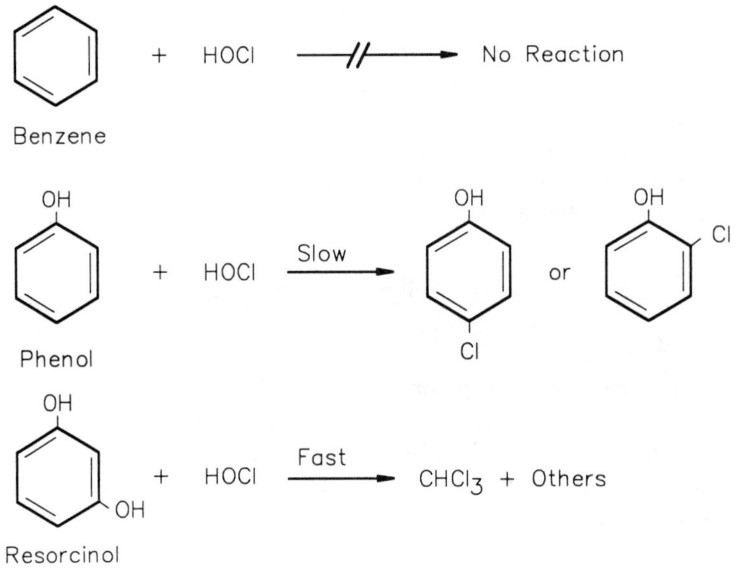

FIGURE 3–2. Effect of activation on chlorine reactions. (Reprinted from *Journal American Water Works,* Vol. 78, No. 4 (April 1986), by permission. Copyright © 1986, American Water Works Association.)

an extent that the benzene ring can be broken, yielding chloroform ($CHCl_3$) and other byproducts (8). This type of reaction is considered to be important in the formation of chloroform and other trihalomethanes in spite of the fact that the resorcinol structure is considerably different from the basic structure of chloroform and might not be an obvious precursor on first inspection.

The key consideration for the significance of resorcinol and similar compounds is the presence of activating sites that permit the reaction to proceed. The lack of such sites in a number of other compounds that may be closer in structure to chloroform often precludes the appropriate reaction path, and chloroform often does not readily form from such compounds. A large number of model compounds other than resorcinol have been evaluated for the tendency to form trihalomethanes. Other possible activating groups include carboxyl (—COOH). The chloroform yield from an array of test compounds varies widely with a number of factors, including the nature and extent of activation (13, 14).

Chloramines

Chloramines are formed by the following substitution reactions in which Cl(+1) is substituted for a hydrogen component, H(+1), in ammonia (NH_3):

$$HOCl + NH_3 = H_2O + NH_2Cl \quad \text{(Monochloramine)} \qquad (3\text{–}3)$$

$$HOCl + NH_2Cl = H_2O + NHCl_2 \quad \text{(Dichloramine)} \qquad (3\text{–}4)$$

$$HOCl + NHCl_2 = H_2O + NCl_3 \quad \text{(Nitrogen Trichloride)} \qquad (3\text{–}5)$$

The distribution among these forms of chloramine depends on other influences such as pH, temperature, the ratio of chlorine to ammonia, and the presence of other compounds, with the ratio of chlorine to ammonia generally being the most significant factor. In disinfection applications, reaction conditions are typically controlled through the chlorine-to-ammonia ratio to ensure that monochloramine is the dominant form because the other two produce taste and odors.

As with HOCl and OCl^-, the reactivity of Cl(+1) is modified by its incorporation into the ammonialike forms. Although the NH_2^- component of the monochloramine, NH_2Cl, has a net charge of −1 and appears to be similar to the HO^- component of HOCl in that regard, differences occur with respect to charge distribution within the molecules. In the case of NH_2Cl, nitrogen in the N(−3) form exerts a much more intense electronegative center than O(−2). As a result of these differences, the Cl(+1) is more strongly bound in chloramines and is much less reactive than in HOCl. As a consequence of this reduced reactivity, chloramines do not readily engage in oxidation reactions and also have a lower disinfection efficiency. Although chloramines can take part in some substitution reactions and can form a number of chlorinated byproducts, the overall extent of such formation is less than for HOCl. Significantly, they are not readily involved in substitution reactions that result in the formation of trihalomethanes, although some pathways have been identified under laboratory conditions using a synthetic organic compound (86).

Chlorine Dioxide

The reactivity of chlorine in chlorine dioxide is substantially different from its reactivity in the other forms. In this case, chlorine no longer occurs as Cl(+1), but is in the form of Cl (+4), an entirely different oxidation state with distinct reaction pathways. Although chlorine dioxide may react with organic material to form some chlorinated substitution products, there is more of a tendency for the formation of unchlorinated oxidation products. Chlorine dioxide also undergoes changes in oxidation state that can form the intermediate inorganic degradation products, chlorite (ClO_2^-) and chlorate (ClO_3^-), prior to ultimate degradation to the inert chloride. Unlike chloride, which is the primary degradation product for both free and combined chlorine, these intermediates are still reactive forms of chlorine, about which health concerns exist.

Ozone

Products of ozone reactions are predominantly the result of oxidation reactions. However, the formation of varying degrees of halogenated products has also been observed (9), probably as a result of indirect reaction pathways involving ozone oxidation of naturally occurring bromides, which subsequently substitute into organic material to form brominated byproducts.

Reactions with ozone (O_3) fall into two general categories:

1. Direct reactions with dissolved ozone.
2. Reactions with a hydroxyl free radical, $OH^{\cdot}$, an important ozone degradation product whose formation is promoted by hydroxide ions (OH^-) in the alkaline pH range. External agents that include ultraviolet light and hydrogen peroxide also can be added to promote such formation of hydroxyl radicals.

In many cases, free radicals are more reactive than dissolved ozone, and the reaction pathways that lead to their formation can have significant consequences in the application of ozone as an oxidant. Because of these alternative pathways, it is possible to oxidize a wide range of organic compounds using ozone. Ozone can also react with bromide to form bromate, an important inorganic byproduct. Bromate has been identified as a carcinogen and has become a significant concern for ozonation of bromide-containing waters. (This is discussed in detail in Chapter 7.)

PRECURSORS AND FORMATION OF DISINFECTION BYPRODUCTS

General Characteristics of Precursors

Naturally occurring precursor compounds that can react with chlorine are found in all surface waters. In most supplies, therefore, the potential for formation of chlorination byproducts is practically unavoidable when chlorine is applied as a disinfectant. The amount of precursor material present depends upon a host of watershed and water quality characteristics. Therefore, wide variations in precursor content are observed from one source water site to another. Variation in precursor level is also observed in many groundwater sources where the background organic content can result in the formation of similar chlorination byproducts. Other groundwater supplies may have negligible organic content, thereby reducing the potential for such formation.

A major precursor group found in most waters is humic material. This material is predominantly an end product of biological decay and tends to be relatively stable in comparison with other biological degradation products. Most humic material is the result of terrestrial decay processes throughout an entire watershed, although some aquatic contribution may also occur. Other components of naturally occurring organic matter include hydrophilic acids, carbohydrates, carboxylic acids, and amino acids. However, humic materials tend to represent the dominant fraction of dissolved organic carbon, most often present at levels of 50 to 90 percent (87). Humic materials have shown significant potential for formation of THMs and other chlorinated byproducts. Other groups exhibit some variation in such formation potential. Carboxylic acids and carbohydrates generally exhibit low byproduct formation potential compared with amino acids and hydrophilic acids (56, 88, 89).

Early studies of precursors focused on the formation of trihalomethanes. Research on chlorination reactions has, however, identified a number of other byproducts. As a consequence, the emphasis is beginning to shift towards scrutiny of a wider variety of byproducts. These can include nonchlorinated organics that are formed by oxidation reactions, as well as other chlorinated species formed by reactions involving the substitution of Cl(+1) and Br(+1) for H(+1) in organic compounds.

Humic materials are diverse in nature. Based more on the analytical methods used for extracting chemical fractions, general characterizations have been developed that segregate these materials into humic acid, fulvic acid, and humin groupings. Under such methods of identification, humic acid has been characterized as the portion of organic matter that is soluble in alkaline solutions but precipitated in acidic solutions. Fulvic acid has been characterized by solubility under both alkaline and acidic conditions. A third class, humins, is not soluble under either acidic or alkaline conditions. Because of low solubility, the reactivity of humins is minimal, and this fraction is not considered a significant class of precursors.

Although the different categories of humic material are not rigorously defined by specific chemical traits, some general characteristics have been observed. Fulvic acids tend to be lower in molecular weight than humic acids and tend to contain more oxygen and less nitrogen when found in both soil and aquatic environments (11).

Humic and fulvic acids contain complex polymerized molecular structures that have not been fully characterized. Specific chemical groups within these structures are thought to be responsible for the reactions with disinfecting chemicals that form byproducts. For example, carboxyl (—COOH) and hydroxyl (—OH) groups associated with benzene rings are proposed as the reactive sites within humic materials for the formation of THMs (12, 13). These groups provide the same activating potential provided by resorcinol in the laboratory-type reactions shown in Figure 3–2.

Aside from the humic products, which are relatively resistant to further biological degradation, other more active biological materials can represent sources of precursors. Such sources can include algae and other aquatic plants (14–18). In laboratory evaluations of pure algal cultures, it was observed that significant levels of trihalomethanes can be formed in chlorine reaction with *Anabena, Scenedesmus,* and *Pediastrum* at biomass levels comparable to those found in many lakes and reservoirs (15, 16). Both algal cells and extracellular products that were excreted into the water column were found to contain precursor material. Characteristics of algal precursor materials were observed to vary depending on species. In some cases, extracellular products produced greater trihalomethane formation, whereas cellular material produced greater yields in other cases. Formation also varied with the particular algal growth phase.

Hoehn et al. (17, 18) evaluated the effect of biological activity on the potential for trihalomethane formation in a reservoir. These data covered variations in primary algal productivity and the level of extracellular products on both a diurnal and annual basis. It was observed that these variations have an effect on the formation and yield of trihalomethanes from algae and algal products. However, because of the number of influences on algal effects and the relative impacts, it was concluded that a direct correlation between THM formation and conventional measures of algal mass, such as chlorophyll *a*, may be oversimplistic.

Several researchers (6, 19, 20) have associated algae and other biologically active sources with the presence of organic nitrogen compounds, such as proteins and amino acids, that lead to the formation of organic chloramines as well as other products. In addition to health concerns, organic chloramines can interfere with analyses to determine free chlorine by yielding false-positive levels, thereby compromising the process control that is necessary to maintain effective disinfection (6). The formation of THMs from proteinaceous material that can be associated with algae has been demonstrated (19). This study concluded that the protein contribution to THM formation may be significant on a seasonal basis when high algal levels are encountered.

Other disinfection byproducts that can be generated from organic nitrogen compounds include aldehydes (21) and haloacetonitriles. Certain ring-structured nitrogen compounds may also be formed that could have a significant health effect potential because of chemical similarities with components of DNA, a property that suggests a strong possibility for mutagenic impact (22).

Man-made sources of precursors can occur in wastewater discharges and may be of significance in some cases. Specific industrial chemicals that have been identified as THM precursors include ethanol, acetaldehyde, methyl ketones, and secondary alcohols (5). However, biological end products are likely to be a more prevalent source of precursors in most municipal wastewater effluents. These can include relatively stable end products such as humic materials (8) that occur as a result of biological degradation processes in wastewater treatment. It should be noted that significant formation of THMs is not normally observed in municipal wastewater disinfection because the presence of ammonia typically leads to the formation of chloramines. However, the potential for THM formation remains and can subsequently be exerted on downstream water supplies where further chlorination can carry the partially chlorinated wastewater through to the breakpoint.

Seasonal and Other Variations of Precursors

Because much of the precursor content in raw water is related to natural biological processes associated with the formation of both humic and other biological materials such as those from algal sources, significant seasonal variations in these predominantly natural phenomena are frequently observed. The effect of these variations should, therefore, be a major consideration in planning for disinfection and the control of disinfection byproducts. Without such consideration, it is possible that the most extreme conditions of disinfection requirements and byproduct formation potential may be overlooked in evaluation.

In some cases, high levels of trihalomethane formation are observed in highly colored waters that occur in association with terrestrial runoff over decayed organic ground cover during the spring and early summer periods (24). In other cases, levels are greatest during the hotter summer period (17). Peak periods of formation may also occur at times during the autumn in areas where leaf fall and decay is significant.

Although higher temperatures tend to increase the rate of trihalomethane formation, one study (25) observed that high trihalomethane formation potentials could occur during flood conditions in the winter for a water system in England. This finding suggests that temperature is not the sole determining factor in certain seasonal variations. Extended wet periods or flood-causing rainfall such as this can sometimes result in an increased organic content in streams due primarily to terrestrial runoff.

Several researchers have observed wide variations in the basic characteristics of precursors throughout the year. For example, the trihalomethane yield reported for a reservoir in Iowa ranged from a low of 0.3 μg of trihalomethane formation potential per mg of total organic carbon (TOC) in December to 20.2 μg of trihalomethane formation potential per mg of TOC in late March and April (24). Variation in the molecular weight distribution of the organic content was also reported over an annual cycle.

The influences of algae and other biologically active sources of precursor material are also likely to be quite variable. Although algal products may have a short-term effect on the total organic content, such products are rapidly biodegraded and do not contribute significantly to the refractory organic content of a water body over extended periods of time (23). Therefore, while algal products may represent seasonal contributors to the precursor pool, long-term contribution on an annual basis should be less significant. In addition to seasonal effects of algae activity, exposure to algal products will also be affected by raw water operating protocols that permit withdrawal at different levels within a water column.

TYPES OF HEALTH EFFECTS

Most of the initial health concerns for disinfection byproducts were essentially related to the findings of carcinogenic potential for chloroform. Additional health issues, however, should be considered for evaluation. These include effects on reproductive capability, teratogenicity (birth defects), damage to specific organs such as the liver or kidney, and damage to systems such as the nervous system (neurological damage) and the circulatory system (hemolytic damage). An example of the latter is the recent concern over possible adverse effects by chlorine dioxide on blood chemistry in the circulatory system (hemolytic effects).

Health impacts can also be characterized by the type of exposure. Acute effects are most often short term in nature, whereas chronic effects have a long-term character. Most often, acute impacts of a particular compound occur at higher dosages and the effects are immediately reversible if exposure is eliminated. However, acute exposures to some chemicals produce effects that have varying latent periods (weeks to years) that are slowly reversible or irreversible and thereby chronic in nature. The more typical chronic effects that arise are in response to exposure to low levels of a substance over long periods, with a resulting progressive deterioration of health. These may or may not be reversible.

The complex nature of cancer causation has led to development of numerous methods for assessing this class of health issues. Basically, cancer is a condition under which the mechanisms for control of cell growth rate are disrupted, resulting in an uncontrolled growth that is damaging and that may ultimately cause death. Cancer can be the result of exposure to conditions or chemicals that cause progressive mutation of the components of cell DNA or chromosomes that control cell reproduction. Chemicals that can cause mutations are considered to have a potential for manifesting carcinogenicity through this type of mechanism. Such mutagenic substances can also be included in a broader group of adverse genetic or genotoxicity concerns.

Cancer can arise from either acute or chronic exposures. With certain kinds of carcinogens (initiators), the response is related to total dose and the effect is somewhat independent of the time frame of exposure. This is the clearest evidence that such effects are irreversible. Most frequently these initiating chemicals are mutagenic.

Other chemicals, termed promoters, can act by nonmutagenic pathways to enhance or promote a mutagenic pathway that results in the onset of cancer. For example, promoters may function by increasing the rate of cell division, thereby increasing the opportunity for a cancer-causing mutation to be replicated in other cells. The effects of promoters are frequently reversible. Consequently, if exposure ceases, the risk of cancer is reduced.

The mechanisms whereby chemicals act are not always simple. Some chemicals, although not directly carcinogenic in their original state, can be modified by human or animal biochemistry to forms that are ultimately mutagenic and potentially carcinogenic. It is also possible for a mutagenic substance to react and be detoxified upon ingestion. Therefore, it should be recognized that a much wider range of considerations may be involved in evaluating the carcinogenic potential of many chemicals.

METHODS FOR EVALUATING HEALTH EFFECTS

Approaches used for evaluation of human health effects generally fall into one of three categories: epidemiological methods, animal studies, and cellular and other short-term bioassay methods. Epidemiological methods involve evaluations to correlate health effects in human populations with characteristics such as the presence of certain contaminants or classes of contaminants. These evaluations frequently involve statistical analyses to determine the mathematical strength of such correlations. A major limitation of epidemiological analyses relates to the difficulty of delineating health effects associated with the specific causal factor under investigation from all other factors to which a population might be exposed. As a consequence, definitive epidemiological evidence for causation is frequently difficult to obtain.

Animal studies are controlled experiments in which test animals, such as rats and mice, are exposed to the contaminants of concern. Because of the desire to obtain a discernible effect within a reasonable period of time and in a relatively small population of animals (typically less than 100), these tests are typically performed using contaminant concentrations that are much in excess of those anticipated in drinking water. Two distinct factors affect extrapolation to estimate effects that might occur in humans. First, humans may not respond to the chemical in a manner similar to test animals. Second, there may be complicating physiological responses of test animals at the high contaminant concentrations used that would not occur either in the physiology of the animal or the human under more typical conditions of exposure to low levels of a contaminant over a lifetime. Moreover, it is possible that detoxification of contaminants by biochemical processes or protection by immune responses can occur in some cases. While these protective processes may take place at the lower dosages of concern, they may be overwhelmed at the higher test dosages, which causes the carcinogenic potential of some substances to be overestimated.

Cellular and other short-term bioassay methods have been developed to establish some general genotoxic properties of test materials. These tests are typically intended to give a rapid indication of potential health effects and have been widely applied for screening chemicals for carcinogenic potential. Because of the much lower amount of effort required for these evaluations, a much larger body of information has been generated on disinfection byproducts by these genotoxic procedures than is available through more definitive animal studies.

At present, the Ames test is the cellular bioassay method that has received the most widespread attention in evaluations of health effects in drinking water. This method uses specifically developed strains of *Salmonella typhimurium* bacteria to determine the tendency of a substance or mixture of substances to cause a mutagenic response. Such a response is taken to indicate possible carcinogenicity of the test substance. Many other bioassay methods are also available, and frequently several different methods are used to provide a diversity of experimental conditions over which to evaluate potential health effects. Some of the more commonly used methods for assessing genotoxic effects are summarized in Table 3–2. Note that each of these methods involves exposure of a test material to cell matter that is well characterized in terms of an identifiable genetic response, known as an endpoint. The genetic responses may involve a general indication of mutation as in the case of the Ames and

TABLE 3–2. Typical Bioassays for Genotoxicity

Test	Test Description	Observed Biological Endpoint
Ames DNA test	Special strains of *Salmonella* bacteria are used that are unable to synthesize the amino acid histidine. The presence of an external source of histidine is required for their growth.	Growth of colonies of test mutation bacteria in the absence of histidine indicates a mutagenic response due to change from the original histidine dependent form. Test materials are indicated to be mutagenic by this response. Degree of mutagenicity is indicated by the number of colonies (or revertants) formed as compared with a normal level of reversion that occurs in blank tests.

(continued)

TABLE 3–2. *(Continued)*

Test	Test Description	Observed Biological Endpoint
Ames test modified by addition of S-9 liver extract	S-9 contains liver extract from various animals, typically test rats. Simulates mammalian enzyme effects on test substances not possible in the Ames bacteria alone.	Same endpoint as Ames test. Tests are commonly performed in conjunction with the normal Ames test, which gives an indication of direct acting mutagenic activity. Test substances activated and inactivated in the presence of S-9 indicate indirect mutagenic characteristics conferred by associated enzymes.
HGPRT test for gene mutation	Mammalian cells treated with the test substance and then exposed to a selected poison that affects normal cells. Only mutant cells can grow in this test. Poisons selected for these tests act on the HGPRT enzyme system. A commonly used poison is 6-thioguanine. Chinese hamster ovary cells are a commonly used mammalian cell.	Growth of cells in the presence of a test substance indicates a gene mutation has occurred to achieve the necessary immunity.
Sister chromatic exchange test for DNA damage in mammalian cells	Selected cells are exposed to a test substance. The cell chromosomes are typically stained, and the two adjoining strands or chromatids that form the total chromosome are examined microscopically.	Exchanges of components of one chromatid to its adjoining chromatid indicate chromosomal changes resulting from DNA damage.
Cellular transformation assays	Selected mammalian cells are exposed to the test substance and are subsequently injected into a test animal. Typically, test cells are selected for sensitivity to cancerlike transformations. The test animals used for subsequent injection include the C3H 10T ½ and BALB/C3T3 strains of laboratory mice.	A positive indication of carcinogenic potential is obtained when a cancerlike change occurs in exposed cells, subsequently resulting in tumor formation upon injection of these cells into the test animals.

HGPRT (hypoxanthine guanine phosphoribosyl transferase) tests or may involve directly observed chromosomal changes as in the case of the sister chromatid exchange test. Cellular transformation assays provide even greater association with carcinogenic effects by evaluating cell changes that can lead to tumor formation upon injection into appropriate strains of laboratory animals.

Conditions for cellular and other short-term testing approaches can generally be characterized as *in vitro* or *in vivo*. *In vitro* tests are performed on cells or tissues that are isolated from a whole animal. This is contrasted with *in vivo* tests, which are performed on a whole animal system. While more complicated, *in vivo* tests have the advantage of exposure under test conditions that involve whole animal physiology. However, while these are on a higher order than *in vitro* tests, they are still limited by differences between conditions of exposure and physiology in humans. These bioassay methods also are less definitive than long-term whole animal studies.

Although genotoxicity in cellular and other short-term bioassays has significant implications for carcinogenicity or other genetic effects, most of the commonly used tests are *in vitro*, and several effects are not characterized by these test methods. For example, test substances might be detoxified or increased in toxicity by human or animal physiology in ways not indicated by these tests. In addition, some substances, such as carcinogenic promoters, are not necessarily genotoxic and may not be properly screened for carcinogenic potential by tests that do not include examination of the promotion potential. Some promoter bioassays have been developed that may be used to fill this need. However, even with such supplemental bioassays the question of correlation with human physiology still remains. Also, as a more complex battery of bioassays is developed, the level of expense and complexity may approach the levels associated with lifetime bioassays in experimental animals. Thus, a major incentive for performing cellular bioassays may be eliminated.

While well-performed animal studies give a much more conclusive basis for decision making, they have required a much greater level of effort. As a consequence, these approaches have been limited in terms of the number of possible byproducts that have been evaluated. They have tended to be reserved for high-priority byproducts, while short-term cellular bioassay methods have been used for screening a broader array in order to assist in identifying potential problem compounds for more detailed study. Uncharacterized mutagenicity observed in these tests also can provide insight into gaps in knowledge for further identifying and characterizing the health effects of disinfection byproducts. However, the significant limitations of cellular bioassay methods need to be acknowledged. For example, many health concerns may not involve carcinogens and may involve nonmutagenic pathways. Also, these methods have not been capable of identifying the important carcinogens that have been identified in drinking water to date. However, cellular bioassay methods cannot be entirely ignored because of the large volume of compounds and attributes that have been evaluated and the importance of some of the questions raised by this work.

BYPRODUCTS

Inorganic Disinfection Byproducts

Even though most attention has been paid to organic byproducts, the formation of inorganic byproducts can also be of concern. Unlike organic byproducts, many inorganic byproducts may not require precursor material for their formation. For example, chlorine dioxide forms two inorganic byproducts, chlorate and chlorite, as a consequence of its degradation. Of the two, chlorite is typically the major degradation product of concern in drinking water. Other significant inorganic disinfection byproducts include bromate and iodate, which are of particular concern when ozone and possibly other disinfectants are added to water containing bromides and iodides. Bromates in particular may be of concern at extremely low levels of 0.01 to 10 μg/l (85).

Cyanogen chloride (CNCl), another potentially harmful inorganic byproduct, has recently been detected under certain disinfection reaction conditions. In the laboratory, this byproduct has been observed largely through reactions of chlorine with humic and amino acids in the presence of ammonia and chloramines and thus appears to have an association with organic precursors (26).

Disinfectants themselves can be inorganic constituents of possible concern. That is to say, disinfectants like chlorine, chloramines, and chlorine dioxide in their unreacted form and in sufficient concentrations can also be harmful.

Organic Disinfection Byproducts

A number of classes of organic disinfection byproducts, summarized in Table 3–3, have been identified by chemical analysis. Table 3–4 presents a survey of byproducts commonly observed in ten water utilities around the country; Figure 3–1 shows their chemical structures. The fact that

TABLE 3–3. Identified Organic Disinfection Byproducts

Chlorine byproducts
Cyanogen chloride
Chloropicrin
Chlorophenols
Organic *N*-chloramines
Haloacetonitriles
Chlorinated benzenes
Chlorinated toluene
Chlorinated xylene
Chlorinated and unchlorinated aldehydes
Chlorinated ketones
Chlorinated alkanes
Chlorinated alkenes
Unchlorinated and chlorinated dicarboxylic acids
Unchlorinated and chlorinated monocarboxylic acids
Halogenated aromatic carboxylic acids
Halogenated thiophenes
Epoxides
Chlorohydrins
Tri (2-chloroethyl) phosphate
Halogenated propenenitriles
Nonhalogenated polycarboxylic acids
Chlorofuranones
Chlorinated cyano-organics
Chlorine dioxide byproducts
Chlorine dioxide
Chlorite
Chlorate
Chlorine
Chloride
Chlorinated and unchlorinated aldehydes
Chlorinated aromatics
Chlorinated and unchlorinated quinones
Carboxylic acids
Epoxy compounds
Chlorophenols
Ketones
Quinones
Aldehydes
Chloramine byproducts
Organic *N*-chloramines
Chlorophenols
Quinones
Aldonic acids
Chlorinated aldehydes
Haloacetic acids

(continued)

TABLE 3–3. *(Continued)*

Cyanogen chloride
THMs (possible limited formation)
Ozone byproducts
Aldehydes
Ketones
Epoxides
Peroxides
Carboxylic acids
Quinones
Phenols
Bromate
Iodate
Halogenated organics (by indirect reactions)

TABLE 3–4. Occurrence of Chlorinated Disinfection Byproducts at Ten Water Utilities

Compound	Number of Locations	Range of Values (μg/l)
High confidence		
Chloroform	10 of 10	2.6–594
Bromodichloromethane	10 of 10	2.6–77
Dibromochloromethane	10 of 10	0.1–31
Bromoform	6 of 10	0.1–2.7
Dichloroacetonitrile	10 of 10	0.2–9.5
Dibromoacetonitrile	3 of 7	0.4–1.2
Bromochloroacetonitrile	7 of 7	0.2–4.0
Chloropicrin	8 of 10	0.2–5.6
Low confidence		
Chloroacetic acid	6 of 10	<10
Dichloroacetic acid	10 of 10	<10–>100
Trichloroacetic acid	6 of 10	10–100
Trichloroacetaldehyde (chloral hydrate)	10 of 10	10–100
1,1,1-Trichloropropanone	10 of 10	10–100
2-Chlorophenol	0 of 10	—
2,4-Dichlorophenol	0 of 10	—
2,4,6-Trichlorophenol	0 of 10	—
Qualitative only		
1,1-Dichloropropanone	0 of 8	—
1,1-Dichloro-2-butanone	0 of 8	—
3,3-Dichloro-2-butanone	1 of 8	—
1,1,1-Trichloro-2-butanone	0 of 8	—
Cyanogen chloride	1 of 7	—
Dichloroacetaldehyde	0 of 10	—

Source: Adapted from Refs. 82, 83.

both of these lists tend to be dominated by byproducts of chlorine is largely the result of much greater abundance of research on chlorination byproducts as compared to those of other disinfectant reactions. Because of this imbalance, direct comparison of the effects anticipated from each of the different disinfectants cannot be made on the basis of the compounds shown in these tables.

To simplify analyses, much of the previous byproduct work has been based on chlorination of model laboratory solutions at higher reactant concentrations than are common to water treatment operations. As a result, some changes or differences in the composition of reaction byproducts appear to occur as a result of the lower constituent concentrations that are more typical of a natural condition. Therefore, compounds identified in Table 3–3 should be considered to give only an indication of byproducts that might result. Actual byproduct formation will vary depending on site-specific conditions.

Identified byproducts of free chlorine and chloramines have tended to be dominated by halogenated byproducts that are formed largely by substitution of $Cl(+1)$. Brominated forms of halogen compounds can also occur as a result of the oxidation of background levels of bromide in the presence of free chlorine. In addition, some nonhalogenated byproducts have been identified. These are primarily formed by oxidation reactions that occur more extensively for free chlorine than for chloramines.

Chlorine dioxide can form halogenated byproducts, as indicated in Table 3–3. Although the percentage of identified halogenated compounds in the table appears to be significant, however, the full range of chlorine dioxide byproducts is more likely to be dominated by the nonhalogenated oxidation compounds, which are more difficult to identify by analytical methodologies.

Ozone forms predominantly oxidation byproducts. Halogenated compounds have also been observed to form, perhaps more as a result of side reactions initiated by ozone (9). The formation of brominated byproducts is of particular concern, as discussed earlier.

ANALYSES FOR BYPRODUCTS

Analysis and Identification of Organic Byproducts

In general, halogenated disinfection byproducts have received the greatest attention as they have been more susceptible to analysis than oxidation byproducts. The lack of sufficient background knowledge of oxidation byproducts has significantly limited understanding of the full range of possible byproducts, but unknowns persist for halogenated byproducts as well. Because of the potential for the formation of a large number of organic compounds, segregation and identification of individual compounds becomes an extremely complex task. This is further complicated by the fact that still-to-be-identified compounds that occur in seemingly minute quantities may still be of health significance.

A common method of analysis for organic compounds is gas chromatography (GC), a technique that involves injection of a sample transported in a gas stream through an adsorptive column, as shown in Figure 3–3. An inert carrier gas, such as nitrogen, argon-methane, helium, or hydrogen, is circulated through the column in order to transport sample substances through the adsorptive media. Flow of organic substances through a column depends on column adsorption phenomena that retard the transport of each compound in a specific manner. Compounds tend to be eluted from the column in individual waves or peaks, whose magnitude is related to concentration.

Injection of a sample that contains several organic compounds will result in a segregation of compounds within a column depending on the retention properties of the adsorptive media for the respective compounds. Columns are generally heated in a specific manner so that effects of temperature on retention and transport rates can be closely controlled. Each compound will exit the column as a concentrated peak at its characteristic time of retention. In fact, compounds can tentatively be identified based on this time of retention. However, some chemicals will have near-

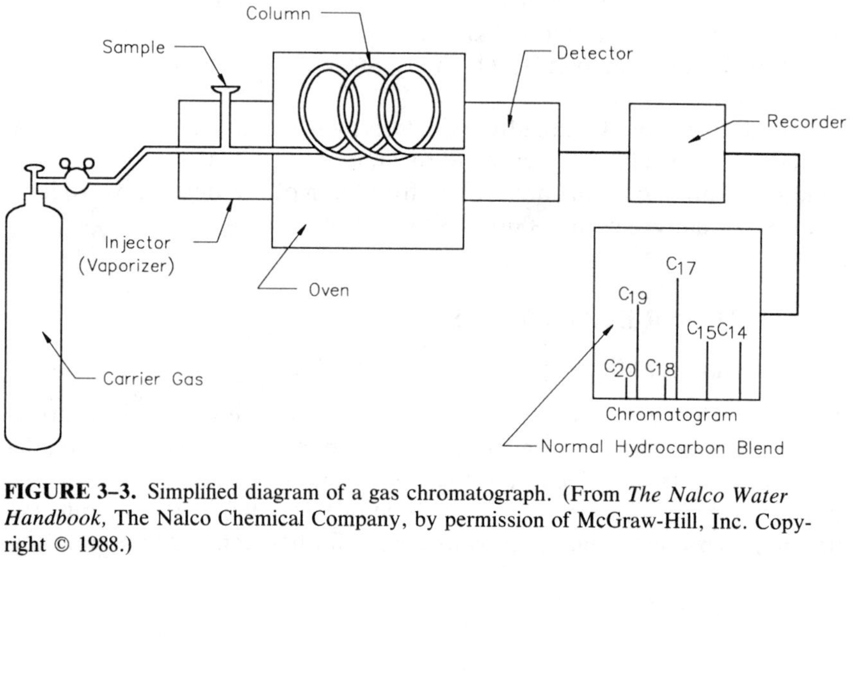

FIGURE 3–3. Simplified diagram of a gas chromatograph. (From *The Nalco Water Handbook,* The Nalco Chemical Company, by permission of McGraw-Hill, Inc. Copyright © 1988.)

identical retention times, so other methods may become necessary to identify the specific chemical in a peak.

Two basic column configurations are available: packed and capillary. In the more common of the packed column configurations, a coating of sticky liquid adsorptive material is applied to the surface of an inert granular solid that forms a packing within the column. Other types of adsorptive packing are also available.

Capillary columns are smaller in diameter, and no packing material is used. Instead, a liquid adsorptive material is coated on the inside of the tubing. These columns are much longer than packed columns. They are typically more complex to use, and for this reason have not been as widely favored for routine analysis in the past. However, improvements have occurred in capillary column technology, and it is beginning to re place packed columns because of greater accuracy for resolving peaks.

In addition to the GC column, which performs the function of segregating organic compounds in accordance with their respective retention times, a detection device must be provided to indicate the presence and quantity of segregated compounds as they are eluted from the column. The flame ionization detector is a commonly used device that responds to combustion of organic molecules as they are eluted. This type of device is suitable for analysis of a broad range of compounds. Other devices, such as the electron capture detector, are more selective in the types of compounds they detect. The electron capture detector, which is highly responsive to halogenated organics, has an advantage of sensitivity that allows analysis of this class of compounds at very low levels. A number of other detectors are available, and selection depends on the specific organic compounds to be analyzed.

As has been discussed, the task of identifying compounds based on column retention times is not always straightforward. In recent years, the capability for identifying compounds has been improved by using mass spectrometers as detection devices to further characterize organic compounds as they are eluted from a GC column. These devices fragment organic molecules into smaller particles containing charges. These charged particles can be identified in the mass spectrometer by their charge/mass ratios. Every molecule yields a characteristic pattern of such charged particles, which allows it to be specifically identified. Use of this approach, which has been termed gas chromatography–mass spectrometry (GC/MS), provides significant additional information that has enhanced the capability for identifying organic compounds.

GC and GC/MS methods are effective for a wide range of compounds that can be extracted from water samples and subsequently transformed into a gaseous form. This is typically accomplished by collecting volatile (low boiling point) organic compounds that are directly released from solution into a gaseous form, or by extracting organic compounds from a water sample into an organic solvent solution that can be subsequently injected into a gas chromatograph under conditions where the solvent and the sample material are converted to gas phase. In some cases, sensitivity for detection of low concentration levels can be enhanced by partially evaporating the organic solvent solutions to concentrate the chemical being analyzed.

While appropriate for many organic compounds, GC and GC/MS methods are ineffective for many nonvolatile (soluble and not converted to a gas) compounds. Such compounds cannot be vaporized into the gas transport stream in the column, cannot readily be recovered when solvent extraction methods are used, or tend to break down at the high temperatures used in GC columns. In some cases, these limitations can be overcome by derivatization methods that alter the character of a compound to a form more susceptible to analysis. An example of a derivatization method is the addition of diazomethane to convert haloacetic acids to methyl esters prior to analysis by gas chromatography. The reason for this approach is that methyl esters are more volatile and hence amenable to gas chromatography. Therefore, haloacetic acids, which are not amenable to direct measurement, are converted by this derivatization in order to facilitate analysis.

Direct sample injection methods are available for analyzing some nonvolative compounds when present at relatively high concentrations. Solvent extraction can be used for some others that can still exhibit a sufficient vapor pressure upon injection into a heated GC column. It is estimated, however, that 80 to 90 percent of organic compounds in drinking water are not readily analyzed by gas chromatography (27, 28), although some greater success may be observed with some specific classes of organics such as halogenated organics. Limitations are caused by thermally unstable (thermally labile) characteristics of compounds that degrade in heated GC environments, lack of efficient separation/extraction from water of many nonvolatile compounds, inadequate vapor pressures in GC environments, and lack of knowledge about the identity of many nonvolatile compounds.

In addition to these limitations, application of GC and GC/MS approaches to broad-spectrum analyses of previously characterized compounds for analysis can still be a complicated undertaking. In many cases, computer library matching techniques can be applied to GC/MS data to identify a large number of compounds. However, simple computer library approaches can be limited in their accuracy for specifically identifying compounds because of the slight variations in response of different types of equipment (29). These approaches represent an initial step of evaluation that may require more refined investigation to specifically identify and characterize suspected contaminants.

An alternative analytical technique, high pressure liquid chromatography (HPLC), has been applied for some analyses of organics in water. In contrast with gas-phase adsorption in a GC column, the HPLC chromatographic column is operated using a liquid stream. Column retention time is used as a basis for identifying compounds as in the case of GC. The need to transfer organic compounds from liquid to gaseous or solvent phases is eliminated by these techniques. Thermal destruction of thermally labile compounds can also be avoided. As such, this technology allows evaluation of many compounds that are not readily assessed by GC or GC/MS methods. However, capability for analysis is frequently limited to specific classes of compounds for any given HPLC procedure. This technology is still being developed, and overall capabilities are being expanded by combining HPLC with MS techniques. Advances are still required for improved reliability and for more affordable equipment.

Other methodologies are also becoming available. These include Fourier transform–infrared spectroscopy, ultraviolet/visible spectrum, and fluorescence spectra methods that can be combined with the chromatographic methods to facilitate compound identification as is now being accomplished with the mass spectrometer (30). Therefore, there appears to be considerable opportunity for expanding the capability for identifying disinfection byproducts.

The inability to routinely identify and quantify major portions of the organic content of a sample represents an area of uncertainty in assessing organic disinfection byproducts and their associated health effects. This is indicated by the fact that concentrates of these unidentified sample fractions can account for much of the mutagenic activity in water samples as determined by bioassay methods such as the Ames test (31, 32).

SURROGATE MEASUREMENTS OF DISINFECTION BYPRODUCT CHARACTERISTICS

Because of problems in evaluating specific disinfection byproducts, surrogate measurements have also been used. Surrogate methods of analysis include measurements of certain chemical properties and application of nonspecific bioassay and animal testing to organic concentrates that can be extracted from disinfected water samples.

Surrogate Chemical Indicators

The total organic halide (TOX) analysis is one of the most widely used surrogate chemical methods for assessing disinfection byproducts. The most common analysis for this surrogate is the carbon adsorbable organic halogen method (CAOX). This method involves the measurement of organically bound halogens (chlorine, bromine, and iodine but not organic forms of fluorine) that are adsorbed by minicolumns of activated carbon. A nitrate wash of the columns is used prior to this analysis to remove any residual inorganic halogen salts that may have been transferred from the sample to the activated carbon. Otherwise, these salts might inadvertently be measured along with the organically bound halogen that is adsorbed by activated carbon. Heat is subsequently applied to the column to break down the organic material. In the process, the adsorbed halogenated organic components are converted to inorganic halides, which are then measured with a halide titration method.

Another surrogate chemical measurement, total organic carbon (TOC), is used as a gross measure of the organic content in a water sample and has application as a general indicator of the presence of organic precursors that could potentially react to form disinfection byproducts. In many cases, a dissolved organic carbon (DOC) modification that examines the TOC remaining after filtration through a 0.45-μm filter is used to estimate the soluble component that may be more directly related to precursor content. Color and ultraviolet (UV) absorbance (at 254 nm wavelength) can similarly be used as general indicators of the precursor organic content that can react to form disinfection byproducts.

Other methods for assessing organic content exist. These methods include generalized broad-spectrum analysis of GC peaks with no specific identification of individual peaks as well as an assortment of class-specific measurements (33). An example of a class-specific method is TOX. Other methods, which have yet to be widely applied in assessing disinfection byproducts, include analyses for organic nitrogen, organic sulfur, several organic amine categories, organic acids, carbohydrates, hydrocarbons, lignins, phenols, surfactants, and oil. Most of these are not specific to disinfection byproducts, so that future application in this role may be limited. However, analyses for phenols, lignins, organic nitrogen, and specific organic amine categories may be applicable as indicators of categories of precursor compounds.

Nonspecific Bioassays

The bioassay methods that have been described for assessing specific compounds can also be applied on a nonspecific basis for general groups of organic contaminants that occur in water samples. Techniques for concentration of organics are typically applied for these tests because normal concentrations are too low for test response. The methods used to concentrate organic materials for evaluation are summarized as follows:

1. *Liquid/Liquid Extraction*—This method involves extraction from water into an organic solvent. Distinct extractions of organic compounds can be performed by using several solvents with different affinities for organic compounds. In this manner, separate categories of extracts can be derived.
2. *Adsorption*—A commonly used adsorption method involves the use of resin beads that have an affinity for organic compounds. The types of organic compounds extracted by this method depend on the nature of the resin and the pH of the liquid sample.
3. *Reverse Osmosis*—This method involves passage of a sample through membrane systems originally developed for rejecting inorganic salts. Many organic compounds can also be accumulated in the reverse osmosis reject stream, which is then collected as a concentrated organic extract. Organic compounds with molecular weights less than 200 are not readily concentrated by this method. This limitation needs to be recognized. It is also possible that the concentration of salts can increase to levels that can interfere with bioassay methods. As a result, reverse osmosis is more commonly used as a preconcentrating approach, followed by extraction using adsorption or liquid/liquid extraction methods that will exclude the salts.
4. *Freeze Drying*—This method involves sample concentration by a controlled freezing process. As the liquid sample freezes, water is removed and a powdered concentrate is produced. Although a number of organics can be concentrated by this method, the more volatile organic compounds tend to be lost from the sample. Also, salts concentrated by this technique can interfere with bioassay methods as in the case of reverse osmosis.

Because of the problems with salt interferences from reverse osmosis and freeze-drying methods, liquid/liquid extraction and adsorption methods have been more commonly used for concentrating samples for nonspecific bioassay evaluations. However, these methods also have limitations since they concentrate only organic compounds with suitable properties for extraction. This limitation can be reduced by using a variety of adsorbents and solvents that have different extraction properties. Extraction properties can also be varied by changing the sample pH.

In many cases, stepwise transfer between solvents may be required if the solvent that is initially used for extraction is toxic or otherwise unsuitable for use with the bioassay test media. Liquid/liquid extraction and selective distillation methods may be required to ultimately transfer the sample material to the desired solvent, which must have a neutral effect on the test.

Factors that can influence test results from bioassays due to these extraction methods include changes in chemical character of organic material during extraction, effects on test results due to background contaminants in adsorbents or solvents, reactions between compounds as they are concentrated, and effects from changing ratios of organic materials that are the result of variable extraction efficiencies of the individual compounds.

In the past, a majority of the nonspecific bioassays for carcinogenic potential have been conducted with the Ames test. Samples applied for this test have frequently been concentrated using XAD resins (a commercial designation for a class of macroreticular resins with affinities for specific organic chemicals, depending upon which XAD resin composition is selected). As in the case of testing for specific organic compounds, inaccuracies in determining carcinogenic potential can occur due to the existence of carcinogenic pathways not evaluated by this test and failure to simulate chemical changes that can activate or deactivate substances exposed to different metabolic pathways available in humans. Moreover, substances that are toxic to the *Salmonella* test bacteria will inhibit growth, resulting in an improper test result due to the reduction or elimination of bacterial colonies that could otherwise indicate mutagenic activity. Nonetheless, the Ames test is reported to give correct responses for predicting carcinogenicity in 60 to 75 percent of the studies of specific compounds (33) and positive test results are taken to be a cause for concern. Other bioassay methods, such as those summarized in Table 3–2, have also been used for nonspecific evaluation.

The role of nonspecific cellular bioassays and other nonspecific methods for assessing disinfection byproducts remains to be determined. Where specific techniques are available to more directly address a concern, they are preferable. However, the disinfection byproducts and associated health concerns involve a complex set of phenomena that may prove difficult to assess by specific measurements alone. At a minimum, nonspecific measurements offer some insights into directions for further areas of evaluation of disinfection byproducts and serve as an indicator of the degree of uncertainty that must be considered in planning for the future. However, it should be noted that a number of compounds that have been subsequently identified as carcinogens have been initially missed in short-term bioassays.

OBSERVED HEALTH-RELATED CHARACTERISTICS OF SPECIFIC DISINFECTION BYPRODUCTS

Although concern for disinfection byproducts was initially related to trihalomethanes, a class that could be readily identified, evidence from a number of analyses have indicated the formation of many other byproducts. Eventually research began to indicate that concerns for disinfection byproducts could not be confined to trihalomethanes. Subsequently, a number of health effects and chemical identification studies have been performed to refine knowledge of disinfection byproducts. These have included studies of health-related properties such as genotoxicity, as well as carcinogenicity and other more specific health effects.

Genotoxic Evaluations Using Cellular Bioassays

Role of Genotoxic Evaluations

While genotoxic evaluations using cellular mutagenic bioassays are not considered to provide definitive information for drawing conclusions about health, information has been generated for a large number of byproducts. Important questions have also been raised regarding portions of mutagenic activity that remain unidentified. In this context, these findings are significant since they point to a number of areas that remain to be scientifically resolved. However, these evaluations serve only to identify certain properties and do not offer a defined characterization of health effects. This area of scientific evaluation, probably involving whole animal testing and evaluations of physiological mechanisms, will need to continue. Also, there is a need for identification and characterization of compounds that have nonmutagenic pathways. These compounds can be highly significant. Therefore, while many important past characterizations have been performed based on genotoxic bioassays, much future work remains to be performed in other areas.

Genotoxic Evaluations in Drinking Water

Several attempts have been made to characterize mutagenic activity found in chlorinated drinking water extracts (34–40). In general, these studies indicated that most of the mutagenic activity occurred in compounds with relatively low molecular weights (molecular weight less than 200 to 500). Many of these compounds tended to be soluble in water and were not readily volatilized. Although some mutagens have been identified by these studies, the identity of significant portions of the mutagenic activity can still prove elusive. This is because of the extreme complexity of identifying mutagens that are only minor components of the overall chemical matrix in these samples.

Genotoxic Evaluations in Model Laboratory Solutions

The greatest success in identification of genotoxic byproducts has been obtained from studies involving model compounds or substances in laboratory solutions. These methods simplify the chemical matrix in which mutagenic substances must be identified and allow experimentation at higher concentrations, thereby simplifying concentrating procedures. Major groups of precursor substances are summarized in Table 3–5. These substances include humic substances, amino acids, peptides, and phenols. Table 3–6 provides a summary of chlorination byproducts that are mutagenic in bacterial tests such as the Ames test. This summary is based on a recent survey of mutagenic evaluations in chlorination of different model solutions (41).

Genotoxicity of Chlorination Byproducts of Humic Materials

Humic substances have been the most widely studied model compounds in disinfection byproduct investigations. They have been recognized as precursors for both trihalomethanes and mutagenic activity generated in the Ames and other bioassay tests. Humic substances also represent the bulk of the organic material in most surface and groundwaters. Trihalomethanes, haloacetic acids, acetonitriles, propanones, propenals, propenenitriles, propenes, phenols, and thiophenes generated in humic reactions were identified with GC/MS after solvent extraction in early studies of the nature of compounds produced after chlorination of humic material (42–44). One study identified the following compounds to be mutagenic in Ames testing: dichloroacetonitrile; 1,1-dichloropropanone; 1,1,1-trichloropropanone; 1,1,3,3-tetrachloropropanone; pentachloropropanone; 3,3-dichloropropenal; and 2,3,3-trichloropropenal. However, these com-

TABLE 3–5. Precursors of Mutagenicity (Chlorination)

Humic acid
Fulvic acid
Lignin
Amino acids
Methionine
Phenylalanine
Tyrosine
Tryptophan
Histidine
Proline

TABLE 3–5. *(Continued)*

Hydroxyproline
Cysteine
Cystine
Glycine
Proteins and peptides
Albumin
Glycyl-phenylalanine
Phenylalanyl-glycine
Acetovanillone
Acetoveratrone
m-Hydroxyacetophenone
p-Hydroxyacetophenone
m-Methoxyacetophenone
p-Methoxyacetophenone
Phenol
Catechol
Resorcinol
3-Methylcatechol
4-Methylphenol
Hydroquinone
Phloroglucinol
Pyrogallol
Guaiacol
Veratrol
p-Hydroxybenzoic acid
3,4-Dihydroxybenzoic acid
Ferulic acid
o-Vanillic acid
p-Vanillic acid
Eugenol
Fumaric acid
Muconic acid
4-Phenylphenol
2,4,6-Trichlorophenol
4,5-Dichlorophenol
2,5-Dichloro-*p*-benzoquinone
2,6-Dichloro-*p*-benzoquinone
Mesityl oxide
Isophorone

Source: Adapted from Ref. 41.

pounds accounted for only 7 to 8 percent of the total mutagenicity observed for one of the Ames *Salmonella* strains and less than 2 percent activity for another strain (43). This work demonstrated that other compounds, not readily analyzed by GC or GC/MS, contribute a significant proportion of the overall mutagenic activity.

TABLE 3–6. Bacterial Mutagens Produced by Aqueous Chlorination

Mutagen	Source[a]
Bromoform	A
Bromochloromethane	A
Bromodichloromethane	A, D
Dibromomethane	A, D
Dibromochloromethane	A, D
Bromomethane	A
1,2-Dichloroethane	A
Iodoethane	A
1-Bromopropane	A
1-Bromobutane	A
Trichloroethylene	D
Tetrachloroethylene	D
Tetrachloropropene	D
Pentachloropropene	D
1,3-Dichloropropanone	B, D
1,1-Dichloropropanone	A, B
1,1,1-Trichloropropanone	A, B
1,1,3-Trichloropropanone	B
1,1,3,3-Tetrachloropropanone	B, D
Hexachloropropanone	D
3,5-Trichloropent-4-ene-2-one	D
Chloral	A
Chloroacetaldehyde	D
2-Chloropropenal	B, D
3,3-Dichloropropenal	B
2,3,3-Trichloropropenal	B
2-Phenyl-2,2-dichloroethanal (PCDE)	C
Chloropicrin	A
Bromochloroacetonitrile	A
Dichloroacetonitrile	A, B, C
Trichloro-1,2,3-trihydroxybenzene	D
Bromo-*p*-cymene	D
Dichloro-*p*-cymene	D
E2-Chloro-3-(dichloromethyl)-4-oxobutenoic acid (E-MX)	A, B, C, D
3-Chloro-4-(dichloromethyl)-5-hydroxy-2 (5H)-furanone (MX)	A, B, C, D
3,4-Dichloro-5-(dichloromethyl)-5-hydroxyfuranone	D

[a] A: chlorinated drinking water; B: chlorinated humic substances; C: chlorinated amino acids; D: chlorinated wood pulp.

Source: Adapted from Ref. 41.

Other research into the chlorination byproducts of humic material has demonstrated the presence of many new products such as chlorinated aromatic acids, chlorinated diacids, and hydroxyamoylchlorides that have not yet been fully evaluated for possible mutagenic or carcinogenic effects (45, 46). Kringstadt (47) detected strong mutagens, 1,3-dichloroacetone and 2-chloropropenal, in extracts from chlorinated pulp liquors (pulp liquors contain high levels of humic material and are therefore of interest relative to possible drinking water effects) as well as some substances with low mutagenicity: bromodichloromethane; dibromochloromethane; trichloroethylene; tetrachloroethylene; pentachloropropene; 1,1,3-tetrachloroacetone; hexachloroacetone; and monochloroacetaldehyde. Later work showed similarities between byproducts formed during chlorination of softwood kraft pulp and humic acid chlorination (48).

A significant outcome of this area of research is the isolation of a very potent mutagen tentatively identified as 3-chloro-4-(dichloromethyl)-5-hydroxy-2(5H)-furanone (49, 50). This compound has become known by the abbreviated designation MX.

MX has been isolated from a humic-rich water that had been chlorinated using a chlorine-to-carbon ratio of 1 : 1 at neutral pH, conditions closer to actual drinking water practice than those used in previous studies at higher chlorine-to-carbon ratios (51). An associated compound, EMX, was also identified. Evaluation of MX and EMX has been facilitated by development of an analytical method applicable in drinking water (52). MX, which may occur at concentrations as low as 0.01 to 0.06 parts per billion in water, was shown to be a major contributor to the mutagenic activity in several waters, in some cases accounting for 40 to 60 percent of the total observed activity. Studies using the Ames test showed MX to be an extremely potent mutagen. These findings are supported by observations that MX can also induce chromosomal changes in Chinese hamster ovary cells in another genotoxic technique (53). However, while there is evidence for a high level of mutagenicity in these relatively simple tests, some higher-order bioassays do not show MX to be significant. Therefore, while MX may explain a significant portion of previously unidentified mutagenicity in relatively simple bioassays, health implications are less clear.

Genotoxic Evaluations of Chlorination Byproducts of Amino Acids

Like humic substances, amino acids have been found to react with disinfectants to form byproducts. For example, research has demonstrated that several naturally occurring amino acids can form chloroform in chlorinated water (54). Amino acids are a category of nitrogen-containing organic acids that are widespread in nature. They serve as building blocks for proteins. Another associated group of compounds includes the polypeptides, which are formed from amino acids and serve as intermediate building blocks for proteins.

The following amino acids are precursors for trihalomethanes and another class of disinfection byproducts, dihaloacetonitriles: aspartic acid, tryptophane, kynurenine, kynurenic acid, and tyrosine (55, 56). Concern for dihaloacetonitriles exists because genotoxicity has been indicated by mutagenic activity in the Ames test, by the production of tumors in mouse skin bioassay, and by abnormal growths in the lungs in mice (57). However, the data base on dihaloacetonitriles is still too incomplete to conclude that they pose a definitive carcinogenic hazard to man. In addition to dihaloacetonitriles, mono- and dichloro-4-hydroxybenzeneacetonitrile have been identified through mass spectrometry in chlorination studies of the amino acid tyrosine.

Indication of mutagenic activity for amino acid byproducts was found in Ames testing of byproducts formed by reaction of chlorine with the amino acids tyrosine, phenylalanine, methionine, tryptophane, histidine, and proline (41). Based on this work, a more in-depth study was carried out in which the extracts of chlorinated amino acids were fractionated to isolate the mutagens (58).

The extracts of chlorinated phenylalanine revealed the presence of 2-phenylethanal benzylcyanide, 2-phenyl-2-chloroethanal, and 2-phenyl-2,2-dichloroethanal (PCDE). PCDE was shown to be mutagenic in the Ames test *Salmonella* strain used in this study and accounted for approximately 30 percent of the activity in the extract. Other recognized mutagens identified included benzoylchloride, benzylchloride, and dichloroacetonitrile.

In the extract of chlorinated tyrosine, only dichloroacetonitrile was detected as a known mutagen. 3-Chloro-4-hydroxybenzylcyanide and 3,5-dichloro-4-hydroxy benzylcyanide were present but were shown to be nonmutagenic to the *Salmonella* test strain used for Ames tests in this study. Using techniques for evaluating MX and EMX, both compounds were shown to be present in one of the chlorinated tyrosine extracts. MX represented approximately 60 percent of the mutagenic activity in this extract.

With respect to peptides and proteins, chlorination studies of several compounds have failed to reveal mutagenic activity. However, one researcher reported that proteins could serve as precursors for trihalomethanes and other chlorinated byproducts (59).

Genotoxic Evaluations of Chlorination Byproducts of Phenolic Compounds

Phenolic compounds (benzene ring–structured organic compounds containing hydroxyl groups, —OH), have received significant attention in evaluations of chlorination byproducts because the phenolic groups in humic materials are thought to be reactive sites for formation of trihalomethanes. As has been discussed, one phenolic compound in particular, resorcinol, has been used as a model compound for reactions that could occur with humic materials. Similarities in the byproducts produced by humic material and another phenolic compound, dihydroxybenzoic acid, have also been reported (13, 45).

One study showed that a wide range of phenols could serve as precursors for mutagen formation under chlorination using high chlorine-to-carbon ratios, which were intended to simulate conditions in wood pulp bleaching (60) (see Table 3–5). At lower chlorine-to-carbon ratios more typical of drinking water practice, the phenolic compound catechol was a precursor for mutagenic activity. Resorcinol and dihydroxybenzoic acid were mutagenic precursors at higher chlorine dosages. Major mutagens identified after chlorination of catechol were *o*-benzoquinone and chloro-*o*-benzoquinone. Although the observed mutagenic activity generated by these reactions was much lower than that encountered after chlorination of the amino acid tyrosine, a study has demonstrated that the following phenolic compounds can serve as precursors in reactions with chlorine that produce MX: phenol, guaiacol, *p*-hydroxybenzoic acid, ferulic acid, and catechol (61).

Genotoxic Evaluations of Chlorination Byproducts of Miscellaneous Precursors

Research demonstrated that certain ketones could be converted to mutagens under conditions similar to those encountered in wastewater and drinking water chlorination (62). In another study, citric acid was reported as a precursor for chlorinated propanones, di- and trichloroacetic acid, and chloroform (63). Other reports discuss precursors of natural origin. One study detected mutagenic activity in chlorinated lake water (64). Whether the activity was due to the humic material or to components chelated in the humic structure is not clear. In other studies, promotion of mutagenic activity was observed in groundwaters and bankfiltered river waters that were uncontaminated with organic pollutants. These conditions were typical of groundwaters from very old aquifers. Anaerobic groundwaters, in particular, have demonstrated this phenomenon (65, 66). Algae and municipal and industrial wastewater effluents have also been observed to contain precursors for trihalomethanes and other halogenated byproducts.

Genotoxic Evaluations of Disinfection Byproducts Formed by Alternative Disinfectants

Ozone, monochloramine, and chlorine dioxide are the most widely applied alternatives for chlorine. As far as mutagenic byproduct formation is concerned, the knowledge about these disinfectants is much more limited, whether they are applied as preoxidants or as postdisinfectants. Several authors have reported no increase in mutagenic activity in the Ames test after ozonation of raw or pretreated water (67–69), while other studies (36, 70–72) have detected mutagenic activity after ozonation. The relation between the applied ozone dose and the observed effects seems complex. The more pronounced effects have tended to occur in water samples exposed to low ozone doses, a condition that often results in low ozone to dissolved organic carbon ratios. Mutagenic findings in these Ames tests have been supplemented by findings of gene mutation in toxicity type tests that included the HGPRT test (73) (see Table 3–2) in mammalian cells.

In general, the potential of ozone for the generation of mutagens appears to be more limited than that of chlorine. However, this general observation may be affected by differences in the effectiveness of prevailing extraction techniques for isolating ozone byproducts, many of which may be more water soluble than those of chlorine. As such, they would not be as easily extracted for testing. Nonetheless, several specific classes of mutagens are thought to be formed by ozonation (74, 75). Specifically identified mutagens formed during laboratory ozonation of a model compound include glyoxal and glyoxylic acid (91). These compounds have been measured in finished water samples as well.

The knowledge about the potential of chlorine dioxide for generation of mutagenic activity is even more limited. Several papers indicate that mutagens can be formed (67, 76), while other studies have found no increase in mutagenic activity after chlorine dioxide application (64, 68, 69). Although it is generally thought that the main precursors for mutagenic activity after chlorine dioxide application are humic substances, it was recently shown that the amino acids tyrosine and hydroxyproline and some peptides exerted mutagenic activity in the Ames test after chlorine dioxide treatment (77).

Little work has been carried out with regard to chloramine. However, at least two studies state that chloramine was able to produce mutagenic activity in the Ames test (69, 76). In addition, a number of other chloramine reaction byproducts of concern have been identified by chemical analysis.

Direct Evaluations of Carcinogenicity

Direct evaluations of the carcinogenic potential of disinfected water have been performed with epidemiological studies and animal studies. Epidemiological studies of the associations between the chlorination of drinking water and the occurrence of cancer have been reviewed in two reports of the National Academy of Science Safe Drinking Water Committee (5, 6).

These studies examined the association between disease outcomes and historical exposure to drinking water chlorination. Because long-term historical data for specific chlorination byproducts are not available, these studies have relied on indirect measures of potential exposure to disinfection byproducts. These indirect measures have included chlorine dose and chlorinated versus unchlorinated water classifications.

In most cases, surface water supplies are chlorinated. Therefore, use of unchlorinated and chlorinated designations tends to segregate study populations by groundwater and surface water sources. As a result there is a potential for effects associated with water quality characteristics other than chlorination. However, at least one study has observed a bladder cancer association with chlorine when comparing the effect of chloraminated waters with chlorinated waters (90). These designations would have less of a tendency to segregate study populations by type of source.

Use of chlorine dose as a measure of potential exposure to disinfection byproducts has limitations. Variation in precursor content between different water sources is likely to have a very significant effect on byproduct formation that is not reflected by chlorine dose as the only parameter of evaluation. Water sources in some regions of the country have a low organic content that may not produce a wide range in disinfection byproduct concentration as chlorine dose is varied. In such cases, significant association between disease and chlorine dose may not be observed, although a relationship to disinfection byproduct content may actually exist (6).

In addition to difficulties in characterizing exposure to chlorination byproducts, a number of confounding factors are encountered in epidemiological studies of long-term exposure. These include the effects of diet, smoking, exposure to cancer-causing agents in the workplace that have no relationship to drinking water quality, exposure to localized contaminants not related to disinfection products, and limitations on capability for characterizing the exposure patterns to water sources as a result of migration of the people within the study population.

In a review of these epidemiological studies by the National Academy of Science Safe Drinking Water Committee (6), early studies were generally observed to suggest low cancer incidences due to chlorination. There was also some inconsistent evidence in the types of cancer that were indicated. However, evidence from these studies suggested a need for a more refined evaluation of bladder cancer, in particular. Further study of colon and rectum cancer also appeared warranted.

The National Academy review stated that later epidemiological studies demonstrated progressive improvement in study design that presented sufficient evidence that chlorination byproducts or some other water quality parameter is associated with cancers of the digestive organs and the urinary tract (6). In the most extensive study, data from the National Bladder Cancer Study were evaluated to determine correlations with exposure to chlorinated water. Smoking was shown to significantly increase the risk for bladder cancer, a factor which masked the effects of chlorination on the sample population that smoked. However, among nonsmokers, the relative risk ratio was 1.3 for members of the sample population who were exposed to chlorinated waters for less than 20 years and was increased to 2.3 for those exposed for 60 or more years (78). To place the significance of these findings in perspective, the relative risk ratios of 1.3 and 2.3 fall into weak and moderate strength of association categories, respectively (79). Therefore, there is some indication of an association between chlorination and bladder cancer in these studies, although the strength of the relationship is not strong. Additional findings of increased bladder cancer were cited in the study that compared chloraminated and chlorinated drinking waters (90). Further study is needed to clarify these issues.

Animal studies showing carcinogenic potential have been limited. Some studies have indicated carcinogenic effects in animals from chloroform, dichlorobromomethane, and bromoform (85). These studies have indicated much higher levels of carcinogenicity for dichlorobromomethane. This yields a potential for more stringent regulation of this specific trihalomethane. EPA has also suggested the possible carcinogenic effects of dichloro- and trichloroacetic acid, chloral hydrate (trichloroacetaldehyde), and trichlorophenol (80, 92). Bromate, a byproduct formed by several disinfectants, with the greatest formation often occurring with ozone, is thought to have potential as a carcinogen at relatively low concentrations (85).

In spite of positive animal test results and the widespread concern that has been expressed for chloroforms and the other trihalomethanes, the overall effect of chlorination of drinking water is not yet clear. Epidemiological evaluations that show a relation between chlorination and cancer have not attempted to delineate the specific effects of trihalomethanes from those of other possible chlorination byproducts, and it is possible that other byproducts may be of greater significance.

Some cellular bioassays have identified MX and several other compounds as byproducts of concern. However, the significance of these findings is unclear since MX may be detoxified by biochemical processes upon ingestion by humans or animals. These types of effects are, therefore, not characterized by simple mutagenic assays where results are usually taken to be suggestive in nature. However, the tedious nature of existing animal testing procedures limits the number of compounds that can be tested, and many of these types of gaps in information will continue to persist as a consequence. Significantly the International Agency for Research on Cancer (IARC), in a review of available information, categorized chlorinated drinking water as not classifiable in its carcinogenicity to humans.

Noncarcinogenic Health Effects

Although carcinogenic effects of organic byproducts were an early basis of concern for disinfection byproducts, other health effects have also become a consideration for establishing future criteria. Significantly, chemicals used for disinfection have strong oxidizing properties and are themselves of potential health concern if present in excess concentrations. This could be a significant factor for some disinfectants if restrictions for residual levels do not allow adequate dosages for achieving criteria for either primary or secondary disinfection goals. In this regard, the desire to minimize adverse health effects from disinfectants has come into potential conflict with the desire to control the adverse health effects of waterborne disease.

In the 1987 review of disinfection by the National Academy of Science Safe Drinking Water Committee (6), the following health concerns were indicated for disinfectants:

Chlorine dioxide and two of its degradation products, chlorate and chlorite, have been observed to affect blood chemistry as a result of oxidative stress on red blood cells. These effects are of concern for people with specific enzyme deficiencies or other factors that place them at greater risk for this type of oxidant stress. Other concerns for chlorine dioxide, chlorite and chlorate relate to thyroid effects observed in laboratory animals that may be due to oxidation of dietary iodide. Neurological effects, for which the causative mechanism is not known, are also of concern.

Chloramines have been of concern in kidney dialysis patients where undesirable oxidation effects have been observed when chloramines are present in tap water used for dialysis baths. Liver toxicity has also been observed in laboratory animals.

Chlorine was observed to have an effect on thyroid function and is also capable of producing several halogenated products upon ingestion. Kidney effects are cited in other reports (85).

Toxicological information on other noncarcinogenic byproducts is limited. Possible liver effects have been noted for chloral hydrate and possible thyroid effects have been noted for cyanogen chloride (85). However, much research remains to determine the noncarcinogenic health effect of disinfection byproducts.

FUTURE CONSIDERATIONS FOR DISINFECTION BYPRODUCTS

Although there has been significant concern and considerable evaluation of disinfection byproducts, understanding of the effect on human health remains fragmented. Available methods of chemical analysis are limited, and the understanding of health effects is evolving. The review of research on disinfection byproducts by the National Academy of Science Safe Drinking Water Committee (6) indicates that a number of chlorination studies have been performed using model laboratory solutions to allow evaluation at high disinfection byproduct concentrations. This type of procedure helps to facilitate chemical analysis, resulting in identification of a wide range of byproducts. However, many of these studies have been performed at higher chlorine-to-organic ratios than are typical of drinking water conditions. These higher ratios are thought to increase the formation of more volatile compounds that are susceptible to chemical analysis by commonly used GC and GC/MS methods. At lower chlorine-to-carbon ratios more typical of water treatment, the ratio of nonvolatile to volatile byproducts may increase, thereby resulting in a somewhat lower level of success in identifying byproducts. These byproducts are less susceptible to GC and GC/MS analysis and have not been fully identified. Cellular bioassays of some of these unidentified fractions indicate that they may represent a potential risk.

A great deal of knowledge has been acquired about the identity of mutagens formed by chlorination of drinking water. It is generally accepted that humic and fulvic acids are significant precursors of mutagenic activity during chlorination. Amino acids and other constituents have also been observed to contribute to the formation of mutagens, but to a lesser degree. The significance of these contributions needs to be determined. Several compounds have been identified that contribute to significant levels of mutagenicity in chlorinated water samples. These include the extremely potent mutagens MX and EMX. In some cases, these two compounds have accounted for a significant part of the mutagenicity in extracts obtained from acidified samples. In spite of this finding, portions of mutagenicity in acidified water samples and the great majority of mutagens in the neutral extracts still remain to be identified.

The background knowledge in the field of mutagen generation and characterization is poorly developed for disinfectants other than chlorine. An overview of the literature indicates a wide variety of effects, but there is a virtual absence of systematic work to characterize precursors and mutagens. Although it is widely believed that these disinfection alternatives tend to generate less genotoxic compounds than chlorine, research in this field is rendered difficult by the fact that many of the reaction products are difficult to analyze.

While THM formation appears to be limited in the presence of chloramines, the formation of several other chlorinated organic compounds is indicated by measurements of TOX and more specific results from studies to identify specific byproducts. The significance of these other compounds was initially obscured by the fact that chloramines did not result in significant formation of THMs, the original disinfection byproducts of concern.

Byproducts of concern have also been identified for ozone. Chemical analyses for ozone byproducts are complicated by the fact that these compounds tend to be nonvolatile and are not as susceptible to analysis by GC or GC/MS methods. Byproducts that are mentioned for possible concern include aldehydes, carboxylic acids, epoxides, peroxides, bromate, and iodate. Formation of halogenated organics, such as bromoform, also appear to occur as a consequence of indirect reactions that involve an initial oxidation of bromide in the presence of ozone. Although these and other possible byproducts need to be given consideration, available studies suggest that the toxicity of ozonated byproducts is less than the toxicity of chlorinated byproducts (6).

In the case of chlorine dioxide, the initial focus for concern has been on chlorine dioxide itself and its degradation products, chlorate and chlorite. However, several other chlorinated and nonchlorinated byproducts have also been identified, including aldehydes and quinones, although much less is known about these byproducts in general.

Future application of a broader range of analytical techniques for identifying disinfection byproducts should facilitate the capabilities for identifying nonvolatiles and other compounds not readily identified by GC and GC/MS, the predominant methods of analysis to date. The development of better liquid chromatography–mass spectrometry couplings and other advanced techniques may lead to improved understanding.

Perhaps the most significant aspect to be determined and defined is the actual health risk that may be expected from exposure to disinfection byproducts. Some recent epidemiological studies have indicated a correlation between chlorination of drinking water and the occurrence of bladder cancer. These studies do not, however, indicate the specific byproducts that might be responsible for this apparent correlation. It is possible that byproducts besides trihalomethanes and other disinfection byproducts currently mentioned for regulation may be of greater importance in explaining this correlation. There is significant potential, therefore, for change in regulatory direction as understanding of causative factors changes over time. Increased epidemiological investigation may also indicate either a greater or lesser degree of concern for disinfection byproducts in general as more information is evaluated. Therefore, a great deal of flexibility is necessary in developing water treatment plant process trains to permit the addition of a range of facilities to deal with potentially harmful disinfection byproducts in the future.

References

1. Rook, J. J. 1974. Formation of haloforms during chlorination of natural waters. *Water Treat. Exam* 23: 234–43.
2. Bellar, T. A., J. J. Kichtenberg, and R. C. Kroner. 1974. The occurrence of organohalides in chlorinated drinking water. *JAWWA* 66(12): 703–9.
3. Symons, J. M., T. A. Bellar, J. Carswell, J. Demarco, K. L. Krop, G. G. Robeck, D. R. Seeger, C. J. Slocum, B. L. Smith, and A. A. Stevens. 1975. National Organic Reconnaissance Survey for Halogenated Organics. *JAWWA* 67(11): 634–47.
4. Brass, H. J., M. A. Feige, T. Halloran, J. W. Mello, P. Munch, and R. F. Thomas. 1977. The National Organic Monitoring Survey: Samplings and analyses for purgeable organic compounds. In *Drinking water enhancement through source protection,* Pojasek, R. B., ed. Ann Arbor, MI: Ann Arbor Science Publishers, Inc., pp. 393–416.
5. National Academy of Science. 1980. The chemistry of disinfectants in water: Reactions and products. In *Drinking water and health,* Vol. 2. Washington, DC: National Academy Press.
6. National Academy of Science. 1987. *Drinking water and health,* Vol. 7: *Disinfectants and disinfection by-products.* Washington, DC: National Academy Press.
7. Sawyer, C. N., and P. L. McCarty. 1967. *Chemistry for sanitary engineers,* 2nd ed. New York: McGraw-Hill.
8. Johnson, J. D., and J. N. Jensen. 1986. THM and TOX formation: Routes, rates and precursors. *JAWWA* 78(4): 156–62.
9. Keuringsinstituut, voor Waterleidingartikelen (KIWA). 1986. *Chlorination by-products: Production and control.* Denver, CO: AWWA Research Foundation.
10. Dempsey, B. A., R. M. Ganho, and C. R. O'Melia. 1984. The coagulation of humic substances by means of aluminum salts. *JAWWA* 76(4): 141–50.
11. Black, A. P., and R. F. Christman. 1963. Chemical characteristics of fulvic acids. *JAWWA* 55(7): 897–912.
12. Rook J. J. 1976. Haloforms in drinking water. *JAWWA* 68(3): 168–72.
13. Boyce, S. D., and J. F. Hornig. 1983. Reaction pathways of trihalomethane formation from the halogenation of dihydroxyaromatic model compounds for humic acid. *Environ. Sci. & Tech.* 17: 202.

14. Oliver, B. G., and D. B. Shindler. 1980. Trihalomethanes from the chlorination of aquatic algae. *Environ. Sci. & Tech.* 14: 1502–5.
15. Briley, K. F., R. F. Williams, K. E. Longley, and C. A. Sorber. 1979. Trihalomethane production from algal precursors. In *Water chlorination: Environmental impact and health effects,* Jolley, R. L., Brungs, W. A., and Cumming, R. B., eds. Ann Arbor, MI: Ann Arbor Science Publishers.
16. Briley, K. F., R. F. Williams, and C. A. Sorber. 1984. Alternative water disinfection schemes for reduced trihalomethane formation. Volume II. Algae as a precursor in chlorinated drinking water. EPA 600/52-84-005.
17. Hoehn, R. C., K. L. Dixon, J. K. Malone, J. T. Novak, and C. W. Randall. 1983. Biologically induced variations in nature and removability by alum treatment of reservoir trihalomethane precursors. Virginia Water Resources Research Center, Blacksburg, VA, Bulletin 127.
18. Hoehn, R. C., C. W. Randall, J. K. Malone, and K. L. Dixon. 1983. Seasonal variations in nature and removability of reservoir THM precursors. Virignia Water Resources Research Center, Blacksburg, VA, Bulletin 127.
19. Scully, F. E. 1986. Significance of organic amino nitrogen compounds in raw water from Thornton, Colorado. Report to City of Thornton, Colorado.
20. Ram, N. M., and J. C. Morris. 1980. Environmental significance of nitrogenous organic compounds in aquatic sources. *Environ. Int.* 4: 397–405.
21. Hrudey, S. E., A. Gac, and S. A. Daignault. 1988. Odorous aldehydes produced by disinfectant reaction with common amino acids. Paper presented at Poster Session, 1988 Annual AWWA Conference, June 1988, Orlando, FL.
22. Johnson, J. D., and R. F. Christman. 1988. Disinfection by-products: Formation and health effects. Presented at workshop on *Disinfection By-Products: Prevention and Control,* 10 March, 1988, at University of North Carolina, Chapel Hill, NC.
23. Wetzel, R. G. 1983. *Limnology,* 2nd ed. New York: Saunders College Publishing.
24. Veenstra, J. N., and J. L. Schnoor. 1980. Seasonal variations in trihalomethane levels in an Iowa river water supply. *JAWWA* 72(10): 583–90.
25. Brett, R. W., and R. A. Claverly. 1979. A one-year survey of trihalomethane concentration changes within a distribution system. *JAWWA* 71(9): 515–20.
26. Hirose, Y., et al. 1988. Formation of cyanogen chloride by reaction of amino acids with hypochlorous acid in the presence of ammonium ion. *Chemosphere* 17: 865–73.
27. Bull, R. J. 1982. Toxicological problems associated with alternative methods of disinfection. *JAWWA* 74(12): 642–48.
28. Tabor, M. W., and J. C. Loper. 1985. Analytical isolation, separation and identification of mutagens from nonvolatile organics of drinking water. *Intern. J. Environ. Anal. Chem.* pp. 281–318.
29. Christman, R. F. 1983. Contaminants in drinking water: What and how we know. Health effects seminar presented by AWWA Research Foundation, Denver, CO.
30. Glaze, W. H. 1990. Confirmation of structure. *Environ. Sci. & Tech.* 24: 271.

31. Kool, H. J., C. F. van Kreijl, and E. de Greef. 1981. Presence, introduction and removal of mutagenic activity during the preparation of drinking water. Presented at *Health Effects of Drinking Water Disinfectants and Disinfection By-Products,* U.S. EPA Symposium, Cincinnati, OH.
32. Jolley, R. L., R. B. Cumming, N. E. Lee, L. R. Lewis, J. E. Thompson, W. W. Pitt, M. S. Denton, and S. J. Hartman. 1982. Nonvolatile organics in disinfected wastewater effluents: Chemical characterization and mutagenicity. EPA-600/2-82-017.
33. AWWA Research Foundation/KIWA. 1988. *The search for a surrogate*. A cooperative research report, published by AWWA Research Foundation, Denver, CO.
34. Kool, H. J., C. F. van Kreijl, and M. Verlaan-de Vries. 1987. *Concentration, fraction, and characterization of organic mutagens in drinking water,* Suffet, I. H., and Malaiyandi, M., eds. Washington, DC: American Chemical Society, pp. 605–25.
35. Fielding, M., and H. Horth. 1986. Formation of mutagens and chemicals during water treatment, disinfection. *Water Supply* 4(3): 103–26.
36. van der Gaag, M., A. Noordsij, and J. P. Oranje. 1982. Presence of mutagens in Dutch surface water and effects of water treatment processes for drinking water preparation. In *Mutagens in our environment,* Sorsa, M., and Vainio, A., eds. New York: Liss, pp. 277–86.
37. Vartiainen, T., A. Liimatainen, S. Jääskelainen, and P. Kauranen. 1987. Comparison of solvent extractions and resin absorption for isolation of mutagenic compounds from chlorinated drinking water with high humus content. *Water Res*. 21(7): 773–9.
38. Ringhand, H. P., J. R. Meier, F. C. Kopfler, K. M. Schenck, W. H. Kaylor, and D. E. Mitchell. 1987. Importance of sample pH on recovery of mutagenicity from drinking water by XAD resins. *Environ. Sci. & Tech.* 21: 382–7.
39. Nazar, W. H., and W. H. Rapson. 1982. pH Stability of some mutagens produced by aqueous chlorination of organic compounds. *Environ. Mutagen.* 4: 435–44.
40. Holmbom, B., and L. Kronberg. 1987. In *Organic micropollutants in the aquatic environment*. Proceedings of the Fifth European Symposium, Angeletti, G., and Bjorseth, A., eds. Dordrecht: Kluwer Academic Publishers, pp. 278–83.
41. Fielding, M., and H. Horth. 1987. In *Organic micropollutants in the aquatic environment*. Proceedings of the Fifth European Symposium, Angeletti, G., and Bjorseth, A., eds. Dordrecht: Kluwer Academic Publishers, pp. 284–98.
42. Kringstadt, K. P., P. O. Ljungquist, F. de Sousa, and L. Stromberg. 1981. Identification and mutagenic properties of some chlorinated aliphatic compounds in the spent liquor from kraft pulp chlorination. *Environ. Sci. & Tech.,* 15(5): 562–6.
43. Meier, J. R., H. P. Ringhand, W. E. Coleman, J. W. Munch, R. P. Streicher, W. H. Kyalor, and K. M. Schenck. 1985. Identification of mutagenic compounds formed during chlorination of humic acid. *Mutat. Res*. 157: 111–22.

44. Coleman, W. E., J. W. Munch, W. H. Kaylor, R. P. Streicher, H. P. Ringhand, and J. R. Meier. 1984. Gas chromatography/mass spectroscopy analysis of mutagenic extracts of aqueous chlorinated humic acid. *Environ. Sci. & Tech.* 18: 674–81.
45. de Leer, E. W. B., J. S. Sinnighe Damsté, C. Erkelens, and L. de Galan. 1985. Identification of intermediates leading to chloroform and C-4 diacids in the chlorination of humic acid. *Environ. Sci. & Tech.* 19: 512–22.
46. Christman, R. F., D. L. Norwood, D. S. Millington, and J. D. Johnson. 1983. Identity and yields of major halogenated products of fulvic acid chlorination. *Environ. Sci. & Tech.* 17: 625–8.
47. Kringstadt, K. P., P. O. Ljungquist, F. de Sousa, and L. Stromberg. 1981. Identification and mutagenic properties of some chlorinated aliphatic compounds in spent liquor from kraft pulp chlorination. *Environ. Sci. & Tech.* 15(5): 562–6.
48. Kringstadt, K. P., P. O. Ljungquist, F. de Sousa, and L. Stromberg. 1983. On formation of mutagens in chlorination of humic acid. *Environ. Sci. & Tech.* 17(9): 553–5.
49. Holmbom, B. R., R. H. Voss, R. D. Mortimer, and A. Wong. 1981. Isolation and identification of Ames mutagenic compounds in kraft chlorination effluents. *Tappi* 64(3): 427–31.
50. Holmbom, B. R., R. H. Voss, R. D. Mortimer, and A. Wong. 1984. Fractionation, isolation, and characterization of Ames mutagenic compounds in kraft chlorination effluents. *Environ. Sci. & Tech.* 18(5): 333–7.
51. Kronberg, L., B. R. Holmbom, J. Hemming, and L. Tikkanen. 1986. In *Proceedings of the 16th European Environmental Mutagen Society,* Léonard, A., and Kirsch-Volders M., eds., pp. 104–9.
52. Hemming, J., B. Holmbom, M. Reunanen, and L. Kronberg. 1986. Determination of the strong mutagen 3-chloro-4-(dichloromethyl)-5-hydroxy-2(5H)-furanone in chlorinated drinking and humic waters. *Chemosphere* 15(5): 549–56.
53. Meier, J. R., W. F. Blasak, and R. B. Knohl. 1987. Mutagenic and castegenic properties of 3-chloro-4-(dichloromethyl)-5-hydroxy-2(5H)-furanone. *Environ. Molec. Mutagen.* 10(4): 411–24.
54. Morris, J. C., N. M. Ram, B. Baum, and E. Wajon. 1980. Formation and significance of N-chloro compounds in water supplies. EPA 600/2-80-031 USEPA, Municipal Environmental Research Laboratory, Office of Research, Cincinnati, OH.
55. Bieber, T. I., and M. L. Trehy. 1983. Dihaloacetonitriles in chlorinated natural waters. In *Water chlorination: Environmental impact and health effects,* Vol. 4. Ann Arbor, MI: Ann Arbor Science, pp. 85–96.
56. Trehy, M. L., R. A. Yost, and C. J. Miles. 1986. Chlorination byproducts of amino acids in natural waters. *Environ. Sci. & Tech.* 20: 1117–22.
57. Bull, R. J., and M. Robinson. 1985. Carcinogenic activity of haloacetonitrile and hapacetone derivation in the mouse skin and lung. In *Water chlorination: Environmental impact and health effects,* Vol. 5. Chelsea, MI: Lewis Publishers, pp. 221–8.

58. Horth, H. 1988. *Identification of mutagens in drinking water.* IWSA Maarten Schalekamp Award Paper, 1988.
59. Scully, F. E., R. Dravitz, G. D. Howell, M. A. Speed, and R. P. Arber. 1985. Contribution of proteins to the formation of trihalomethanes on chlorination of natural waters. In *Water chlorination: Chemistry, environmental impact and health effects,* Vol. 5, Jolley, R. L., Bull, R. J., Davis, W. P., Katz, S., Roberts, M. H., and Jacobs, V. A., eds., Chelsea, MI: Lewis Publishers, pp. 807–20.
60. Rapson, W. H., M. A. Nazar, and V. Butsky. Mutagenicity produced by aqueous chlorination of organic compounds. *Bull. Environ. Contam. Toxicol.* 24: 590–6.
61. Holmbom, B. R., L. Kronberg, J. Hemming, M. Reunanen, P. Backlund, and L. Tikkanen. 1990. Formation and properties of MX, a potent mutagen in chlorinated waters. In *Water chlorination: Environmental impact and health effects, chemistry,* Vol. 6, Jolley, R. L., et al., Chelsea, MI: Lewis Publishers, pp. 125–36.
62. Cheh, A. M. 1986. Mutation production by chlorination of methylated, alpha, beta-saturated ketones. *Mutat. Res.* 169: 1–9.
63. Streicher, R. P., and H. Zimmer. 1986. *Anal. Lett.* 19: 5–6, 681–96.
64. Guttman-Bass, N., M. Bairey-Albuquerque, S. Ulitzur, A. Chartrand, and C. Rav Acha. 1987. Effects of chlorine and chlorine dioxide on mutagenic activity of Lake Kinnereth water. *Environ. Sci. & Tech.,* 21(3): 252–60.
65. Noordsij, A., L. M. Puyker, and M. A. van der Gaag. 1985. The quality of drinking water from bank-filtered river water in the Netherlands. *Sci. Total Environ.* 47: 273–92.
66. Kool, H. J., and C. F. van Kreijl. 1988. *H_2O* 21(12): 316–18.
67. Kool, H. J., and C. F. van Kreijl. 1984. Formation and removal of mutagenic activity during water preparation. *Water Res.* 18: 1011–16.
68. Backlund, P., L. Kronberg, G. Pensor, and L. Tikkanen. 1985. Mutagenic activity in humic water and alum flocculated humic water treated with alternative disinfectants. *Sci. Total Environ.* 47: 257–64.
69. Daignault, S., W. B. Anderson, E. Savage, D. W. Rector, P. M. Huck, R. C. von Borstel, G. A. Irvine, and D. T. Williams. 1987. Drinking water treatment alternatives as evaluated chemically and biologically at pilot scale. Presented at the AWWA Annual Conference, 13–18 June, 1987, Kansas City, MO.
70. van Hoof, F. 1983. Influence of ozonation on direct-acting mutagens formed during drinking water chlorination. In *Water chlorination: Environmental impact and health effects,* Vol. 4, Jolley, R. L., et al., eds. Ann Arbor, MI: Ann Arbor Science, pp. 1211–20.
71. Cognet, L., Y. Courtois, and J. Mallevialle. 1986. Mutagenic activity of disinfection byproducts. *J. Environ. Health Perspect.* 69: 165–75.
72. van Hoof, F., J. G. Jansens, and H. van Dijck. 1985. Formation of mutagenic activity during surface water preozonation and its removal in drinking water treatment. *Chemosphere* 14(5): 501–510.

73. Hartemann, P., C. Danglot, M. M. Bourbigot, L. Pottenger, Z. Elias, and J. L. Paquin. 1987. Cellular toxicity and mutagenicity assays from on-site sampling of drinking water treatment plants using multistage ozonization. *Ozone: Sci. Eng.* 9: 179–94.
74. Marley, K. A., R. A. Larson, P. L. Stapleton, W. J. Garrison, and C. M. Klodnycky. 1987. Ozonolysis of naphthalene derivatives for water and in kerosene films. *Ozone: Sci. Eng.* 9: 23–36.
75. Duguet, J. P., A. Ellul, E. Broadard, and J. Mallevialle. 1983. In *Ozonization: Environmental impact and benefit.* Proc. IOA Symposium, Brussels, September 1983, pp. 424–42.
76. Lykins, B. W., Jr., W. E. Koffskey, and R. G. Miller. 1986. Chemical products and toxicologic effects of disinfection. *JAWWA* 78(11): 66–75.
77. Tan, H., W. B. Wheeler, and W. Cheng-i. 1987. Reaction of chlorine dioxide with amino acids and peptides: Kinetics and mutagenicity studies. *Mutat. Res.* 188(3): 259–66.
78. Cantor, K. P., R. J. Heover, P. Hartgi, T. J. Mason, P. T. Silverman, and L. I. Levin. 1985. Drinking water source and risk of bladder cancer: A case-control study. In *Water chlorination: Chemistry, environmental impact and health effects,* Vol. 5, Jolley, R. L., Bull, R. J., Davis, W. P., Katz, S. J., Roberts, M. H., and Jacobs, V. A., eds. Chelsea, MI: Lewis Publishers, pp. 145–52.
79. Craun, G. F. 1985. Epidemiological considerations for evaluating associations between the disinfection of drinking water and cancer in humans. In *Water chlorination: Chemistry, environmental impact and health effects,* Vol. 5, Jolley, R. L., Bull, R. J., Davis, W. P., Katz, S. J., Roberts, M. H., and Jacobs, V. A., eds. Chelsea, MI: Lewis Publishers, pp. 133–43.
80. Orme, J., and E. V. Ohanian. 1988. Potential health risks of drinking water disinfection byproducts. Presented at AWWA Water Quality Technology Conference, November 1988, St. Louis, MO.
81. Akin, E., et al. 1987. The (U.S. EPA) Office of Research and Development health research program on drinking water disinfectants and their by-products: An issue paper prepared for a science advisory board program review.
82. Stevens, A. A., L. A. Moore, C. J. Slocum, B. L. Smith, D. R. Seeger, and J. C. Ireland. 1990. By-products of chlorination at ten operating utilities. In *Water chlorination: Chemistry, environmental impact and health effects,* Jolley, R. L. et al., eds. Chelsea, MI: Lewis Publishers, pp. 579–604.
83. Rice, R. G. 1988. *Emerging technologies for compliance with disinfection and disinfection by-products regulations.* EPA Workshops 1987–1988. Ashton, MD: Rice Inc.
84. Krasner, S. W., et al. 1989. The occurrence of disinfection by-products in U.S. drinking water. *JAWWA* 81(8): 41–53.
85. Bull, R. J., and F. Kopfler. 1991. *Health effects of disinfectants and disinfection by-products,* AWWARF Report. Denver: AWWA.
86. Topudurti, K. V., and C. N. Haas. 1991. THM formation by transfer of active chloric from monochloramine to phloroacetophenone. *JAWWA* 83(5): 62–66.

87. Thurman, E. M. 1986. Dissolved organic compounds in natural waters. In *Organic carcinogens in drinking water,* N. M. Rametal, ed. New York: John Wiley, pp. 55–92.
88. de Leer, E. W. B., and C. Erkelens. 1984. Pathways for the production of organochlorine compounds in chlorination of humic materials. In *Biohazards of drinking water treatment,* Larson, R. A., ed. Chelsea, MI: Lewis Publishers, pp. 97–106.
89. Larson, R. A., and A. L. Rockwell. 1979. Chloroform and chlorophenol production by decarboxylation of natural acids during aqueous chlorination. *Environ. Sci. & Tech.* 13: 325–9.
90. Craun, G. F. 1988. Surface water supplies and health. *JAWWA* 80(2): 40–152.
91. Bablon, G., et al. 1991. Fundamental aspects. In *Ozone in water treatment: Application and engineering,* Langlais, B., et al., eds. Chelsea, MI: Lewis Publishers.
92. U.S. Environmental Protection Agency. 1991. *Status report on development of regulations for disinfectants and disinfection by-products.* USEPA-OGWDW, Washington, DC, June 20, 1991.

4

Free Chlorine

HISTORY OF CHLORINE USE

Following the discovery that certain diseases were transmitted by waterborne bacteria, early attempts to control these bacteria were directed to physical removal by filtration. Although filtration produced high removals, such removals were not complete or absolute. Residual bacteria in the filtered water still posed a potential threat of disease. Chlorine was eventually recognized as a method of reducing this disease potential and was applied to filtered water as a disinfectant as early as 1904 in the United States (1).

For all practical purposes, the steady expansion of filtration and disinfection in the United States eliminated waterborne diseases such as typhoid and cholera. For example, in Niagara Falls, New York, in 1911, 185 deaths out of 100,000 were caused by typhoid. By 1915, following introduction of filtration and disinfection, the death rate was reduced to nearly zero (1).

When chlorine was initially introduced in the United States in 1904, it was fed into drinking water as liquid hypochlorite. Use of chlorine gas, compressed and stored in steel containers, became popular following the development in 1913 by Wallace and Tiernan of equipment to dissolve measured amounts of chlorine gas in water. By midcentury most water treatment plants employed chlorine gas. However, recent concern about the risks associated with transport and handling of chlorine gas in congested areas has prompted a return to the use of liquid hypochlorite in some locales (1).

CHEMICAL FORMS OF FREE CHLORINE

Free chlorine is toxic to most forms of pathogenic bacteria and other microbes harmful to human health. The term *free chlorine* is used in reference to molecular (gaseous) chlorine (Cl_2) and its derivatives—hypochlorous acid (HOCl) and hypochlorite ion (OCl^-). Free chlorine in these forms has a strong tendency to gain electrons to obtain a more stable minus one (−1) oxidation state, as found in chloride. In this reaction, free chlorine serves as an oxidizing agent, and chloride is the ground state that is no longer very reactive. Many of the reactive properties of free chlorine are a result of the strong tendency to return to this ground state. The level of reactivity, oxidizing power, and associated disinfecting capability vary according to the individual species of free chlorine and the proportion of each species in water. These effects are important to the application of free chlorine and will be discussed later in the chapter.

COMMERCIAL FORMS OF CHLORINE

Commercial forms of free chlorine include molecular chlorine (chlorine gas), liquid sodium hypochlorite, and granular hypochlorites. On-site generation is an alternative to purchasing these commercial sources of chlorine.

Chlorine Gas

Chlorine gas is pressurized to liquid form for delivery in special containers. Release of pressure at the point of application returns liquid chlorine to the gaseous form for use in gas feeding equipment (1).

Impurities in some sources of manufactured chlorine gas have resulted in measurable levels of contaminants reported in finished water (1). Impurities can also cause operational problems. For example, excessive moisture causes corrosion and organic impurities cause fouling of feed equipment. Adherence to quality standards for chlorine gas established by the American National Standards Institute (ASTM-E410, E412, E647, E806, and D2022) and the American Water Works Association (B-301) are necessary to prevent such contamination and operational problems.

Sodium Hypochlorite

Generally, sodium hypochlorite liquid is commercially available in strengths of 12 to 16 percent as available chlorine. Selection of solution strength and location of storage can be affected by freezing properties, with a minimum freezing point of about −20°F occurring for a concentration of approximately 18 percent. Freezing occurs at approximately 10°F and 22°F in 10 and 5 percent solutions, respectively (2).

The rate of sodium hypochlorite degradation is a consideration in the selection of solution strength; degradation tends to increase as solution strength is increased. Besides solution strength, elevated temperatures and metal impurities such as iron, copper, nickel, and cobalt can accelerate deterioration. Storage in sunlight should be avoided since photochemical decay also increases the rate of deterioration (1).

Sodium hypochlorite solution is usually not economically competitive with chlorine gas, but is selected where safety in transport and handling are prime considerations. Chlorine is contained in solution as hypochlorite, thereby reducing risks of accidental release of chlorine gas. Sodium hypochlorite is also selected at many smaller installations since it can be fed using relatively simple methods that include solution feed pumps, hydraulic eductors, or simply gravity flow.

Granular Hypochlorite

Granular hypochlorite is typically dissolved in batch solution in tanks located near the point of application and is then fed as a liquid. Available forms include calcium hypochlorite ($Ca(OCl)_2$) and lithium hypochlorite ($LiOCl$). Although calcium hypochlorite is widely used, it may produce precipitates, which can foul metering equipment. Lithium hypochlorite, a less widely available form, has an advantage in this regard because it minimizes the formation of such precipitates (1).

On-Site Generation

On-site generation of free chlorine employs electrolytic processes for conversion of sodium chloride. These systems are similar to those used for commercial production of chlorine. The generated chlorine is commonly allowed to react with sodium hydroxide, a byproduct of generation, to form liquid sodium hypochlorite.

In on-site generation, sea water or brine solutions ($NaCl$) are used as the chloride source. Sea water systems tend to be less efficient, thereby resulting in excess sodium in the hypochlorite solution; brine solutions are preferable, especially where sodium levels must be limited in treated water (1).

The advantage of on-site generation is that delivery, handling, and bulk storage are not required, thereby affecting safety and allowing use in more remote situations such as sea-going vessels. However, considerable cost and complexity of operation can be encountered in many municipal water treatment installations. Therefore, the use of electrolytic generation systems has usually been reserved for special applications.

CHEMISTRY OF CHLORINE

Chlorine is generated from chloride compounds by the addition of sufficient energy from chemical or electrochemical reactions to displace electrons from the parent chloride. An illustrative chemical reaction is the one used by Karl W. Scheele, a Swedish chemist, who discovered chlorine in 1774 by heating hydrochloric acid with manganese oxide (1):

$$4HCl + MnO_2 = 2H_2O + MnCl_2 + Cl_2 \tag{4–1}$$

Electrochemical methods, developed by 1800, now are widely used for manufacture of caustic soda (NaOH) and molecular chlorine (Cl_2):

$$2NaCl + 2H_2O + \text{electrical energy} = H_2 + 2NaOH + Cl_2 \tag{4–2}$$

Under normal conditions chlorine reacts in water to form hypochlorous acid (HOCl):

$$Cl_2 + H_2O = HCl + HOCl \tag{4–3}$$

In Equation 4–3, one of the molecular chlorine atoms is reduced to chloride, which is relatively inert. The other atom changes its oxidation state in forming hypochlorous acid. Hypochlorous acid is highly reactive and becomes an active disinfecting agent. Hence, only half the original molecular chlorine takes part in disinfection. However, it is standard practice for chlorine dose to be expressed in terms of an equivalent level of molecular chlorine added (i.e., as Cl_2), regardless of the ultimate species.

At pH values greater than 7, hypochlorous acid begins to dissociate to form hypochlorite ions (OCl^-):

$$HOCl = H^+ + OCl^- \tag{4–4}$$

As pH is increased above 8, hypochlorite ions become the predominant chlorine species and begin to replace hypochlorous acid as the active disinfecting agent. The relationship between pH and the formation of hypochlorous acid and hypochlorite ions is illustrated in Figure 4–1. Note that in the acidic pH region, chlorine tends to remain in the molecular Cl_2 form.

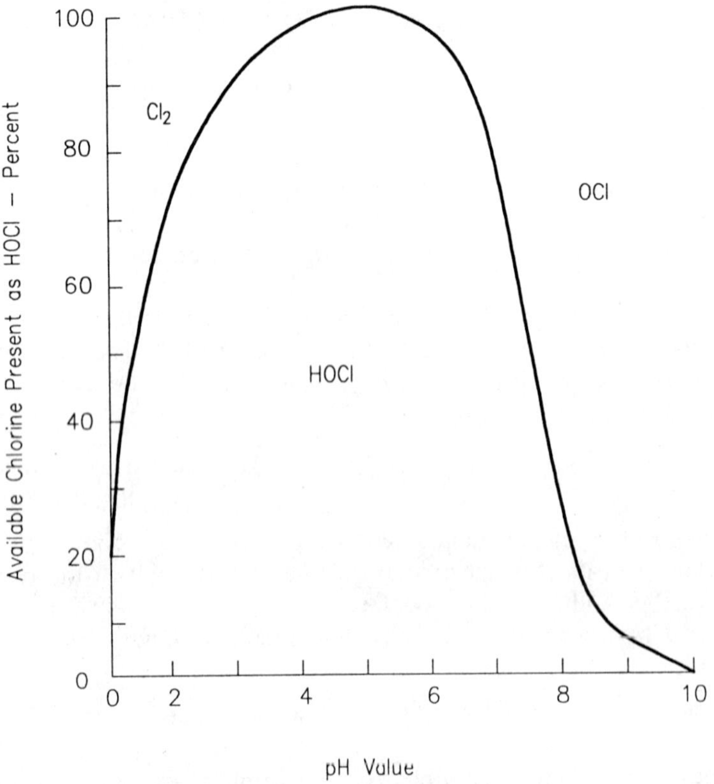

FIGURE 4–1. Distribution of chlorine species with pH. (Reprinted from *Journal American Water Works*, Vol. 78, No. 4 (April 1986), by permission. Copyright © 1986, American Water Works Association.)

Molecular chlorine (Cl_2), hypochlorous acid (HOCl), and hypochlorite ion (OCl^-) are the major species of free chlorine. Under certain conditions, transient chlorine species are also formed. These include H_2OCl^+, Cl^+, and Cl_3^-. The most significant of these is thought to be H_2OCl^+, which may be important for the catalysis of reactions that involve HOCl as the major species (3).

Free chlorine species can react in two general ways: (1) in oxidation reactions in which the oxidation state of the chlorine changes by losing electrons to form chloride (Cl^-), and (2) in substitution reactions in which the chlorine remains in the (+1) oxidation state while substituting into other chemical constituents. Although chlorine (+1) occurs in all of the free chlorine species, its reactivity varies significantly. For example, the tendency for substitution of chlorine (+1) can be characterized as follows (4):

$$Cl^+ > H_2OCl^+ > Cl_2 > HOCl > OCl^-$$

Among the more common free chlorine species, both Cl_2 and HOCl have strong tendencies for both substitution and oxidation, whereas OCl^- is much less reactive. Since pH affects the degree of formation of all of these free chlorine species, it thereby affects the tendency for reaction as well.

Substitution and oxidation reactions can be illustrated by the stepwise reactions of hypochlorous acid with ammonia (NH_3). The first reaction substitutes chlorine for one hydrogen atom in the ammonia to form monochloramine (NH_2Cl):

$$HOCl + NH_3 = H_2O + NH_2Cl \quad (4\text{–}5)$$

Monochloramine can be maintained as a relatively stable compound, leaving chlorine in its original oxidation state at this point in the reaction. Upon further addition of hypochlorous acid, chlorine substitutes for an additional hydrogen atom to convert monochloramine to dichloramine ($NHCl_2$):

$$HOCl + NH_2Cl = H_2O + NHCl_2 \quad (4\text{–}6)$$

Dichloramine is then susceptible to degradation by oxidation of nitrogen and reduction of chlorine to chloride through a reaction that can be generally represented as follows:

$$NHCl_2 + NH_2Cl = 3H^+ + 3Cl^- + N_2 \quad (4\text{–}7)$$

As a result of the chlorine reduction that occurs in Equation 4–7, the reactive chlorine residual decreases by the amount of chlorine that is converted to inert chloride. In fact, once this reaction begins with the onset of dichloramine formation, continued addition of hypochlorous acid results in further oxidation of ammonia and depletion of residual chlorine until the oxidation of nitrogen is completed. Only at this point are the chloramines fully dissipated, thereby allowing a reliable free chlorine residual to begin to be established. The overall reaction that results in the oxidation of ammonia to nitrogen gas through the above reaction sequence can be expressed as follows:

$$3HOCl + 2NH_3 = 3H_2O + 3HCl + N_2 \quad (4\text{–}8)$$

The changes in chlorine residual resulting from reactions of chlorine with ammonia are illustrated in Figure 4–2. Initially, chlorine residual increases in the monochloramine region up to a chlorine-to-nitrogen weight ratio of 5. With further chlorine addition, chlorine residual decreases with the formation of dichloramines until a theoretical chlorine-to-nitrogen weight ratio of 7.6 is reached. (Actual weight ratio is likely to be slightly higher than theoretical ratio due to additional reactions in which chlorine is involved.) The location of the break from a trend of decreasing chlorine residual immediately before achieving complete oxidation of ammonia to a trend of increasing chlorine residual upon completion of this oxidation is termed the *breakpoint*. Chlorination past the breakpoint to yield free residual chlorine is termed *breakpoint chlorina-*

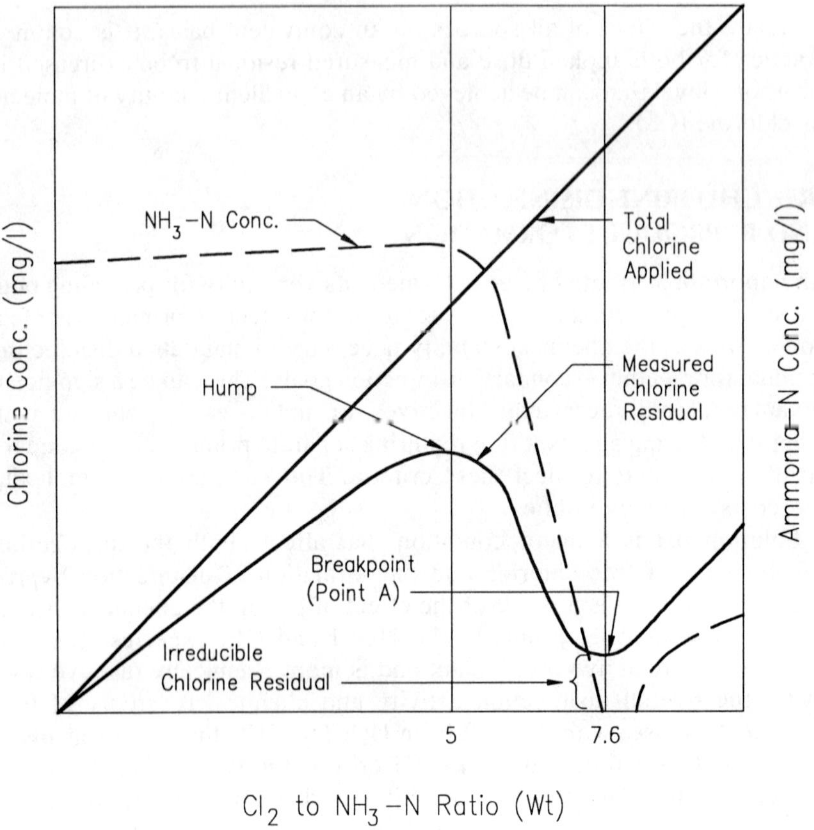

FIGURE 4–2. Theoretical breakpoint curve. (From Ref. 1, by permission. Copyright © 1986, Van Nostrand Reinhold Co., Inc.)

tion. It is this point that delineates free chlorination from chloramination. As a consequence, free chlorination can be viewed as the process that occurs largely beyond the breakpoint.

The foregoing discussion illustrates some of the basic chemical properties of free chlorine. In considering these properties, note that the original source of free chlorine species can vary. For example, sodium hypochlorite can serve as a source through the following reactions, which vary with solution pH just as for a molecular chlorine (Cl_2) source:

$$NaOCl = Na^+ + OCl^- \quad (4\text{–}9)$$

$$H^+ + HOCl + Cl^- = H_2O + Cl_2 \quad (4\text{–}10)$$

$$H^+ + OCl^- = HOCl \quad (4\text{–}11)$$

To relate the effect of all sources on an equivalent basis, it is common practice for both applied dose and measured residual to be expressed in terms of a level that can be achieved by an equivalent quantity of molecular chlorine (Cl_2).

FREE CHLORINE DISINFECTION AND BYPRODUCT FORMATION

An important attribute of free chlorine is its versatility for providing both the strong disinfecting properties required for effective primary disinfection as well as the chemical stability necessary to maintain a disinfecting residual for meeting secondary disinfection goals. This can be a significant advantage, since these dual objectives are not as easily achieved with other disinfecting agents, often requiring separate primary and secondary disinfecting agents to meet these criteria. This can increase complexity and costs for many utilities.

Solution pH is a major condition that affects both the disinfection effectiveness of free chlorine and the formation of disinfection byproducts. In part, this is a result of the effect of pH on the chemical speciation of free chlorine, primarily the HOCl and OCl^- species. Because HOCl is a more active disinfectant and is more chemically reactive than OCl^-, the overall disinfection activity and chemical reactivity of free chlorine decreases with the shift from HOCl to OCl^- that occurs as pH is increased. This is reflected in EPA CT criteria for disinfection of *Giardia* by free chlorine. These criteria exhibit a marked increase with increased pH. CT data for viruses did not exhibit as definitive a trend in the pH range of 6 to 9.

In some applications, reduction in the disinfection activity of OCl^- can be partially offset by the greater stability afforded by its lower chemical reactivity, a condition that can allow a residual to be maintained over a longer period. Although this may not completely offset the diminished disinfecting activity of OCl^- in primary disinfection applications, it can have a value in cases where free chlorine is used as a secondary disinfectant for providing residuals over extended periods.

The general effect of pH on the formation of halogenated byproducts is illustrated by the nonpurgeable TOX data in Figure 4–3. These data exhibit a trend of decreased TOX formation with increased pH, an effect that would be anticipated based on conversion to the less chemically reactive OCl^- species. Data for chloroform, also shown in Figure 4–3, exhibit an opposite trend where increased formation occurs with increased pH. Some research suggests that the increased formation of chloroform at high pH actually occurs due to reactions in which other TOX compounds become more likely to convert to chloroform (6, 7). The conversion reaction is increasingly favored as pH is increased, thereby resulting in the opposite trend for chloroform formation, which is actually an indication of shift in byproduct composition, not in the level of overall byproduct formation. It is important to recognize that although formation of chloroform can be reduced at low pH, other halogenated byproducts are not avoided and their formation can be enhanced by this condition. This is illustrated by the results of humic acid chlorination in laboratory tests, shown in Figure 4–4 (8). Note that chloroform ($CHCl_3$) increases with pH, whereas TOX decreases as before. Also shown in this figure are data for another major byproduct, trichloroacetic acid (TCAA). Note that its concentration reaches a maximum in the acidic pH range and is depleted with the increased pH condition that favors formation of chloroform.

Increasing awareness of the above phenomena has resulted in a wider outlook from the original narrow focus on chloroform and other trihalomethanes. In a recent study, the occurrence of different byproducts was evaluated for 35 water utilities around the country (9). This study evaluated THMs, halocentonitriles, haloketones, haloacetic acids, chloropicrin, chloral hydrate, cyanogen chloride, 2,4,6-trichlorophenol, formaldehyde, and acetaldehyde. Widespread occurrence of these compounds was observed, particularly THMs, which accounted for about half of the total byproducts measured, and haloacetic acids, which accounted for about 25 percent. Most of the other compounds occurred at lower levels. In the alkaline pH range, shifts in the occurrence of some byproducts were observed. These included declining levels of haloacetonitriles, haloke-

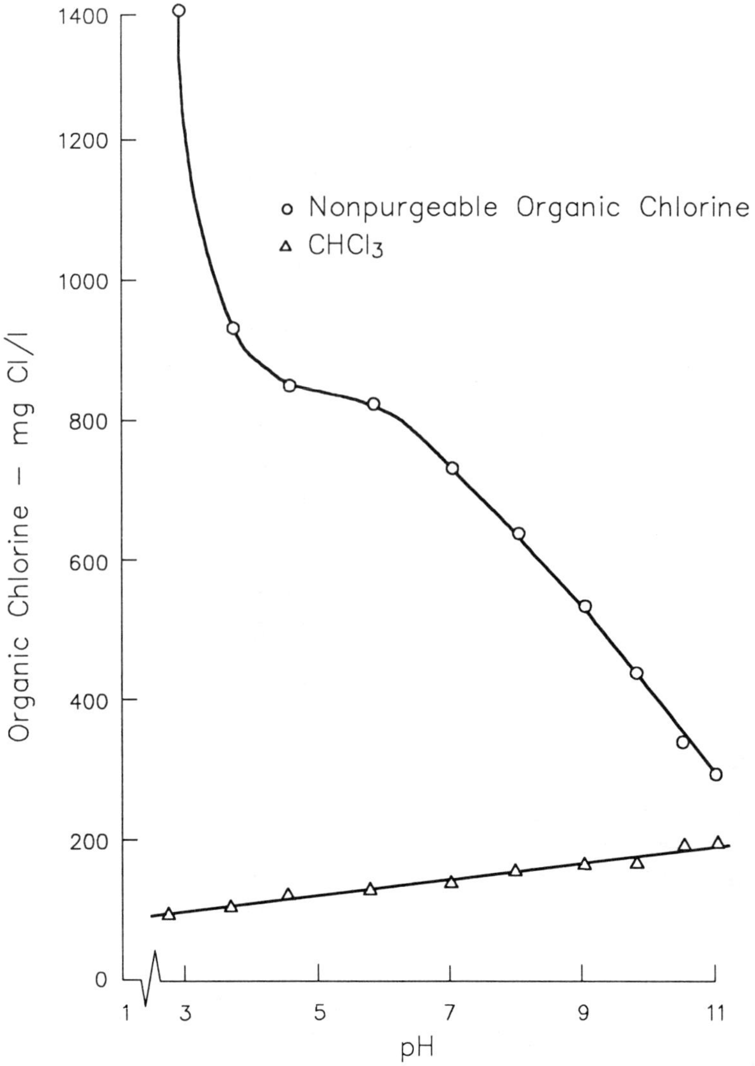

FIGURE 4–3. Effect of pH on the formation of organic chlorine by free and combined chlorine. (From Ref. 5. Reprinted from *Journal American Water Works,* Vol. 75, No. 3 (March 1983), by permission. Copyright © 1983, American Water Works Association.)

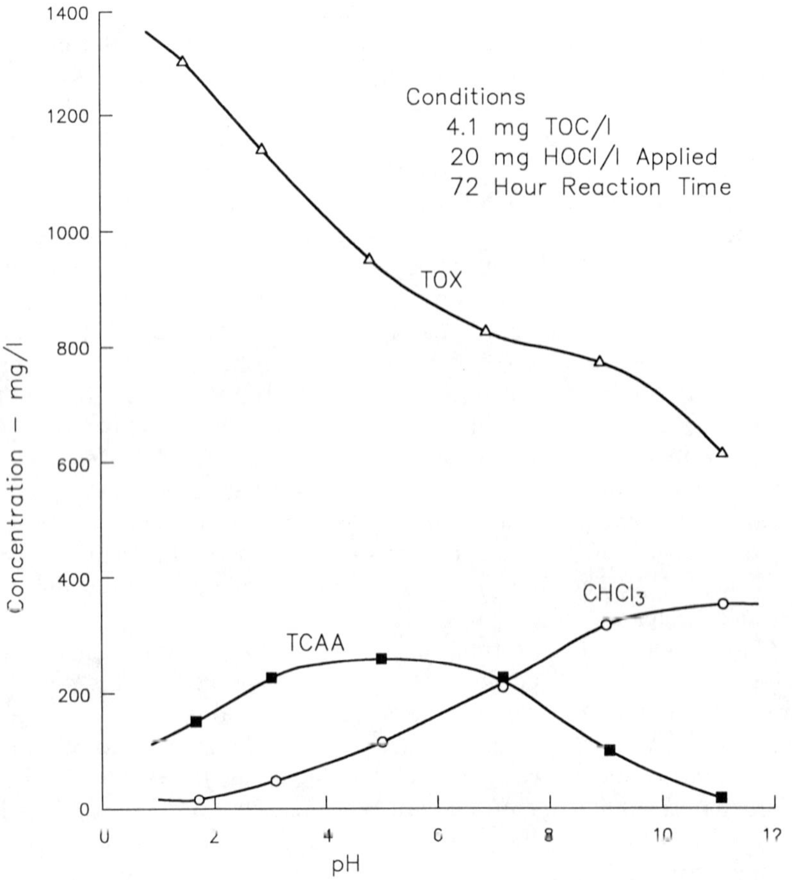

FIGURE 4–4. Organic halide yields from Black Lake fulvic acid as a function of pH. (From Ref. 8. Reprinted from *Journal American Water Works,* Vol. 76, No. 4 (April 1984), by permission. Copyright © 1984, American Water Works Association.)

tones, chloral hydrate, and possibly cyanogen chloride with the occurrence of increased levels of chloroform and some other compounds. Also, formaldehyde and acetaldehyde were observed to be formed as a result of chlorination, although they are not chlorine-containing byproducts. These formations would be due to chlorine oxidation reactions that do not involve chlorine substitution.

In addition to pH, bromide has been observed to affect the formation of chlorination byproducts. When bromide ions are present, the overall formation of THMs can be accelerated, and the extent of formation of brominated THM species is increased as well (10). Although this effect of bromide has been widely observed for THM formation, the effect on overall organic halide formation may be much less. For example, one study has indicated that bromide did not significantly increase the extent of overall organic halide formation (11). Instead, the speciation appeared to be changed through the formation of brominated intermediates that more readily degrade to THMs instead of non-THM species. Other effects on speciation have been reported. For example, one study of reactions with fulvic acid under laboratory conditions indicated that the formation of the haloketone, 1,1,1-trichloropropanone, could be suppressed by the formation of chlorobromopropanones and other compounds at sufficient bromide concentrations (31). Although the total quantity of organic halides may not be significantly changed by bromides, the effect on the distribution of byproducts may be important. This is illustrated by a greater concern for carcinogenicity for some brominated THMs, particularly dichlorobromomethane, as discussed in Chapter 3.

Other phenomena can also affect byproduct formation. For example, one study has shown that copper ions could increase THM formation in humic acids (12). The effect was variable and did not occur for some other precursor compounds.

Chlorine can react to form a number of mutagenic substances, as discussed in Chapter 3. The formation of low levels of MX, a chlorinated furanone compound, has explained a significant portion of this mutagenic activity. Other sources of mutagenicity exist and may need to be considered. Some studies have shown that reducing agents, such as sodium sulfite, can remove some of the mutagenic activity (31). The applicability for this type of treatment, however, remains to be demonstrated because of unclear relationships between mutagenic activity and cancer.

In addition to the reactions with organic material that have dominated concerns for disinfection byproducts, there are concerns about chlorate (ClO_3^-) as an inorganic degradation product that occurs in chlorine solution. Formation increases with elevated pH levels and long reaction times, conditions that are common in storage of sodium hypochlorite (32). This alternative represents a significant increased potential for chlorate formation as compared with molecular chlorine, which is stored as a gas, where no reaction is possible during storage.

NONDISINFECTION USES OF CHLORINE

Aside from its use in disinfection, free chlorine is widely used for other water treatment purposes, such as oxidation of iron and manganese, control of tastes and odors, removal of color, enhancement of coagulation and filtration, and control of biological growths throughout water treatment plants. Hence, in evaluating alternative or substitute methods to replace chlorination for disinfection, consideration must also be given to the means for replacing nondisinfection benefits of free chlorine that may be necessary at the water treatment plant in question.

Removal of Iron and Manganese

Iron and manganese may occur in both surface and ground supplies. In surface waters, iron and manganese contained in lake or reservoir sediments can be chemically reduced to soluble forms that are released to the overlying water column. This release is generally seasonal, following a period of water stratification when oxygen is depleted in the lower depths over the iron- and manganese-bearing sediments. In ground waters, iron and manganese may be released from subsurface formations throughout the year.

The presence of iron and manganese in potable water can cause esthetic problems such as discoloration, staining, and taste. For this reason, the EPA secondary drinking water standards set maximum concentrations at 0.3 mg/l for iron and 0.05 mg/l for manganese.

Iron and manganese treatment commonly employs a chemical oxidant early in the process to oxidize iron (Fe^{2+}) and manganese (Mn^{2+}) to species that can then react to form oxide and hydroxide precipitates for removal by sedimentation and filtration processes. An alternative to this approach is the use of coatings on filter media or the use of other filter media, such as greensand, to adsorb and subsequently catalyze the oxidation of iron and manganese.

Theoretical doses for oxidation by chlorine are 0.64 mg of chlorine per mg of iron oxidized and 1.30 mg of chlorine per mg of manganese oxidized (14). Actual dose requirements can be significantly higher due to the presence of other sources of chlorine demand. Therefore site-specific testing is required to establish actual dosage requirements.

Depending on required reaction time for complete iron and manganese oxidations, a detention period may be necessary immediately following chorine feed. This detention can be provided in raw water pipelines, storage basins, or specially designed tanks. Where colloidal particulates may be generated, such as in the case of manganese precipitates, the oxidation reaction should normally be completed ahead of floc-forming processes so that the colloidal manganese can be enmeshed in the floc for enhanced removal. An exception to this practice is where coatings on filter media or alternative greensand media oxidize and adsorb iron and manganese where separate steps ahead of filtration are not used.

Reaction rates for both iron and manganese are reduced as water temperature decreases, with more significant reductions as temperatures approach 2 or 3°C (14). The effect of temperature may be offset by the use of longer detention times, increased chemical dosage, or both. For surface waters affected by iron and manganese generated only during impoundment stratification in warm weather, however, design can often be based on warmer temperature conditions.

While the effects of pH on reaction rate also need to be considered, the reaction of chlorine with iron is relatively rapid in the 6.5 to 8.0 pH range most often encountered in water treatment. Reaction rate with manganese, more sensitive to pH, is much slower at pH values below 8 (14).

The effectiveness of iron and manganese oxidation is influenced by the presence of natural organics such as humic and fulvic acids. In the case of iron oxidation, natural organics exert a competitive chlorine demand and can also form organic iron complexes, thereby adversely affecting the overall oxidation process (14). Although organic complexation of manganese has been cited by some (13), others report that dissolved manganese is not well complexed by naturally occurring organics (14). They suggest that difficulties in oxidizing manganese in the presence of organics derive more from a competitive oxidant demand. Under this concept, oxidation of manganese would not proceed to any significant extent until sufficient chlorine is added to overcome the competing demand of natural organics. Following chlorine oxidation, a chlorine residual should be generally maintained through subsequent processes to prevent reducing conditions that can lead to resolubilization of precipitates.

As alternatives to the use of chlorine for iron and manganese removal, other oxidants have been employed to achieve faster reaction rates and to minimize undesirable byproducts. Stronger oxidants include chlorine dioxide and ozone. The special character of potassium permanganate make this oxidant useful for treating manganese. However, residuals for these chemicals can dissipate more rapidly than chlorine, which is more effective in maintaining an oxidant residual through subsequent water treatment processes (15). Under some conditions, depleted residuals that occur with other oxidants can increase the likelihood for subsequent resolubilization of manganese from sludge layers in downstream sedimentation units, thereby resulting in incomplete control of manganese.

The elimination of prechlorination at one plant illustrates a problem that may result with use of alternative oxidants. In this case, potassium permanganate and chlorine dioxide were used to replace chlorine for manganese oxidation. With chlorine, residuals had been maintained throughout the plant. However, the alternative oxidants, while they may have been effective at the point of addition, did not provide a reliable method for maintaining a continuous residual throughout the plant. Before mechanical devices were installed in this plant, sludge was collected in sedimentation basins for extensive periods prior to manual cleaning. Sludge became anaerobic in the absence of consistent oxidizing/disinfecting residuals. Periodic flotation of sludge and solubilization of previously removed manganese occurred as a consequence. While this case was somewhat extreme, similar problems with manganese release have been observed in other plants, even where sludge collection equipment is available. The extent of such release appears to depend on the frequency of sludge collection and is significantly reduced, although not always eliminated, when collection is practiced on at least a daily basis. Other problems of solubilization of both iron and manganese have also been reported in the recycling of supernatant from processes involving concentration of sludges from sedimentation basins and recovery of filter backwash (15, 17).

Because many plants do not fully achieve the desired level of manganese removal in preoxidation coagulation/sedimentation sequences, a supplemental removal across filters is often important. With chlorine, this removal process often involves a coating of oxidized manganese that accumulates at the surface of the media filter media. This coating catalyzes the oxidation and adsorption of iron and manganese in the filter itself. Many plants have inadvertently been employing this approach through a prefiltration chlorination practice that also provides the oxidizing residual necessary for developing an adsorptive coating on the surface of filter media.

The principal features that enhance the development of media surface coatings are a near neutral or slightly alkaline pH and maintenance of an oxidizing condition by using chlorine at concentrations greater than 1 mg/l (16). Of the two, maintenance of oxidating conditions is the more important. While regeneration of the oxidized coating by periodic chlorination of the filters is possible, operating experience at some locations indicates that a continuous chlorine residual is most effective for preventing resolubilization of manganese from these coatings (19, 20). Recognizing the importance of oxidized coatings, at least one plant reported the use of aged filter media that was mixed with fresh media in order to retain manganese adsorption capabilities in its filters (21).

Process control for manganese removal across filters can require consideration of potentially conflicting objectives. For example, a pH of 6 is frequently adequate to achieve the necessary level of oxidation once a coating is established, although a higher pH is better. However, as pH is increased, the disinfecting efficiency of chlorine decreases and the potential for the formation of trihalomethanes increases. A higher pH can also adversely affect filtration by redissolving aluminum from alum floc. Therefore, some compromise is required.

Introduction of alternate oxidants in these filtration processes can result in manganese removal by formation of a colloidal manganese oxide as opposed to adsorption to the coated filter media. This can result in a significant change in removal characteristics. In such instances, the extent of manganese reduction depends on the effectiveness of filtration in removing the colloidal particles (14, 18). These particles may prove to be difficult to filter, resulting in carryover and a manganese problem in the finished water unless a prefiltration coagulation process is provided (13). Therefore, care should be taken before selecting alternative oxidants when removal of manganese by filtration is an objective. Extreme caution should be exercised to ensure full control over manganese if free chlorine is being eliminated from the treatment system as a strategy for addressing disinfection byproduct concerns.

Control of Tastes and Odors

Undesirable tastes and odors may occur in water from a wide range of sources, including algae, sulfides and other inorganic constituents (e.g., copper, iron, zinc, manganese, sodium, and potassium) (22), and industrial compounds. Chlorination has been used successfully to control tastes and odors in many water supplies. However, chlorination is not a universally successful approach, and aeration, activated carbon, potassium permanganate, ozone, and chlorine dioxide can be used as alternatives.

Algal tastes and odors are a widespread problem, particularly in supplies that are obtained from lakes or reservoirs. These problems normally occur on a seasonal basis, depending on the type of algae generated and the extent of algal growth. Many of these taste and odor events are successfully controlled using free chlorine, but some cannot be easily controlled, and others require chlorine doses of 5 mg/l (1) or more (1, 23). In cases where these high dosages might be required, there may be a conflict with goals to limit formation of chlorine byproducts.

Chlorine is also used to control odors from sulfides. Several end products are possible from reactions between chlorine and sulfides, including elemental sulfur and polysulfides (1). Elemental sulfur forms a colloidal precipitate, which must be removed by filtration. However, polysulfides may create a problem if they are not controlled since they can be reduced to hydrogen sulfide, which returns sulfide to the water.

A combination of processes is generally required to control sulfide products. For example, chlorination can be followed by filtration to remove colloidal sulfur and by a sulfur dioxide/rechlorination sequence to convert any residual polysulfides or colloidal sulfur to sulfates. Chlorination can also be used to supplement sulfide removal by gas stripping (1).

Tastes and odors can also be caused by various industrial compounds. The applicability of chlorine for removal of these tastes and odors depends upon the specific chemical characteristics of the causative compound and other general characteristics, such as pH. With phenols, partial chlorination using low doses of chlorine can actually intensify taste and odor problems through the formation of chlorophenols. These considerations often make chlorination inappropriate for phenol-related tastes and odors, although at increased chlorine doses these problems can be overcome.

Hrudey et al. (24) found that chlorine can also create problems associated with tastes and odors that derive from formation of aldehydes. Both chloramines and free chlorine were observed to react with amino acids to form taste- and odor-causing aldehydes. This phenomenon was associated with seasonal taste and odor problems during spring thaw on the North Saskatchewan River in Edmonton, Alberta, that resulted in high levels of nitrogen.

Removal of Color

Chlorine can play an important role in bleaching or decolorizing highly colored waters (15). In some cases, replacement of chlorination as a decolorizing agent can involve complex trade-offs. For waters low in color or where color removal can be achieved with aluminum or iron coagulants, replacing a decolorization role of chlorine may not be difficult. However, even where coagulants can be successful in color removal, chlorine frequently enhances the process (1). In highly colored waters, coagulation processes may not achieve the desired color reduction when used alone. These situations may require a substantial oxidant dose, and replacement of chlorine may be more involved under these conditions. Ozone, chlorine dioxide, and, in some cases, powdered activated carbon (PAC) represent possible alternatives. However, assigning a role for color reduction to these chemicals may significantly alter their dose requirements from those associated with other treatment goals for which they are applied. In some situations, high dosage requirements for alternative oxidants can significantly increase the cost for color reduction as compared with free chlorine (15).

Enhanced Coagulation

Prechlorination has enhanced coagulation and filtration processes at numerous water treatment plants by reacting with source water organic matter and by inhibiting biological growths in the treatment train. In many cases, application of prechlorination prior to coagulant addition has reduced the required coagulant dose. While the basis for this reduction is not understood entirely, it is likely that chlorine oxidizes organic compounds that would otherwise interfere with coagulation.

Control of Biological Growth

Chlorine can frequently be used to control algal species and slime growth that can cause tastes and odors and cause filter clogging. Algal growth would normally occur in uncovered settling basins and filters. Slime growth, on the other hand, can occur in both covered and uncovered treatment units. Filter clogging can be a significant seasonal problem depending on the species and the extent of proliferation of the biological growth. Maintaining a chlorine residual or use of chlorine in shock treatment can assist in minimizing mud-ball formation, prolonging filter runs, avoiding buildup of organic matter at the surface of filters, and, in general, reducing loss of filter media and achieving improved bacterial quality of filtered water (1).

As an alternative to maintaining a continuous chlorine residual, the use of shock chlorination has been employed widely to control biological growths in wells, raw water pipelines, aeration facilities, basins, filters, distribution systems, and other facilities. In shock treatment, a relatively high dosage of chlorine is applied and held for a short time.

GASEOUS CHLORINE SYSTEMS

Since gaseous chlorine is delivered as a pressurized liquid-gas mixture, and since gas can be vaporized from the liquid if pressure is relieved, systems can withdraw chlorine directly from containment tankage as either a gas or a liquid. The choice of withdrawal method depends upon feed rates needed to meet maximum chlorine demands. Natural vaporization can commonly sustain gas withdrawal rates up to about 400 lb/day from a single ton container. For higher rates, the vaporization from the liquid form is not sufficiently rapid at normal ambient temperatures. Under these conditions, liquid is drawn directly into an evaporator, which employs heat to accelerate the change from liquid to gaseous chlorine. The addition of heat also prevents the freezing phenomenon associated with formation of chlorine hexahydrate and the consequent clogging that could otherwise occur at excessively high liquid-to-gas evaporation rates (1).

Gaseous chlorine flow is controlled and metered in a chlorinator (feeder) and then can be fed either directly as a gas for mixing with the treatment stream or indirectly via an injector, which uses a separate stream of dilution water to form a concentrated chlorine solution for subsequent mixing with the treatment stream. Direct feed generally is limited to rates less than 300 lb/day and most often is used for standby or emergency purposes. The most common injector systems employ a hydraulic injector that uses water flow under a venturi principle to create a vacuum, which draws gaseous chlorine through the chlorinator and supply piping. These devices also achieve mixing of the chlorine gas in the dilution water stream to create a chlorine solution.

Several arrangements for handling and feeding gaseous chlorine are available, which consist of the principal elements shown schematically in Figure 4–5. These include the following:

- Containment tankage
- Storage and weighing facilities
- Evaporators
- Piping arrangements to and from chlorinators
- Chlorinators
- Injectors

Containment Tankage

Containment tanks for chlorine gas in a pressurized liquid state are made of steel in the various capacities listed in Table 4–1. This tankage consists of cylinders, containers, tank trucks, and railroad tank cars, which are

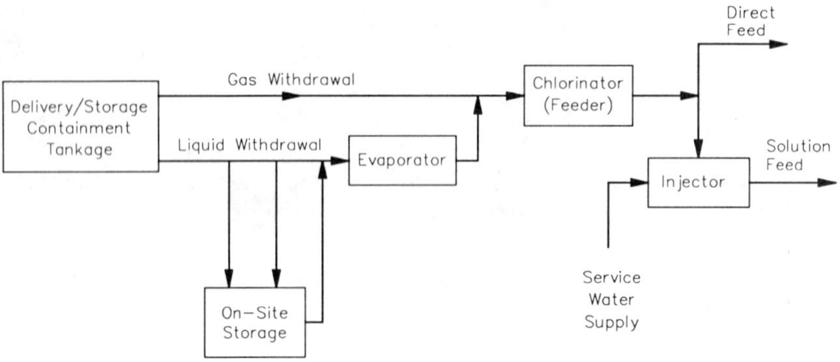

FIGURE 4–5. Gaseous chlorine system alternatives.

TABLE 4–1. Gas Chlorine Tankage Available

Type of Container	Net Weight	Approximate Tare Weight	Gross Weight	Approximate Gas Draw-off Rate (lb/day)[a]
Cylinders	100 lb	63–105 lb	163–205 lb	
	150 lb	85–140 lb	235–290 lb	50
Ton container	2,000 lb	1,300–1,650 lb	3,300–3,650 lb	400
TMU-ton	15 tons	—	—	
container car	16 tons	—	—	
Single-unit	16 tons	—	—	
tank cars	30 tons	—	—	
	55 tons	—	—	
	85 tons	—	—	
	90 tons	—	—	

[a] (Minimum Room Temperature − 10°F) × J = withdrawal rate, where J = 1 for 150-lb cylinder and 8 for ton container.

Source: Wallace & Tiernan, Inc.

normally provided with fittings and valves for connection to chlorine feed systems. Hence, containment tankage may be used both for transport and for on-site storage for feeding.

Only a gas outlet is provided on cylinders 150 pounds and less in capacity because they are too small for practical use in liquid withdrawal systems. Ton containers are provided with two outlet valves on the same end. When the container is positioned with one valve above the other, the option exists for using the upper valve as a gas outlet or the lower valve as a liquid withdrawal outlet. Vapor pressure usually is adequate in ton containers to force liquid from containers when using liquid withdrawal in conjunction with evaporation systems.

In the case of tank trucks and railroad tank cars, provisions are made for liquid withdrawal, including the option for transfer to pressure storage tanks located at water plants. When liquid is withdrawn at high rates, an air padding system that adds pressure to the storage tank is needed to aid in the withdrawal of chlorine, especially under cold weather conditions. Chlorine Institute Pamphlet 66 (33) describes the necessary components for air padding.

Containment tankage is designed specifically to protect against accidental release of chlorine, including provisions to protect against puncture and damage to valves and connections. Cylinders and containers are provided with fusible plugs, which melt and release pressure to allow cooling and thereby prevent rupture under overheated conditions.

Tank trucks and railroad tank cars are equipped with special check valves to contain the contents and prevent major spills in the event of a severe accident that may shear off the dome that encloses the valve connections. A specially automated shut-off system is provided for lower-level leaks that would not be sufficient to activate the special check valve (1). A pressure-relief valve is also provided to protect against rupture due to excessive pressure.

Storage and Weighing Facilities

Ideally, storage should be adequate to provide thirty days of average chlorine usage or twenty days of the highest usage condition. Peak chlorine usage is often associated with periods of peak water demand, such as during the summer. However, peak use can occur at other times, such as during spring runoff or when other conditions require high chlorine doses to overcome a high chlorine demand.

Adequate space should be provided adjacent to the chlorine storage area for truck turning and for handling full and empty cylinders and containers. The minimum vertical clearance for a monorail or crane hook should be 6.5 feet above the floor to permit lifting one ton container over another. About 12 feet of clearance should be provided above ground level to allow for the height of the delivery vehicle. If possible, the hoist should be able to reach over a portion of the delivery vehicle and should be capable of lifting two to three times the container capacity to allow for a tare weight of 1,600 pounds and to minimize structural lateral strain from swinging containers. The container-supporting structures should provide for eccentric loading to allow for different arrangements of full and empty storage tanks or containers. Ton containers are usually placed on a horizontal rack equipped with rollers that permit the containers to be easily rotated and properly positioned for valve connection. Scales should be provided to maintain an inventory of chlorine in connected cylinders and containers. Either load cells or balance type scales with digital or analog dials are available.

Evaporators

Evaporators are not required in cases where maximum rates of gaseous chlorine withdrawal are adequate to meet the full range of chlorine usage. Typical maximum rates of withdrawal for gaseous chlorine are listed in Table 4–1. Excessive rates of gas withdrawal can produce evaporative heat losses sufficient to cause freezing of liquid chlorine in the containment tankage. At these withdrawal rates, chlorine must be withdrawn as a liquid. At the most common ambient temperatures, a practical limit for gaseous withdrawal is about 400 lb/day per ton container, but containers can be manifolded to allow total gas withdrawals of 1,200 to 1,500 lb/day.

When liquid withdrawal is required, the liquid stream is conveyed to a heated evaporator, where it is changed to the gaseous state prior to discharge to a chlorinator. Evaporators may also be employed when there is a need to stabilize withdrawal rates under widely varying ambient temperatures that may create control problems with gas withdrawal systems.

General Arrangements of Feeders

Piping arrangements for gas withdrawal from cylinders or ton containers would be similar for most system capacities up to about 500 lb/day. Arrangements may be designed to use cylinders or containers as individual units, as multiple units acting as a single unit in a manifold arrangement, or as two units (or two manifolded units) in a manifold arrangement with automatic or manual switchover from one unit to the other.

Pipe used to carry chlorine, liquid or gas, under pressure is usually schedule 80, seamless carbon steel. Isolation valves are provided at each cylinder or container, at each connection to manifolds, and at other strategic locations to permit equipment to be removed from service with minimum exposure to chlorine remaining in the system. When equipment and piping layouts are designed, complete backup requirements of the EPA Surface Water Treatment Rule must be considered.

The discharge piping from evaporators is typically provided with a pressure-regulating valve that closes automatically at low temperatures in order to prevent freezing and damage to equipment. Filters are provided in the evaporator discharge line to remove particulate impurities from the gaseous chlorine that could clog or damage chlorinator equipment.

Automatic switchover from empty to full storage units is a common practice to ensure a continuous chlorine supply for high reliability. When the chlorine in the first unit (lead unit) is depleted, the second unit (lag unit) is placed in service automatically. The switchover is generally activated by low pressure in the piping leading from the lead storage unit. Control can be achieved by settings on pressure or vacuum regulating valves, depending on the type of system.

As in the case of evaporator piping, a filter is frequently placed in the gas manifold piping to remove impurities. In addition, an external pressure-reducing valve is provided to minimize the possibility of reliquification since both conditions can foul equipment. Pressure-relief valves also serve to prevent pipe ruptures. Discharge lines from these pressure-reducing valves are routed either to remote locations where chlorine can be dispersed into the atmosphere without harm or to absorption systems where chlorine is contained and neutralized.

In vacuum feed systems, piping from containment storage is under pressure up to the vacuum control assemblies. Vacuum control valves are located near the containment tankage when no evaporators are used, otherwise they are located directly after the discharge of the evaporators. Vacuum-type systems operate under vacuum from the vacuum control point through the feeders to the injection device. The vacuum within this length of piping is actually created in the injection device by aspirating water at high velocity through a venturilike device.

In small installations, chlorine feeders are often connected directly to cylinders or containers, as shown in Figure 4–6. These installations typically also use a vacuum system with vacuum regulators mounted near the containment tank to provide a controlled transition to vacuum conditions in the gas piping. Simple, cylinder-mounted chlorine feeders for low application rates combine vacuum regulation with feed control in a single unit.

Larger installations may include simple manifold piping arrangements for cylinders and containers as shown in Figure 4–6. Somewhat more complex systems may be used for ton containers as well as the smaller cylinders to meet the feed requirements for the particular application requirements.

The vacuum control assembly should be as close as possible to the containment tankage to minimize the length of pressurized pipe. However, there are limitations on distance between the vacuum control valve and the feeder due to friction losses in excessively long pipe runs. Although distances vary with specific feeders, generally the vacuum loss in the piping between the vacuum regulator and the feeder should be limited to no more than 5 inches of water. All piping should be arranged for duplicate routing and adequate isolation valves to allow each piece of equipment to be removed while still feeding chlorine.

Chlorinators

The main function of chlorinators is to control the rate of chlorine feed. Chlorinators consist essentially of a metering orifice with an adjustable opening to vary feed rate and a rotameter to measure the gas flow. A differential vacuum-regulating valve commonly is used in vacuum-type systems to provide a controlled pressure gradient across the metering orifice, thereby achieving stable or steady-state flow control. Some chlorinators eliminate the need for this valve by operating at sonic velocities where rate is governed only by the size of the orifice. Several arrange-

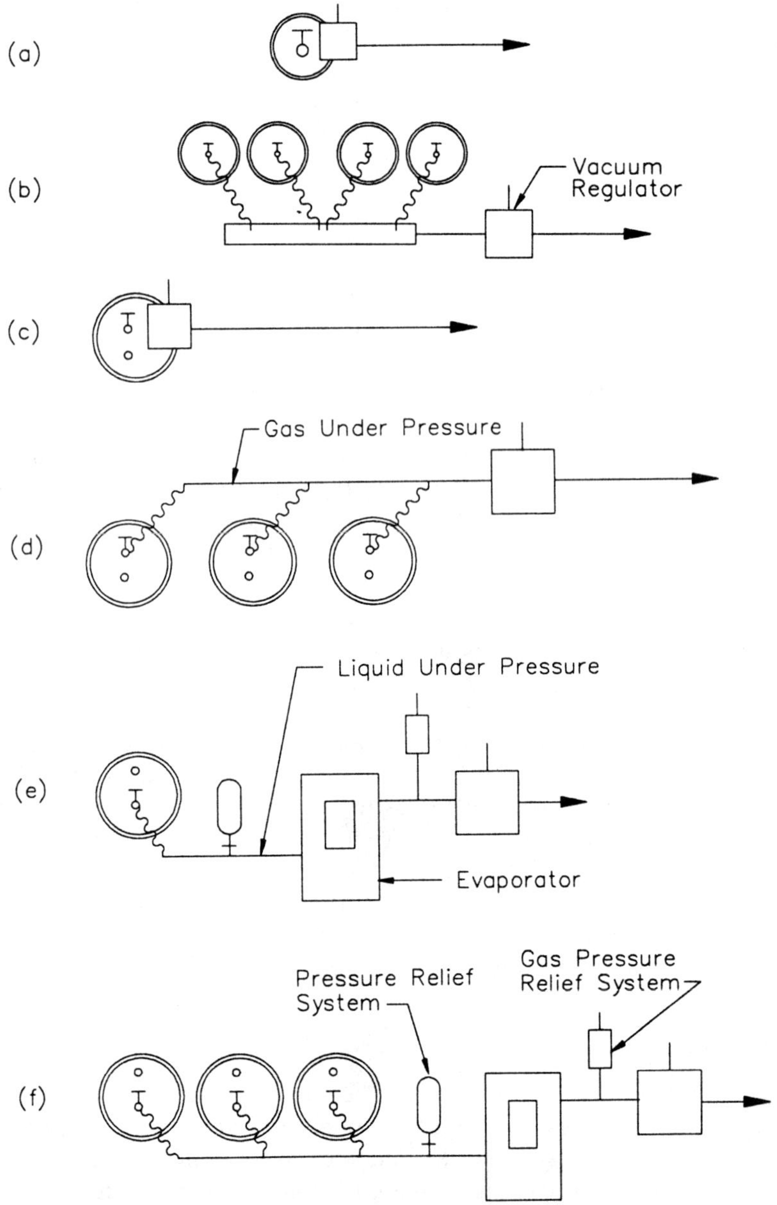

FIGURE 4–6. Alternative storage arrangements: (a) vacuum regulator mounted on single cylinder; (b) manifold mounted vacuum regulator with cylinders; (c) vacuum regulator mounted on single ton container; (d) manifold mounted vacuum regulator with ton containers; (e) liquid tap from ton container; (f) liquid taps to manifold for ton containers.

ments of chlorinators with injection devices can be used, as shown in Figure 4–7.

Chlorinator capacities are rated in terms of both console capacity and rotameter capacity. Console capacities limit the maximum capacity of the overall installation, while rotameter capacities are selected within the console capacity for specific operating conditions. Several rotameters may be provided with a chlorinator so that operators can select the one that will operate at desired rates at mid and upper ranges where accuracy is better than at lower readings.

A chlorinator rotameter normally will have a working range of 10 to 1 or 12 to 1 (maximum-to-minimum flow rate). However, lower readings may be accurate only to 5 percent of the maximum scale reading. This can result in errors of up to 50 percent at low rotameter readings. Therefore, care should be exercised at the lower end and, in these cases, consideration should be given to using a smaller rotameter to improve accuracy.

Injectors

Injection systems are typically used to disperse chlorine gas into a dilution water stream. These systems include a service water supply to the injector, the injector itself, the injector vacuum line from the chlorinator, and the injector discharge or chlorine solution line. The maximum concentration of the resultant chlorine solution is limited by a solubility of 3,500 mg/l. Where pertinent, this limitation needs to be considered for determining the required service water quantities.

The solution line transports the chlorine solution from the injector to a diffuser installed at the point of application. Typical materials used for solution piping include PVC with threaded or solvent-weld joints, flexible polyethylene, rubber, or rubber-lined steel pipe.

Injectors may be located either near the point of application or near the chlorine supply. In the first case, the vacuum line is longer; in the latter, the solution line is longer. Where the injector is located near the feeder and some distance from point of application, it may be necessary to provide a source of high pressure. It is often more attractive to run longer vacuum lines than it is to run long solution lines, since no special pressure boosting equipment is needed as might be the case for greater pressure drops encountered in liquid stream piping. However, total vacuum pipe loss from the feeder to the injector should not exceed 20 inches of water near sea level, with lower losses at higher elevations.

The potential for leaks must be minimized in both types of lines. In this regard, vacuum systems offer a safety advantage since air will be drawn into a leaking vacuum line, thereby inhibiting release of chlorine to the

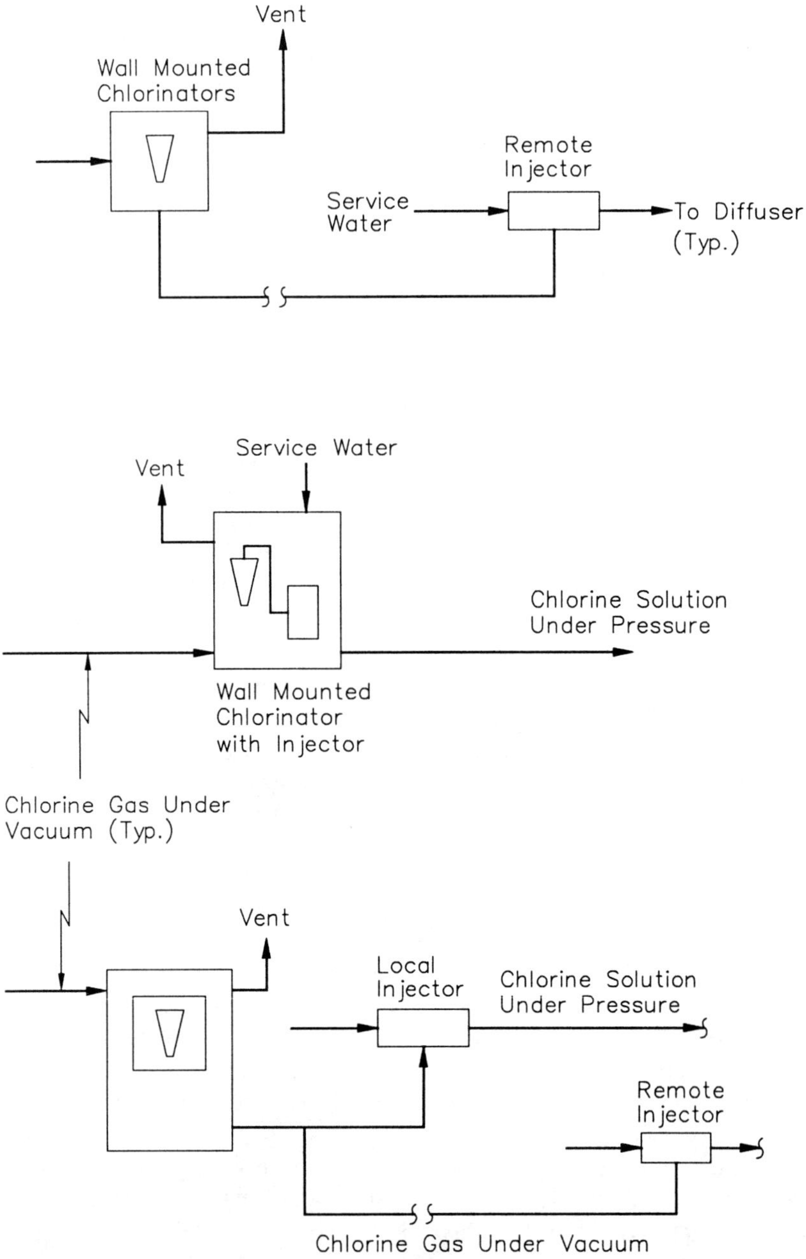

FIGURE 4–7. Arrangements of chlorinators and injectors.

external environment. Also, complete rupture of a vacuum line will typically shut down a chlorinator due to loss of vacuum, whereas a ruptured solution line on the injector can still allow flow through the injector, which will continue to maintain a vacuum.

HYPOCHLORITE SYSTEMS

In the hypochlorite form, free chlorine is obtained from either a liquid or a solid source. This is less hazardous than using gaseous chlorine, a form that can be more directly emitted into the surrounding air through leaks or breaks.

Sodium hypochlorite and calcium hypochlorite are the predominant forms in use. Sodium hypochlorite is available as a liquid in a wide range of delivery sizes that include 5- and 13-gallon small plastic or glass carboys, 30-gallon rubber-lined drums, and bulk deliveries in 1,300- to 3,600-gallon tank trucks (26). Although very large facilities might also consider delivery by rail in large tank cars, rail delivery of sodium hypochlorite is prohibited in some areas (1).

Typically, calcium hypochlorite is available either as tablets or as granular material that contains at least 70 percent available chlorine. It can be shipped in drums of up to 100 pounds, in 3- to 5-pound cans, and in 2- to 9-pound plastic containers (26).

Chlorinated lime, a form that is similar to calcium hypochlorite, is also available. This form contains both calcium and hypochlorite, but the available chlorine content is only 25 to 37 percent. Chlorinated lime is relatively unstable and can be more readily degraded (26). Therefore, its use is less common.

Basic components of hypochlorite systems include provisions for delivery and unloading, storage facilities and feed tanks, and solution feed equipment and piping. Dilution tanks may be desired where low dosages would otherwise reduce the feed volume below levels that can be reasonably controlled with available metering equipment. Granular forms, such as calcium hypochlorite, will also require a dissolving tank.

Hypochlorite feed rate is typically controlled using either pumping or gravity-driven systems. Eductor systems, which use water-driven devices to draw the feed stream into solution under vacuum, can also be used (1).

Hypochlorite solutions tend to be alkaline, which can produce a scaling potential in waters with excessive hardness levels. For example, serious scaling was experienced in solution piping and diffusers in Detroit where slightly hard water was used for service water. Addition of a polyphosphate to the hypochlorite solution alleviated the problem.

Gravity-driven systems can be applied at plants where the hypochlorite tanks are located at an elevation above the point of application. These systems can use modulating valves to control feed rates, thereby eliminating the need for maintaining chemical metering pumps. However, gravity feed will not be appropriate unless sufficient elevation is available. In addition, gravity feed systems usually do not provide sufficient head to be suitable for application to pressurized piping.

In cases where positive displacement, diaphragm-type pumps are used, design should consider needs for dampening the pulsing feed characteristics of this type of equipment. Otherwise, an uneven chlorine feed will occur, resulting in erratic disinfection performance. Pulsation-dampening devices are available for these pumping systems.

In design and operation of hypochlorite systems, several factors need to be considered:

Corrosivity

Hypochlorites can be extremely corrosive to wood and most metals. As such, solutions are normally stored in plastic, fiberglass, or rubber-lined containers or tanks. Piping and pumping equipment should also be made of corrosion-resistant materials.

Degradation

All hypochlorites degrade over time, resulting in a reduction in solution strength. Therefore, periodic monitoring is required to make necessary adjustments in feed rates that will compensate for this effect. Several factors can affect the actual rate of hypochlorite degradation and should be considered in facility design and operation:

1. *Solution impurities*. Hypochlorite degradation can be accelerated in the presence of certain impurities, particularly iron, copper, nickel, and cobalt. Care should be taken in selecting a source of hypochlorite that has minimum levels of these impurities. White (1) suggests that copper and iron should not be present at levels greater than 0.5 mg/l and 1.0 mg/l, respectively.
2. *Storage time*. Many sodium hypochlorite suppliers recommend a maximum shelf life of 60 to 90 days (27). However, this is only a general rule of thumb since storage conditions have a significant effect on degradation rate and can alter the desired storage time. As long as they are maintained in a solid form, hypochlorites will have a longer shelf life. For example, calcium hypochlorite has a recommended shelf life of 1 year (26).

3. *Sunlight*. Hypochlorites should be protected from sunlight, particularly from the ultraviolet wavelengths. Otherwise, the life of hypochlorite solutions will be significantly reduced. Although protection can be provided by completely shielding solutions from light, household bleach is sometimes delivered in amber-colored bottles that provide sufficient shielding from the wavelengths of primary concern.
4. *Solution concentration*. Sodium hypochlorite can be obtained in various solution strengths or diluted concentrations. Typical bulk solution concentrations for sodium hypochlorites are 12 to 16 percent, but lower concentrations are available. Calcium hypochlorite is normally mixed at solution concentrations of 3 percent or less because of practical solubility considerations (26).

   At facilities where large quantities of sodium hypochlorite are used, cost considerations may favor the use of the most concentrated solutions that reduce the volume of solution that must be delivered and handled. Otherwise selection of concentration may involve a balance between the higher rate of degradation in more concentrated solutions and the freezing problems that can be encountered at low solution concentrations.
5. *pH*. The stability of hypochlorite solutions is significantly reduced as pH is reduced below 11. Therefore, the pH of sodium hypochlorite solutions is frequently controlled to this level in order to improve solution stability. Calcium hypochlorite typically provides an alkaline pH, thereby simplifying operations by eliminating the need for pH adjustment in small plants (28).
6. *Temperature*. Degradation of hypochlorite solutions increases rapidly with increased temperature. Exposure to excessively high temperatures should, therefore, be avoided. A common practice is to try to limit temperatures to 80°F or less. With respect to lower temperature constraints, a 12 to 16 percent sodium hypochlorite solution does not readily freeze. It is still liquid at temperatures down to 1°F and only begins to freeze at −20°F. Therefore, this higher-strength solution can be stored outside in many areas (26). Freezing constraints will be more restrictive at lower solution concentrations.

Spontaneous Combustion

Spontaneous combustion is not a problem for liquid hypochlorite. However, it is a major consideration for storage of dry granular calcium hypochlorite, which spontaneously combusts at temperatures greater than 350°F. Reactions with organic materials, including cardboard boxes or containers that may be contaminated with grease or other organics, can also generate heat that may lead to spontaneous combustion. Care should be taken, therefore, to eliminate possible heat sources in areas of dry material storage and to avoid the possibility of violent reactions with organics by confining calcium hypochlorite within appropriate containers and using clean scoops for material transfer.

Dangerous Chemical Reactions

As long as the pH of a hypochlorite solution is sufficiently alkaline, free chlorine is stored as the hypochlorite ion (OCl^-) and is relatively innocuous. However, if the pH is lowered, conversion to hypochlorous acid (HOCl) occurs, with a subsequent potential for conversion to molecular chlorine (Cl_2) by the following reaction sequence:

$$OCl^- + H^+ = HOCl \tag{4–12}$$

$$H^+ + HOCl + Cl^- = Cl_2 + H_2O \tag{4–13}$$

Molecular chlorine is released from solution as a gas and presents the same hazard encountered with gaseous chlorine systems. Therefore, care must be taken to prevent accidental mixing of acidic chemicals with hypochlorite solutions.

Violent reaction can also occur if certain chemicals are put in contact with hypochlorite. These can include strong reducing agents, such as bisulfite solutions, that may be used for dechlorination at some water treatment plants (1).

CHLORINE DISPERSION AND CONTACTING

Dispersion

The objective of dispersion is to achieve complete distribution of chlorine in the process stream. Incomplete dispersion can result in localized areas of low chlorine content in which disinfection or desirable reactions may be reduced. Localized areas of high concentration may result in greater formation of undesired chlorination byproducts.

Diffusers that extend across a diameter of a pipe are frequently used to achieve chlorine distribution through a series of orifices in the diffuser tube. High velocities are used through the orifices to promote good dispersion. Diffusers may not be needed in small-diameter pipes if chlorine is injected at the center of the pipe at the location of highest turbulence (1).

Diffusers are also used in open channels where they may be placed in a horizontal position across the channel. Good locations include those downstream from flow-measuring flumes and weirs where turbulence is generally high. Adequate submergence (a minimum of 6 inches) should be provided to minimize off-gas release from the surface of channel flow.

Adequate back pressure should be provided to avoid a negative pressure condition in a solution pipe. A siphon breaker is not desirable in a chlorine solution feed line, since it will introduce air, which eventually will draw out the chlorine. When dispersion is in a pressure pipe, it may be necessary to add a back siphon or check valve to prevent back flow of water to the chlorinator system.

In many cases, chlorine is dispersed in rapid mix basins and filter channels. With rapid mix basins, dispersion is achieved by the mixing device. The chlorine solution should be injected at a location that maximizes the dispersion efficiency of the mixing device (usually close to the eye of the mixing impeller).

Contacting

In many systems, chlorine is added at two or more locations. Chlorine demand is typically essentially satisfied at upstream application points where an initial level of disinfection is achieved, while the final application completes the in-plant disinfection process and achieves control over the chlorine residual maintained in finished water as it enters the distribution system. Where disinfection byproducts may be a problem, upstream chlorination may be located after coagulation/sedimentation processes. This allows for removal of some of the precursors by coagulation processes. Chlorine demand can also be reduced by these processes, thereby lowering chlorine dosage requirements. Both conditions can combine to significantly reduce byproduct formation.

Long retention times are normally available in tankage used for sedimentation basins, clearwells, and finished water storage tanks. In the past, this type of tankage was not designed specifically for chlorine contacting. Imperfections in flow distribution patterns in existing treatment plant tankage must now be taken into account to comply with EPA disinfection guidelines, as discussed in Chapter 2.

Internal baffling might be added to existing storage tanks to minimize short-circuiting and improve the residence time distribution characteristics. In new plant design, consideration should be given to tank configuration and baffling arrangements to attain the necessary residence time distribution for adequate disinfection contact. In some cases, the addition of separate chlorine contact chambers may provide more efficient contacting tankage for both existing plant improvements and new plant designs. Under some conditions, these chambers could provide greater control over the time of chlorine contact and yield benefits for improved control of disinfection byproducts as a consequence.

CHLORINE MONITORING AND CONTROL

Recent EPA criteria, associated with the Surface Water Treatment Rule, require continuous monitoring of disinfectant residuals in finished water (30). Several alternatives are available for monitoring chlorine, including amperometric, electrochemical, and colorimetric methods such as DPD-FAS. Devices employing these methods are reliable when maintained properly. Even with proper maintenance, all chlorine monitoring devices will require periodic calibration and cleaning (1).

Chlorination efficiency can be maximized by using an automatic control system to regulate chlorine residual. However, water treatment applications do not often experience rapid variability in chlorine demand, so simpler control methods may be used. Flow pacing is one simple automated control approach that can be used as an alternative to chlorine residual control.

For some facilities, manual control may be the preferred mode of operation, especially where routine electronics maintenance support cannot be provided. In any event, emergency or standby manual control should be provided even where automatic control is installed.

CHLORINE LEAK CONTROL

All systems should provide features to deal with accidental chlorine leaks. Detection systems should be provided in chlorine storage and feed areas. If leaks are detected, automatic controls should shut off chlorine flow from storage containment and close the normal ventilation system to divert exhaust air through an emergency ventilation system. This emergency system may be designed to discharge chlorine-laden air directly to the atmosphere or indirectly through a scrubber system designed to neutralize the chlorine. Some adsorption systems are being marketed as an alternative to the scrubber. In general, some form of chlorine neutralization can be extremely desirable from a safety standpoint. Cost is a consideration and specific safety considerations or requirements often dictate whether or not these systems are installed.

Ventilation systems for chlorine should always be independent from general plant systems. Care must be used in locating the exhaust in relation to other buildings and air intakes, taking into consideration the fact that chlorine is heavier than air and will collect in low-lying pockets. It may be desirable to employ interlocks within the plant instrumentation that will close elements of normal ventilation systems during a chlorine emergency. It also may be desirable to have emergency controls for general plant ventilation systems energized manually in response to alarms so that the situation can be assessed by an operator before any action is taken.

Generally, ventilation systems for chlorine feed and storage facilities are designed to keep the area under a slight negative pressure. When a chlorine leak occurs, the chlorine greatly expands and, under a major leaking condition, could result in the storage area being pressurized. The emergency ventilation system should have the capacity to maintain the negative pressure in the area or to allow only a slight positive pressure.

Neutralization systems for a chlorine-laden air exhaust generally employ an air-scrubbing system that uses sodium hydroxide (caustic soda), which produces the following reaction:

$$Cl_2 + NaOH = NaOCl + HCl \tag{4–14}$$

The rate of reaction is affected by temperature increases that result from the reaction itself.

Neutralization can be accomplished using either single-pass or recycling systems. A single-pass system will normally keep the room under a slight negative pressure and consist of a two-component system utilizing a venturi scrubber followed by a packed tower. The recycle system, which would normally allow some pressure to build up in the storage area, usually includes only a venturi scrubber. In either case, the ventilation ductwork should be equipped with dampers that open in case of excessive pressure.

The emergency scrubber can be designed to discharge either directly to the atmosphere or back to the storage or feed area for subsequent air recycle through the scrubber until the chlorine content is entirely neutralized. Recycle systems are used to achieve economy since scrubbers and related components can be made smaller. There is, however, a disadvantage due to recirculation of a chlorine-laden mist that can increase corrosion damage and impede emergency response.

Chlorine leaks often occur during the change of cylinders or containers as a result of leaky or broken pipes and valves or leaky containment tankage. Piping leaks are usually readily controlled by closing isolation valves and proceeding with repairs. Uncontrolled leaks may be limited in rate and quantity to the amount of gas that can escape from containment tankage before evaporative heat loss causes the chlorine to freeze.

A pipe break in the vacuum piping downstream from the vacuum control valve will typically automatically close the chlorine supply and limit leakage to piping from the valve. If pressure piping includes an evaporator (in a liquid chlorine system), up to 125 pounds of chlorine could be released just from liquid storage in the evaporator (1). If a liquid chlorine line breaks upstream from the evaporator, the entire contents of the connected containment tankage could be released. Under these circumstances, isolation of the break by properly trained and adequately equipped plant personnel would be necessary to reduce the volume of leakage.

Venturi ejector scrubbers usually are selected for emergency systems. The system requires on-line storage of sodium hydroxide in sufficient quantity to react with the chlorine gas released. The system must be maintained adequately so that it is always ready for chlorine leak emergencies.

In theory, an activated carbon contact tank would be an alternative to a caustic scrubber and would offer some advantage in readiness and reliability of chemical. However, to date none have been installed because of the possibility of combustion of the dry material within the carbon storage vessel.

The Chlorine Institute Pamphlet 74 (29) describes methods for calculating the amounts of chlorine likely to result from major leaks and the areas likely to be affected. These data should be used in the design of leak-protection facilities.

TYPICAL PLANT REQUIREMENTS

The principal purpose of this section is to present basic information to consider in developing capital and operating cost estimates for chlorination systems. For this purpose, the major elements required are shown in Table 4–2. Costs for these elements are best estimated based on consultation with equipment and chemical suppliers in conjunction with engineering experience.

Operating costs, in addition to the cost of chlorine, are those required for heating and ventilating the space and for energy required to boost the solution water pressure. Chlorine cost can vary depending upon the location and the quantity used, and local vendors should be contacted to supply prices for various bulk quantities.

Using sodium hypochlorite solution can reduce the basic (capital/operation) cost for smaller plants in many cases. For these facilities, two covered and vented hypochlorite tanks should be included, each with a mixer. The chemical pumps should be arranged so that either pump could use either tank. The piping should include back pressure and antisiphon

TABLE 4–2. Elements to Include in Cost Estimates for Typical Gas Chlorination Facilities

1. Structure	8. Feeders
2. Special HVAC	9. Evaporators
3. Hoisting and weighing equipment	10. Automatic switchover
4. Process piping	11. Automation
5. Scrubber	12. Safety equipment
6. Sodium hypochlorite tank	13. Chlorine gas detector
7. Feed pumps	

valves. Materials for handling hypochlorite solutions are rubber and plastics.

References

1. White, G. C. 1986. *Handbook of chlorination.* New York: Van Nostrand Reinhold Company.
2. ASCE. 1990. *AWWA water treatment plant design.* New York: McGraw-Hill.
3. Morris, J. C. 1978. The chemistry of aqueous chlorine in relation to water chlorination. In *Water chlorination: Environmental impact and health effects,* Jolley, R. L., ed., pp. 21–33. Ann Arbor, MI: Ann Arbor Science Publishers.
4. Morris, J. C. 1967. Kinetics of reactions between aqueous chlorine and nitrogen compounds. In *Principles and applications of water chemistry,* Faust, S. D., and Hunter, J. V., eds. New York: John Wiley & Sons.
5. Fleischacker, S. J., and S. J. Randtke. 1983. Formation of organic chlorine in public water supplies. *JAWWA* 75(3): 132–8.
6. Morris, J. C., and B. Baum. 1978. Precursors and mechanisms of haloform formation in chlorination of water supplies. In *Water chlorination: Environmental impact and health effects,* Vol. 2, Jolley, R. L., Gorcher, H., and Hamilton, D. H., eds. Ann Arbor, MI: Ann Arbor Science Publishers.
7. Boyce, S. D., and J. F. Hornig. 1980. Formation of chloroform from chlorination of diketones and polyhydroxybenzenes in dilute aqueous solution. In *Water chlorination: Environmental impact and health effects,* Vol. 3, Jolley, R. L., Brungs, W. A., Cumming, R. B., and Jacobs, V. A., eds. Ann Arbor, MI: Ann Arbor Science Publishers.
8. Reckhow, D. A., and P. C. Singer. 1984. The removal of organic precursors by preozonation and alum coagulation. *JAWWA* 76(4): 151–7.
9. Krasner, S. W., M. J. McGuire, J. J. Jacangelo, N. L. Patania, K. M. Reagan, and E. M. Aieta. 1989. The occurrence of disinfection by-products in U.S. drinking water. *JAWWA* 81(8): 41–53.
10. Cooper, W. J., R. G. Zika, and M. S. Steinhauer. 1985. Bromide-oxidant interactions and THM formation: A literature review. *JAWWA* 79(4): 114–21.

11. Symons, J. M., P. L. K. Fu, R. C. Dressman, and A. A. Stevens. 1987. The influence of bromide ion on organic chlorine and organic bromine formation during free chlorination. *JAWWA* 79(9): 114–18.
12. Conyers, B., and F. E. Scully. 1988. The influence of metals on the formation of trihalomethanes. Paper presented at Annual Meeting of Virginia Section AWWA, Fairfax, VA.
13. Trace Inorganic Substances Committee. 1987. Committee report: Research needs for the treatment of iron and manganese. *JAWWA* 79(9): 119–22.
14. Knocke, W. R., et al. 1990. Alternative oxidants for the removal of soluble iron and manganese. Report for the AWWA Research Foundation, Denver, CO, March 1990.
15. Singer, P. C. 1986. THM control using alternative oxidant and disinfectant strategies: An evaluation. Paper presented at Annual AWWA Conference, Denver, CO, June 1986.
16. Knocke, W., S. Occiano, and R. Hungate. 1990. Removal of soluble manganese from water by oxide-coated filter media. Report from AWWA Research Foundation, Denver, CO, March 1990.
17. Hoehn, R. C., J. T. Novak, and W. E. Cumbie. 1987. Effects of storage and preoxidation on sludge and water quality. *JAWWA* 79(6): 67–75.
18. Knocke, W. R., J. R. Hamon, and C. P. Thompson. 1980. Soluble manganese removal on oxide-coated filter media. *JAWWA* 80(12): 65–70.
19. Bailey, Tom. 1988. Personal communication.
20. Weng, C., D. L. Hoven, and B. J. Schwartz. 1986. Ozonation: An economic choice for water treatment. *JAWWA* 78(11): 83–9.
21. Osborne, T. Z., and R. E. Shaw. 1971. A multi-purpose water program. *The American City,* April 1971.
22. Anonymous. 1985. *Standard methods for examination of water and wastewater,* American Public Health Association, 16th ed. American Water Works Association, and Water Pollution Control Federation.
23. Lalezary, S., M. Pirbazari, and M. J. McGuire. 1986. Oxidation of five earthy-musty taste and odor compounds. *JAWWA* 78(3): 62–9.
24. Hrudey, S. E., A. Gac, and S. A. Daignault. 1988. Odorous aldehydes produced by disinfectant reaction with common amino acids. Paper presented in Poster Session of Annual AWWA Conference, Orlando, FL, June 1988.
25. Mitcham, R. P., M. Shelley, and C. M. Wheadon. 1983. Free chlorine versus ammonia-chlorine: Disinfection, trihalomethane formation and zooplankton removal. *JAWWA* 75(4): 196–8.
26. Anonymous. 1987. *AWWA standards for hypochlorites, B-300-87.* Denver, CO: American Water Works Association.
27. Anonymous. 1973. *Water chlorination: Principles and practices, manual M20.* Denver, CO: American Water Works Association.
28. Montgomery, J. M. 1985. *Water treatment: Principles and design.* New York: John Wiley & Sons.
29. Chlorine Institute Inc. 1982. Manual No. 74, *Calculating the area affected by chlorine releases.* Washington, DC.

30. *Guidance manual for compliance with the filtration and disinfection requirements for public water systems using surface water sources*. October 1989. U.S. EPA Science and Technology Branch, Criteria and Standards Division. Washington, DC: U.S. Environmental Protection Agency, Office of Drinking Water.
31. Croue, J. P., and D. A. Reckhow. 1989. Destruction of chlorination by-products with sulfite. *Environ. Sci. & Tech.* 23: 1412.
32. Gordon, G. 1991. Control strategy 3: Inorganic disinfection by-products removal. Presented at 1991 AWWA conference preconference seminar: *Controlling Disinfection By-Products; Utilities Experiences and Future Research Needs*, Philadelphia, PA, June 1991.
33. Chlorine Institute Inc. 1979. Manual No. 66, *Chlorine tank car loading, unloading, air padding, and hydrostatic testing*, Washington, DC.

5

Chloramination

HISTORY OF CHLORAMINATION

Chloramination of drinking water was first practiced during 1916 and 1917 in Ottawa, Canada, and Denver, Colorado (1). In fact, chloramination has been a long-standing practice for the Denver Water Department, which has yielded benefits for controlling tastes and odors in addition to achieving disinfection. The Denver system obtains water from a high-quality source and has been closely monitored for bacterial quality to assure effectiveness. Distribution system monitoring and a routine flushing program have been practiced to provide further assurances of bacteriological quality (2).

In the time since these initial applications, the history of chloramination has been somewhat varied. Early attention centered on a capability for eliminating certain taste and odor conditions that occurred in the presence of free chlorine. Chloramines were also found to provide a more stable residual in water distribution systems. Subsequently, the practice of chloramination increased until the end of the 1930s, with 16 percent of the utilities employing chloramination, as indicated in a nationwide survey in 1938. Thereafter, the use of chloramination declined as ammonia availability declined during World War II and as the understanding of breakpoint chlorination improved. By the early 1960s, use of chloramination had declined to less than 3 percent of the surveyed water suppliers (1).

Another factor that has contributed to the decline in use of chloramination is concern for relative disinfecting capability as compared with free chlorine. In fact, a few states do not allow the use of chloramines at all, while others have restricted it only from use as a primary disinfectant (3). The prospect for use as a primary disinfectant has been reduced by very restrictive EPA CT criteria for *Giardia* and enteric viruses. However, renewed interest in chloramines has emerged as a result of a capability for meeting secondary disinfection goals for providing a protective residual in water distribution systems, while minimizing the formation of trihalomethanes and other disinfection byproducts that occur with the use of free chlorine.

If a conversion to a chloramine approach is being considered, some effects on end users need to be anticipated. For example, adjustment may be necessary for kidney dialysis equipment in medical facilities and by fish hobbyists who maintain aquariums. A public information program to notify users of this type of change and possible effects is a good practice.

CHLORAMINE REACTIVITY

Chloramines can be viewed in some respects as chemical "cousins" to the two common free chlorine species: hypochlorous and hypochlorite ion. The chlorine component of all of these chemical species occurs in a +1 oxidation state. This is illustrated by the following breakdown of valences for the respective compounds:

Free Chlorine	
Hypochlorous acid	$H^{+1}O^{-2}Cl^{+1}$
Hypochlorite ion	$(O^{-2}Cl^{+1})^{-1}$
Chloramines	
Monochloramine	$N^{-3}H_2^{+1}Cl^{+1}$
Dichloramine	$N^{-3}H^{+1}Cl_2^{+1}$
Nitrogen trichloride	$N^{-3}Cl_3^{+1}$

The main distinction of chloramine chemistry results from binding of chlorine (+1) in an ammonialike structure (NH_x—) as opposed to the hydroxide (HO—) and oxygenated (O—) structures of the free chlorine species. As a consequence of binding chlorine to an ammonia structure, its availability for chemical reaction is modified by reducing its reactivity, especially as compared with hypochlorous acid. This modified reactivity has provided benefits for several utilities where formation of certain taste and odor compounds resulting from reactions with free chlorine is avoided and a disinfecting residual that can be more persistent in water distribution systems due to slower degradation reactions is provided. Recently, chloramination has also been a subject of widespread interest because this less active state of chlorine limits the formation of trihalomethanes and many other disinfection byproducts of concern.

The status of chloramination for meeting disinfection requirements has undergone changes in recent years. Under past regulations, it has often been acceptable simply to provide criteria for primary disinfection of coliform bacteria. However, the relatively weak disinfecting properties of chloramines for inactivation of viruses and protozoan pathogens will affect its role under future regulations. For example, under most conditions specified in the EPA Surface Water Treatment Rule, criteria for primary disinfection of viruses and *Giardia* will be difficult to meet with chloramines. On the other hand, even when primary disinfecting criteria cannot be met, chloramines can still be acceptable for providing a persistent disinfecting residual for secondary disinfecting protection against microbial growth in distribution systems.

COMMERCIAL CHEMICALS TO FORM CHLORAMINES

Chloramines are not delivered as a single manufactured chemical. Instead, they are formed at the site of application by reactions between chlorine and ammonia, as illustrated by the following general reaction sequence in which X and Y represent constituents to which chlorine and ammonia can be bound in their original chemical form.

$$\underset{\text{Chlorine Source}}{XCl} + \underset{\text{Ammonia Source}}{YNH_3} = \underset{\text{Monochloramine}}{NH_2Cl} + X + Y + H^+ \qquad (5\text{–}1)$$

The reaction can be further illustrated by the following specific examples:

$$\underset{\text{Hypochlorous Acid}}{HOCl} + \underset{\text{Ammonia}}{NH_3} = NH_2Cl + H_2O \qquad (5\text{–}2)$$

$$\underset{\text{Sodium Hypochlorite}}{2NaOCl} + \underset{\text{Ammonium Sulfate}}{(NH_4)_2SO_4} = 2NH_2Cl + 2H_2O + 2Na^+ + (SO_4)^{2-} \qquad (5\text{–}3)$$

Since discussions of sources of chlorine have been presented in Chapter 4, this chapter will focus on sources of ammonia.

Ammonia is a chemical that is produced in large quantities and is widely used for industrial and agricultural purposes. The most common method of manufacture is the Haber-Bosch process. Under this process, nitrogen and hydrogen gases are contacted at high temperatures and pressures in the presence of a catalyst to yield the following reaction:

$$3H_2 + N_2 = 2NH_3 \tag{5–4}$$

Ammonia can also be derived as a byproduct of the destructive distillation of coal or coke (4). However, the possible presence of impurities should be considered before applying this source of ammonia in water treatment.

Subsequent to its manufacture, ammonia can be converted to several commercial forms that have varying costs and operational considerations. The most commonly encountered commercial forms are as follows:

Chemical Name	Chemical Formula	Percent Available Ammonia as NH_3	Commercial Form
Anhydrous ammonia	NH_3	Almost pure	Liquefied gas
Ammonium hydroxide or aqua ammonia	NH_4OH	Normally 29–30, but lower concentrations available	Solution of ammonia dissolved in water
Ammonium sulfate	$(NH_4)_2SO_4$	Approx. 25	Dry chemical
Ammonium chloride	NH_4Cl	—	Dry chemical

The anhydrous or liquefied gas form is the least expensive and most widely used source of ammonia. This form consists of molecular ammonia that is compressed into cylinders. Anhydrous ammonia is a hazardous substance that is handled in specially designed storage devices similar to those required for gaseous chlorine. It is available in 100- or 150-pound cylinders and in an 800-pound container that is similar in dimension to the 1-ton container used for chlorine. The lower carrying capacity for ammonia in this container is a result of the fact that anhydrous ammonia has roughly half the density of chlorine. Another commonly used container is a 4,600-pound tank that can be provided by some ammonia suppliers. Larger, bulk shipments can be handled in 80-ton rail tank cars, 25-ton rail tank cars, and 20-ton tank trailers (5). Storage facilities can be provided for the delivered containers in smaller facilities, and customized storage tanks of any size can be provided for receiving bulk shipments and providing in-plant storage at larger facilities.

Bulk anhydrous ammonia typically comes in two grades: commercial and refrigeration. Commercial grades typically contain a small amount of moisture that can result in corrosive conditions. Refrigeration grade, which is moisture free, is recommended for water treatment applications (4).

Ammonium hydroxide solution, or *aqua ammonia*, as it is more commonly known, is another widely used form. It is formed by the dissolution of ammonia in water:

$$NH_3 + H_2O = NH_4OH \quad (5\text{–}5)$$

Aqua ammonia is sold in a standard commercial strength as a solution that is approximately 29 to 30 percent ammonia. It can, however, also be purchased in lower concentrations in some locations. It is available in 55-gallon drums and bulk tank truck shipments. Care should be taken to obtain an appropriate source of aqua ammonia that is free of undesirable levels of impurities. Food-grade aqua ammonia is often required to meet this criterion.

The dry forms of ammonia, ammonium sulfate and ammonium chloride, are generally the most expensive to purchase and tend to be less widely used. However, when these forms are applicable, ammonium sulfate is more commonly used than ammonium chloride because of its lower cost.

Ammonium sulfate is available in several different grades. Consideration should be given to the level of purity in selecting the appropriate grade since ammonium sulfate is often produced as a byproduct material that can contain impurities. It is also available in a more expensive, food-grade form that results from the reaction between ammonia and sulfuric acid. Some states require this food-grade quality for application to potable water (6); otherwise AWWA Standard B302 should be consulted to evaluate acceptable levels of impurities.

Cost and safety are the major factors in selecting the source of ammonia for particular applications. The dry forms are the most costly to purchase but may be more safe, which should provide a possible advantage in smaller systems where operator safety and training in the handling of the anhydrous and aqua ammonia forms are a concern. Aqua ammonia is safer than anhydrous ammonia because pressurized systems are not involved. However, because anhydrous ammonia is compressed into a smaller volume, cost for purchase and delivery can be significantly reduced. In some cases, this cost saving can be offset by greater capital cost and operational complexity as compared to aqua ammonia feed systems. For example, simple metering pump systems can be used for aqua ammonia; more complex gas feed systems are required for anhydrous ammonia. In fact, some utilities have found that overall costs for aqua ammonia can be lower in spite of the higher purchase cost for chemicals. This results from greater equipment costs for storing, handling, and feeding anhydrous ammonia (7). These factors vary, and selection will depend on considerations that include the relative costs for purchase of the different chemicals in a given area.

CHEMISTRY OF CHLORAMINATION

Chlorine-Ammonia Reactions

Reactions between chlorine and ammonia are the underlying foundation of the chemistry of chloramination. These reactions have already been introduced in the discussions of breakpoint chlorination chemistry in Chapters 3 and 4. However, because of their significance for formulating decisions for chloramination, these reactions are discussed here in greater detail with emphasis on aspects that are pertinent to application of chloramines.

Under an idealized breakpoint chlorination reaction, chlorine (Cl_2) oxidizes ammonia (NH_3) to molecular nitrogen (N_2) as indicated by the following representation of the overall reaction:

$$3Cl_2 + 2NH_3 = 6H^+ + 6Cl^- + N_2 \qquad (5\text{–}6)$$

However, the reaction does not proceed directly as shown here, but actually requires a sequence of steps. An idealization of this sequence can be generally represented as four reactions, as follows:

1. Formation of hypochlorous acid (HOCl) from molecular chlorine (Cl_2):

$$Cl_2 + H_2O = HOCl + Cl^- + H^+ \qquad (5\text{–}7)$$

2. Reaction between hypochlorous acid and ammonia (NH_3) to form monochloramine (NH_2Cl):

$$HOCl + NH_3 = NH_2Cl + H_2O \qquad (5\text{–}8)$$

3. Reaction between hypochlorous acid and monochloramine to form dichloramine ($NHCl_2$):

$$HOCl + NH_2Cl = NHCl_2 + H_2O \qquad (5\text{–}9)$$

4. Degradation of dichloramine to oxidize nitrogen to molecular nitrogen gas and reduce chlorine to chloride:

$$2NHCl_2 + H_2O = N_2 + HOCl + 3H^+ + 3Cl^- \tag{5-10}$$

The above reaction sequence involves several changes in the oxidation state of chlorine as well as its substitution into the ammonia molecule to form the chloramine species. It begins with conversion of chlorine from the 0 oxidation state in molecular chlorine to the +1 oxidation state in HOCl. This oxidation state is then retained in the next two steps of reaction as chlorine (+1) substitutes into the ammonia structure to form mono- and dichloramine. These forms of chlorine are still relatively reactive and can provide a degree of disinfecting capability under chloramination approaches. However, once adequate chlorine is added, the dichloramine degradation reaction begins, and chlorine again changes its oxidation state, this time to form chloride, a −1 oxidation state. In this form, chlorine is relatively inert to further chemical reaction and provides no disinfecting potential. Therefore, one of the keys to chloramination is to provide an adequate chlorine-to-ammonia ratio that allows chloramine formation to occur while avoiding excess quantities that will trigger the degradation reaction.

The dichloramine degradation reaction is the step that delineates chloramine chemistry from free chlorine chemistry. Prior to this step, substitution of chlorine (+1) in ammonialike structures is the dominant feature. Following this step, nitrogen is oxidized by the dichloramine degradation reaction from its relatively reactive −3 oxidation state, as found in both chloramines and ammonia, to the relatively inert molecular nitrogen form (0 oxidation state). Because of the completion of nitrogen oxidation at the breakpoint, it is no longer available for reaction with chlorine, thereby ending the diversion of free chlorine into chloramines. Once this point is reached, further addition of chlorine will result in free chlorine.

The basic reaction sequence explains the general shape of the breakpoint curve discussed before and shown in Figure 5–1. During this sequence, chlorine remains in a chloramine form until the dichloramine degradation step is reached. Because chlorine is more readily substituted into ammonia molecules to form monochloramine, dichloramine is not extensively formed at lower chlorine doses, and the degradation step does not occur to an appreciable extent under this low-dose condition. As a consequence, an initial rise in the chloramine component of a total chlorine (+1) residual is observed. When monochloramine formation is nearly complete, further chlorine addition leads to dichloramine formation and begins the subsequent degradation reaction in which chlorine (+1) is con-

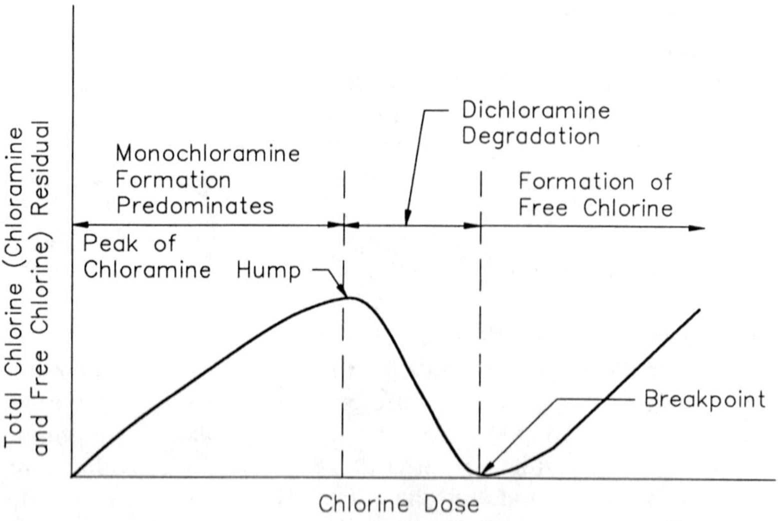

FIGURE 5–1. Idealized breakpoint curve for reactions with ammonia.

verted to chloride, thereby dissipating the chloramine residual. This accounts for the observed decline in the chlorine (+1) residual prior to the breakpoint.

The dichloramine degradation reaction is complex, involving several intermediate reaction steps. Saunier and Selleck have discussed the theories associated with this degradation in detail (8). From a practical standpoint, however, it is important only to understand the major implications:

1. The dichloramine formation step is required for the reaction to proceed.
2. Hydrogen ions are reaction products, thereby linking the reaction to pH.
3. Most of the chlorine is converted to chloride, and the chlorine (+1) residual is lowered as this reaction proceeds to breakpoint.
4. The nitrogen found in chloramines is oxidized to molecular nitrogen.

This idealization of the overall reaction provides a basis for characterizing the chlorine dosage required to react with a specified amount of ammonia, and yields a theoretical chlorine-to-ammonia molecular ratio of 3 to 2 at the breakpoint, as shown in the following representation of the overall reaction sequence:

$$3Cl_2 + 2NH_3 = 6H^+ + 6Cl^- + N_2 \tag{5–11}$$

The resultant free chlorine (Cl_2)-to-ammonia (N) weight ratio is 7.6 for this condition.

In reality, the idealized reaction sequence provides only a general characterization of breakpoint chlorination phenomena. Experience indicates that actual ratios are somewhat higher even in laboratory solutions that are relatively free of demand-causing substances other than ammonia. The following specific aspects, which are important considerations for chloramination practices, provide insight into the reasons for deviations from the theoretical ratio.

Incomplete Degradation of Chloramine Species

The dichloramine degradation reaction that leads to the formation of molecular nitrogen can proceed at different rates. Note that this reaction results in the formation of H^+ as an end product. In alkaline pH solutions, H^+ can rapidly react with OH^- to form water, thereby providing a ready mechanism for accommodating the excess H^+ into solution. However, the reaction proceeds more slowly as the solution becomes acidic, and residual levels of dichloramine can remain in these solutions for extended periods. Note also that the formation of dichloramine requires a chlorine-to-ammonia molecular ratio of 2 to 1 if chlorine is maintained in this form and does not ultimately degrade through the dichloramine degradation reaction. This results in a weight ratio of 10 : 1 compared to the ratio of 7.6 : 1 for the breakpoint reactions. Therefore, the ratio is increased by any of the chlorine that is retained in the dichloramine form. The reason for the decrease in chlorine required for breakpoint can be seen in the dichloramine degradation reaction (Equation 5–10) in which a portion of the chlorine that begins in the dichloramine form is converted back to HOCl and becomes available for further reaction.

In addition to slowed degradation, buildup of dichloramine in the acidic pH range can also occur as a consequence of the following reaction (9):

$$2NH_2Cl + H^+ = NH_4^+ + NHCl_2 \qquad (5\text{–}12)$$

This reaction involves a conversion of monochloramine in the presence of hydrogen ions to form both dichloramine and an ammonium ion (NH_4).

Another possible product, nitrogen trichloride (NCl_3), can also occur under appropriate conditions, and result in further alterations of the chlorine-to-ammonia ratio. This compound can be formed by the following reaction between dichloramine and hypochlorous acid:

$$NHCl_2 + HOCl = NCl_3 + H_2O \qquad (5\text{–}13)$$

The reaction tends to be relatively slow in comparison with formation of monochloramine and dichloramine (10) and would not proceed to an appreciable degree without the prolonged availability of dichloramines that occurs as the solution pH becomes more acidic. An additional pH effect is associated with the fact that nitrogen trichloride tends to degrade more rapidly in basic solutions, thereby reducing its tendency for buildup when these conditions exist (10). Accelerated nitrogen trichloride degradation has also been observed in the presence of excess ammonia, a condition that would occur at lower chlorine-to-nitrogen ratios.

The impacts of all of these deviations from ideal breakpoint conditions are illustrated in Figure 5–2. Note that the ratio of chlorine to ammonia at the breakpoint is greater than the theoretical ratio of 7.6 in all cases, particularly for the breakpoint curve at pH 6.0. Very little residual remained at the breakpoint at pH 8.0 and 7.0, indicating a relatively complete reaction. However, a measurable residual occurred at the breakpoint of pH 6.0. This effect would be anticipated based on both the slower rate of dichloramine degradation and the increased formation of nitrogen trichloride as pH is lowered.

The occurrence of dichloramine and nitrogen trichloride under different conditions is also indicated in Figure 5–2. These variations have significance for application of chloramination since the different chloramine forms have different properties. For example, both dichloramine and nitrogen trichloride are less desirable due to associated tastes and odors. Of the two, nitrogen trichloride produces the most severe effects and is the least desirable (4). As indicated in Figure 5–2, the occurrence of dichloramine is favored by decreased pH and is maximized near the hump in the breakpoint curve. Nitrogen trichloride begins to occur at chlorine-to-nitrogen ratios beyond the breakpoint, especially as pH is decreased.

In past practice, chlorine-to-ammonia ratios used to form chloramines were commonly in the range of 3 : 1 to 4 : 1. This placed the operating range before the hump, in a region where monochloramine predominates. White (4) indicates that these ratios were selected because they often achieved the best-tasting water. However, a full range of effects needs to be considered in selecting the appropriate ratio. For example, a 5 : 1 ratio is needed to achieve the theoretical ratio for full conversion of ammonia to monochloramine, a condition that would minimize the availability of unreacted ammonia for undesirable nitrification as discussed in the section Biological Nitrification Phenomena Associated with Chloramines. Other characteristics, such as pH, can have an influence on the appropriate ratio since pH affects the distribution of chlorine among the various chloramine species, as indicated in Figure 5–2. The most desirable pH

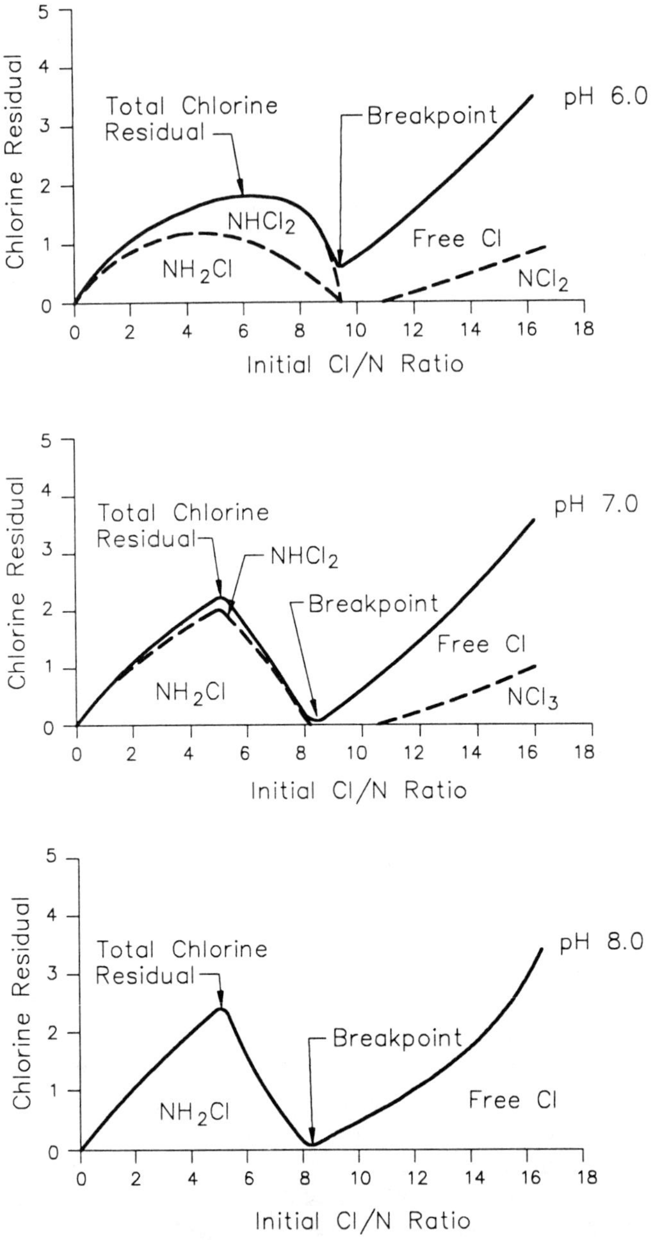

FIGURE 5–2. Distribution of chlorine compounds at initial ammonia concentration of 0.5 mg/l as N. (Adapted from A. T. Palin, "Chemical Aspects of Chlorination," *Journal of the Institute of Water Engineers* 4: 565–81, 1950.)

is near neutral to avoid the increased formation of dichloramine and nitrogen trichloride that occurs at lower pH levels.

Chloride ions are a characteristic that can increase nitrogen trichloride formation in acidic solutions, presumably due to catalytic effects (10). This type of variability is another indication of the need for specific testing to characterize the breakpoint curve for a particular set of conditions.

Alternative Nitrogen End Products

Deviations can occur as a result of nitrogen end products other than molecular nitrogen. An example of this is the reaction pathway that leads to the formation of nitrate instead of molecular nitrogen (11). The overall reaction alters the theoretical molecular ratios of chlorine to nitrogen at breakpoint from 1.5 : 1 for formation of molecular nitrogen to 4 : 1 for formation of nitrate:

$$4Cl_2 + NH_3 + 3H_2O = NO_3^- + 9H^+ + 8Cl^- \qquad (5\text{-}14)$$

The reaction involves hydrogen ions as end-products, thereby introducing a pH effect in which the reaction becomes increasingly favored in the alkaline pH range with an associated increase in hydroxide ion availability for assimilating the hydrogen ions into solution.

Other oxidation products that have been proposed to form to a lesser extent include $H_2N_2O_2$, N_2O, NH_2OH, NO, and NO_2^- (4). Compared with molecular nitrogen, however, neither nitrate nor any of these other possible oxidation products are likely to be dominant end products in the pH range typical of water treatment practice. Nonetheless, they can form to a certain extent, thereby having some influence on chlorine-to-nitrogen ratio at breakpoint.

Chlorine Reactions with Organic Nitrogen Compounds

Organic nitrogen compounds, particularly organic amino compounds, can compete with ammonia in reactions with chlorine. The result is the formation of organic chloramines, a group of reaction products that are analogous to the inorganic chloramines formed by reactions with ammonia. Basic amino compounds can be characterized by the following general representations:

RNH_2	Primary amines
R_2NH	Secondary amines
R_3N	Tertiary amines

In these representations, R denotes the organic groups that are attached to nitrogen. Note that as amines progress from primary to tertiary structures, there is a progressive replacement of hydrogen by the organic groups (R).

As in the case of ammonia, chlorine (+1) from HOCl can substitute for a hydrogen in an organic amino group, as indicated by the following reaction between hypochlorous acid and a secondary amino compound:

$$HOCl + R_2NH = ClNR_2 + H_2O \qquad (5\text{–}15)$$

A number of amino-type organic compounds, with varying affinities for chlorine, can take part in these reactions. Those most commonly encountered include the amino acids and the higher-order compounds they can form through biological pathways. A spectrum of these organic nitrogen species can be characterized by the following sequence of progression from simple amino acids to larger proteins, which are ultimately formed by biological building processes using amino acids as basic building components:

$$\text{Amino Acids} \longrightarrow \text{Dipeptides} \longrightarrow \text{Polypeptides} \longrightarrow \text{Proteins}$$

Within this sequence, a variety of organic nitrogen compounds can be encountered. Therefore, a varied range of reaction possibilities for chlorine can exist. In fact, chlorine affinity for some amino acids can be quite high, and these reactions can proceed more readily than the formation of the ammonia-related inorganic chloramines (12). Because these are parallel substitution reactions that compete with the inorganic chloramine reaction, formation of the inorganic chloramines can be impeded in some cases.

The potential to form organic chloramines depends on the presence and type of organic nitrogen compounds. These compounds can occur in water supplies in association with algae and other plant life. In a review of the effects of organic nitrogen compounds, it was observed that an organic nitrogen content of 0.5 mg/l was not uncommon in many source waters, and one source reported a level as high as 21.7 mg/l in association with a bloom of blue-green algae (12). Dissolved organic nitrogen can frequently comprise over 50 percent of the total soluble nitrogen content in fresh waters (13). Amino forms of nitrogen typically constitute more than half of the dissolved organic nitrogen content. Because they can be rapidly degraded by bacteria, low concentrations of free amino acids are often encountered in fresh water, and much of the amino content may frequently be comprised of the higher-order amino nitrogen compounds that degrade more slowly. For example, two-thirds of the amino nitrogen may occur as higher-order amino compounds such as polypeptides, with one-third occurring as free amino acid compounds (13). This can affect the tendency of a given water to produce organic chloramines since the amino acids are typically more reactive than the larger peptide molecules.

Based on these observations, a number of factors are involved in determining the quantity and types of organic nitrogen compounds. A high degree of variation can occur in response to variations in biological productivity and the extent of amino acid degradation. As a consequence, site-specific and seasonal characterization of effects are a consideration. In lakes and reservoirs where the level of biological activity varies within the water column, organic nitrogen concentrations can also be affected by depth (13). Therefore, raw water intake levels can be an important consideration in avoiding formation of these organic compounds.

The formation of organic chloramines is typically undesirable, since such formation can significantly reduce the disinfection capability afforded by chlorine. However, the extent of these effects can depend on a variety of factors. For example, the disinfection capability of some organic chloramines can vary with pH. In one study (14), it was reported that one form, chlorinated glycine, exhibited an acidic disinfecting capability at pH 4, while chlorinated taurine and gelatin exhibited alkaline disinfecting capability at pH 9.5. Effectiveness declined for all of these compounds as the pH shifted towards more neutral pH conditions. Some other organic chloramine compounds are under consideration as disinfectants that can provide greater long-term stability than free chlorine, thereby indicating that effective disinfection is possible with some amino compounds (15). Therefore, a depleted disinfecting capability is not necessarily a universal outcome of the formation of organic chloramines.

An illustration of the complex effects of organic chloramines on disinfection was observed in the disinfection of a treated drinking water supply where severe organic chloramine interference was suspected (12). When ammonia and chlorine were added separately to the reservoir water, disinfection proceeded more slowly than when ammonia and chlorine were mixed together to preform the chloramine solution prior to addition. It was postulated that the deteriorated performance of the separate addition method resulted from the immediate diversion of chlorine into organic chloramines before it could react with ammonia. To an extent, this problem was avoided when the chloramines were preformed prior to contacting with the reservoir water. However, after a period of contact, it was noted that the preformed chloramines appeared to dissipate by progressive transfer of the chlorine to form organic chloramines. The following two reaction sequences were considered to offer possible explanations for this phenomenon:

Sequence 1, involving formation of protonated monochloramine (NH_3Cl^+):

$$NH_2Cl + H^+ = NH_3Cl^+ \tag{5-16}$$

$$NH_3Cl^+ + RNH_2 = RNHCl + NH_4^+ \tag{5-17}$$

Sequence 2, involving degradation of monochloramine back to ammonia and hypochlorous acid:

$$NH_2Cl + H_2O = NH_3 + HOCl \tag{5-18}$$

$$HOCl + RNH_2 = RNHCl + H_2O \tag{5-19}$$

It was noted that a significant difficulty in assessing the effects of organic chloramines on disinfection results from the fact that organic chloramines are not distinguished from ammonia chloramines by the conventionally used analytical techniques of amperometric titration or DPD-FAS titration. As a consequence, both organic and ammonia chloramines are typically measured as a combined residual with no basis for delineating the specific categories. More advanced techniques involving high pressure liquid chromatography have been developed and have the capability for making these distinctions (16). However, these methods are not widely applied.

In addition to adverse effects associated with organic chloramines, amino acids also can react to form certain taste and odor compounds. For example, it has been observed that several odor-related aldehydes could be formed by reactions between both chlorine and chloramines and certain amino acids (17). By comparison, the extent of such formation was lower with ozone and did not occur at measurable levels with chlorine dioxide. Although the potential for these undesirable chloramine reactions were indicated by specific studies, the significance of these findings is not clear due to the reliance on laboratory solutions.

It is evident that possible reactions with organic nitrogen compounds should be taken into account when practicing chloramination, and possible adverse effects should be minimized. The formation of organic chloramines can be reduced by the addition of ammonia at dosages that achieve a significant increase in the ratio of ammonia nitrogen to organic nitrogen, thereby increasing the likelihood of reactions with ammonia. In some cases, formation of an adequate concentration of inorganic chloramines for disinfection requires a chlorine dose high enough to satisfy reactions for both ammonia and organic nitrogen. It is noted that organic chloramines can still persist beyond the breakpoint and are not entirely removed, even by this process. Therefore, some account for this effect is appropriate even when free chlorine disinfection is practiced (12).

Effects of Other Reactions

Several other chlorination reactions may exert a demand that diverts chlorine from the formation of chloramines. These reactions can include oxidation of reduced forms of iron, manganese, and other inorganics such as hydrogen sulfide. Although reactions to form chloramines are generally more rapid than these other reactions, frequently an initial consumption of chlorine causes a shift in the breakpoint curve as shown in Figure 5–3. Note that chloramine formation can be retarded until some of the initial demand is satisfied. Further shifting can occur at other locations along the curve as well. Reactions with organic compounds other than the nitrogen-containing species are also possible, causing further deviations from the ideal curve.

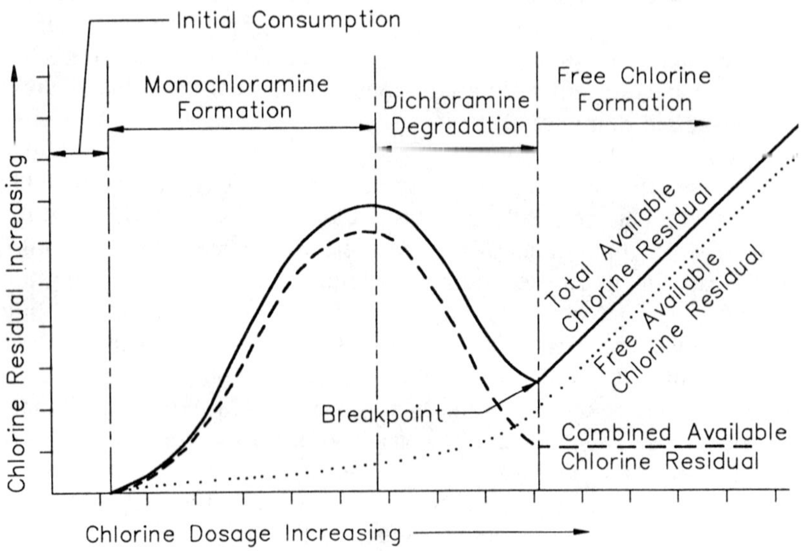

FIGURE 5–3. Breakpoint chlorination. (Reprinted from *American Water Works Opflow*, Vol. 8, No. 10 (October 1982), by permission. Copyright © 1982, American Water Works Association.)

In addition to these competing reactions, the reaction sequence can be modified by chlorine oxidation of bromide (where present) to form hypobromous acid:

$$HOCl + Br^- = HOBr + Cl^- \quad (5\text{–}20)$$

Subsequent reactions with hypobromous acid can then lead to the formation of bromamines. Oxidation reactions between monochloramine and bromide can also lead to the formation of bromamines. This is a pH-dependent reaction that begins to proceed at pH 7 and is increasingly favored as pH is reduced (18). Although these bromamine reactions alter disinfecting properties, disinfecting capability is not eliminated since bromamines can also be effective disinfecting agents.

CHLORAMINE DISINFECTION

While chloramines have a generally lower disinfecting capability than free chlorine, there is some capability for achieving significant disinfection of bacteria. The effectiveness of chloramines for the inactivation of protozoan and viral pathogens, however, can be very low. As a consequence, CT criteria in the EPA Surface Water Treatment Rule for primary disinfection of *Giardia* and viruses are extremely difficult to meet using chloramines, although a high CT approach may still be a consideration. Otherwise, use of chloramines may be more appropriate for secondary disinfection to maintain a protective residual in the distribution system. Both EPA and certain state regulations will allow for site-specific testing alternatives to demonstrate chloramines as an acceptable primary disinfectant at lower CT levels.

Although free chlorine has a greater disinfecting capability, chloramines offer a particular advantage of greater stability, frequently allowing residuals to be maintained for longer periods of time. This characteristic can be significant for secondary disinfection goals by providing an increased capacity for maintaining a disinfecting residual throughout a distribution system. In fact, in some distribution systems, where free chlorine residuals are difficult to maintain, conversion to chloramines can provide a more reliable residual that improves control of bacterial indicator organisms. This also can be a result of a greater capability of chloramine to penetrate biofilms, whereas the more reactive chlorine is more easily dissipated in such penetration. However, caution should be exercised before switching to chloramines, since much remains to be learned about biofilm control.

A disadvantage of chloramine use for secondary disinfection is associated with erratic microbial growths that occur in some systems. These growths appear to result from biological nitrification in response to the ammonia available in chloramines. Nitrifying bacteria may then serve as a food source for other microbes, and elevated levels of heterotrophic plate count are sometimes observed during these events. Corrective action typically involves a temporary conversion to free chlorine to burn out the system (47). These phenomena are discussed in more detail in the section Biological Nitrification Phenomena Associated with Chloramines.

Another possible disadvantage of chloramine use for secondary disinfection is a low disinfecting capability for *Legionella* bacteria, a significant regrowth pathogen that can occur in some areas of plumbing systems. However, the EPA Surface Water Treatment Rule does not consider this feature and only specifies a minimum disinfecting residual of 0.2 mg/l entering the distribution system with the maintenance of a measurable residual throughout, irrespective of the secondary disinfecting agent. In fact, the use of free chlorine, the much stronger secondary disinfecting agent, also does not provide complete protection against *Legionella* at this residual level, and supplemental control methods may be required in either case, as discussed in Chapter 2.

Although the EPA Surface Water Treatment Rule does not distinguish between free chlorine and chloramine residuals for meeting secondary disinfection criteria, several states have more stringent standards for chloramines that can supersede these EPA criteria. Therefore, specific state criteria should be confirmed in each disinfection situation.

CHLORAMINE BYPRODUCT FORMATION

Reduced formation of halogenated disinfection byproducts is one of the most widely cited advantages of chloramination. This was demonstrated in a recent survey of a number of utilities, which examined the occurrence of selected disinfection byproducts in the following chemical categories: trihalomethanes, chlorinated acetic acids, haloacetonitriles, haloketones, chlorophenols, aldehydes, chloropicrin, chloral hydrate, and cyanogen chloride (19). In general, the occurrence of these byproducts was significantly reduced in systems that used chloramines instead of free chlorine. An exception occurred in the case of cyanogen chloride, which was slightly elevated when chloramination was used. However, its occurrence was relatively low for both disinfectants.

Both trihalomethanes (THMs) and other halogenated byproducts can increase as chlorine-to-ammonia ratios increase toward the breakpoint and are lower in the chloramine portion of the curve. However, some differences can occur in specific dose ranges. Figure 5–4 shows an example of the formation of total organic halide (TOX) and THMs at points

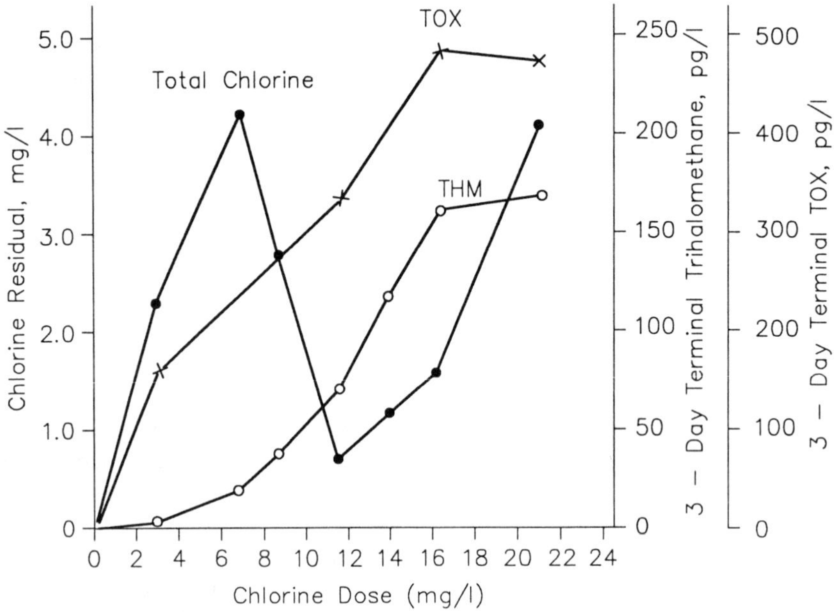

FIGURE 5–4. THM and TOX formation characteristics along breakpoint curve in Thornton Co. raw water. (Reprinted from *Treatment Alternatives for Controlling Chlorinated Organic Contaminants in Drinking Water*, 1987, by M. A. Speed, et al., with permission of U.S. EPA.)

along a breakpoint curve for a raw water in Thornton, Colorado (20). Note that although some THM formation occurs, it tends to be suppressed until the chlorine dose approaches the breakpoint. However, a number of other halogenated organic compounds are formed prior to the breakpoint, as indicated by significant formation of TOX that begins in this portion of the curve. THMs begin to comprise a more significant portion of the halogenated organic chlorine at doses greater than the breakpoint. This increase in THMs suggests some shifting in the composition of halogenated byproducts along the breakpoint curve.

In general, less is known about reaction byproducts formed in the chloramine portion of the breakpoint curve. Significant levels of total organic halides are typically observed with chloramines, and some byproducts have been identified, as discussed in Chapter 3. There is a greatly reduced tendency to form THMs with chloramines, as shown by these data. One recent study showed that a degree of THM formation could occur in a laboratory reaction between monochloramine and a model precursor compound, phloroacetophenone. It was hypothesized that reaction occurred as a result of transfer of Cl^{+1} from monochloramine to phloroacetophenone (48). Although a measurable chloroform formation occurred in this reaction, the level of chloroform production was much lower than in comparable reactions with free chlorine.

While reaction pathways such as this exist, THM formation by monochloramine is often quite low in many natural waters and can be less than detectable in some cases. However, significant THM formation still occurs in many chloramination processes due to a period of contact with free chlorine that results from the practice of separate addition of chlorine and ammonia to form chloramines. Although chloramines can form in a relatively short time, this method of addition allows a brief period of contact with free chlorine that heightens the formation of THMs. These phenomena will be further discussed later in this chapter, in the section Basic Chloramine Formation Conditions.

Although the data in Figure 5–4 indicate a reduced concern for THMs in the chloramine portion of the breakpoint curve, possible concerns for other byproducts are still indicated by the presence of TOX. In fact, there have been some indications of significant mutagenic and carcinogenic activity in association with the use of chloramines (21). However, a recent review of mutagenic studies of drinking water (22) indicates that while mutagenic activity can be observed in chloraminated water, it is typically less than that observed in chlorinated water. No final conclusions can be drawn from this information, however, since mutagenic studies of this type do not give a complete understanding of potential health effects, and uncertainties about chloramine byproducts still remain.

Biological Nitrification Phenomena Associated with Chloramines

The complete biological nitrification process is a two-step process involving an initial oxidation of ammonia to nitrite by *Nitrosomonas* bacteria (Equation 5–21), followed by a conversion of nitrite to nitrate by *Nitrobacter* bacteria (Equation 5–22):

$$\underset{\text{Ammonia}}{2NH_3} + 3O_2 = \underset{\text{Nitrite}}{2NO_2^-} + 2H^+ + 2H_2O \qquad (5\text{–}21)$$

$$2NO_2^- + O_2 = \underset{\text{Nitrate}}{2NO_3^-} \qquad (5\text{–}22)$$

One undesirable effect can occur when partial nitrification results in an accumulation of nitrite. Although partial biological nitrification to nitrite is not normally encountered in most aquatic systems, this phenomenon has been observed in some water distribution systems in which chloramination is practiced. For example, in 1978, the City of Thornton, Colorado, eliminated a practice of chloramination when nitrite levels approaching 2 mg/l were observed at some points in a distribution system. Nitrite formation also has been reported at other locations that include several utilities in South Florida (37, 47) and the Metropolitan Water District of Southern California (38). The presence of nitrite in a water supply is a health concern. For example, where a nitrite level of 1 mg/l exists, infants can be especially susceptible to methemoglobinemia, a condition under which the oxygen transfer capability of the blood can be reduced.

Deterioration in microbial quality in association with either complete or partial biological nitrification is more commonly reported than problems with excess nitrite. A general increase in heterotrophic plate count is often observed with the onset of either partial or complete nitrification (38, 47). Two conditions are thought to contribute to this phenomenon: (1) production of bacterial byproducts from nitrifying bacteria where these autotrophic bacteria, which do not require organic material for growth, could serve as organic food source for other heterotrophic bacteria, and (2) depletion of chlorine residual caused by chemical demand exerted by chemical oxidation of nitrite to nitrate under circumstances of partial biological nitrification.

Phenomena that lead to nitrification in water distribution systems are not fully understood. However, the addition of ammonia for chloramination serves to provide the nitrogen source that can be converted under the proper conditions. The chlorine-to-ammonia ratio has been observed to have a possible influence. Note that ammonia is not completely reacted at typical chlorine-to-nitrogen ratios of 3 : 1 to 4 : 1, common in past practice, which results in excess ammonia that could serve as a source for nitrification. Research (50) has demonstrated the benefit of increasing the ratio to 5 : 1, the theoretical ratio for full conversion to monochloramine. Also, residual levels of approximately 2 mg/l or more in the distribution system have been found to assist in limiting nitrification. Monitoring of free ammonia levels should be performed to make sure excessive levels are not encountered in the distribution system. However, even with these approaches, periodic burnout with free chlorine appears to be required to kill off a nitrifying population. In fact a number of utilities periodically practice a free chlorine burnout on a planned basis.

Burnout involves applying free chlorine to the distribution system intermittently. During these periods, moderately elevated concentrations of free chlorine may be required to overcome accumulated chlorine demand that can build up in a chloraminated system. The free chlorine feed period may be accompanied by an intense flushing program to help distribute residuals to remote areas and to clean out the system.

Nitrification is also probably influenced by physical distribution system characteristics that can include dead ends subject to stagnation, accumulation of sediment and tubercles that could partially shield bacteria from disinfectants, and finished water reservoirs where long detention times and accumulation of sediments may offer bacterial growth sites. Therefore, control measures, such as management of system storage to reduce detention times and routine system maintenance in the form of pipe flushing and cleaning, may be an adjunct to proper control of the dose and the chlorine-to-ammonia ratio. Another factor that appears to be important is the flow pattern in finished water reservoirs. A through pattern that minimizes dead areas is desirable. However, many reservoirs and tanks have single inlet/outlet pipes or other configurations that yield poor flow-through patterns. Consideration can be given to modification of existing facilities in some cases. New facilities should give consideration to the flow pattern (50).

NONDISINFECTION USES OF CHLORAMINES

One of the major distinctions between chloramines and free chlorine results from the fact that chloramines do not readily oxidize other chemical constituents. This has a significant effect on the use of chloramines for nondisinfection purposes. For example, the lack of this capability eliminates the potential for carrying out many of the oxidation reactions that can frequently be achieved by free chlorine for removal of color, iron, manganese, sulfides, and certain taste- and odor-related compounds. Therefore, methods for achieving nondisinfection goals must be carefully evaluated when considering chloramines in place of free chlorine in different locations within a treatment process.

If there is a need for oxidation reactions to achieve nondisinfection goals, other oxidizing chemicals, such as potassium permanganate, may be required in conjunction with chloramines. A period of contact with free chlorine might also be provided prior to ammonia addition. Under this approach, ammonia is subsequently added to form chloramines, thereby ending the period of exposure to free chlorine.

In many cases, especially those where a prechlorination contact period is not provided prior to ammonia addition, the somewhat ineffective primary disinfecting capabilities of chloramines will only allow replacement of the secondary disinfection function of free chlorine. Under these conditions, either chlorine dioxide or ozone can be considered as replacements of free chlorine for achieving primary disinfection and might also provide some of the alternative oxidizing capabilities. Evaluations for these situations should consider sequencing and operating conditions required to combine these chemicals with chloramines to achieve the full range of both disinfection and nondisinfection goals. In some situations, chlorine dioxide and ozone feed requirements can be significantly increased by nondisinfection goals. In these cases, other chemicals, such as potassium permanganate, might be more cost-effective oxidants, even when chlorine dioxide or ozone are applied for primary disinfection at locations later in a plant process. Under such conditions, chlorine dioxide or ozone would be primarily optimized for disinfection, while the other oxidants would be optimized for nondisinfection goals and to reduce the primary disinfectant demand.

Although oxidation-related uses are not available with chloramines, biocidal properties for control of biological growth can still be provided. Some utilities also have specifically used chloramines to replace free chlorine to avoid the formation of certain chlorinated taste and odor byproducts that occur in the presence of free chlorine.

Control of Biological Growths

In water treatment, biocidal uses involve control of microorganisms just as in the case of disinfection. However, this use is distinguished by the fact that it is intended primarily for control of nuisance organisms that can cause operational problems. These problems include formation of slimes; tastes and odors; interference with processes such as coagulation and filtration; and reduction in the hydraulic capacity of raw water pipelines. Chloramines can also provide biocidal-related benefits for preventing biological activity in open tanks and in filter media.

Chloramines can have a distinctive advantage for biocidal uses over reactive disinfectants such as ozone and chlorine dioxide, both of which can dissipate rapidly. Because of its slower dissipation feature, chloramines are often more available for control of biological activity throughout an entire treatment plant process train.

Specific biocidal applications indicate that chloramines have been effective in the control of algae as well as several other types of biological growths. In fact, for some organisms, chloramines can be more toxic than free chlorine (2). However, the relative orders of toxicity can depend on the species of concern, and site-specific considerations become important factors in determining the relative effectiveness of chloramine. This was demonstrated in evaluations of alternatives for control of zooplankton involving three species of small crustaceans at the Langford Water Treatment Plant of the Essex Water Company in the United Kingdom (23).

These small crustaceans were of principal concern with respect to filter clogging. Although both chloramines and free chlorine were capable of killing these organisms, the relative effectiveness varied. Chloramines were more effective for a Copepoda species (*Cyclops*), whereas free chlorine was more effective for the two Cladocera species (*Daphnia* and *Bosmina*).

While experience has indicated that chloramines can be effective as biocides, some aspects of their application require caution. For example, White (4) suggests care when using chloramines before filtration due to the potential for growth of nitrifying bacteria in the presence of excess ammonia. Steps recommended to avoid this problem include an adequate chlorine-to-ammonia ratio and maintaining a filtered water chloramine residual of 0.5 to 1.0 mg/l.

Biocidal uses of chloramines are not confined to treatment plants, and they have also been used in raw water pipelines. For example, one study (24, 25) investigated the effectiveness of chloramines for control of the Asiatic clam in raw water pipelines used by the Coastal Water Authority in Houston, Texas. These clams, which now inhabit many of the rivers throughout the southern half of the United States, can cause a significant problem by clogging raw water piping and causing taste and odor problems. Chloramines were found to provide an effective method for control of these problems when applied on either an intermittent or a continuous basis. Higher concentrations were required for colder water temperatures and for intermittent applications.

Other biocides considered in this work included free chlorine, potassium permanganate, copper sulfate, bromamine, and chlorine dioxide. Copper sulfate was not effective, and bromamine, which was partially effective, was not considered due to formation of brominated THMs. Potassium permanganate, which was also observed to be ineffective in this particular study, has been reported to be effective at other locations (26). Chlorine dioxide was observed to meet criteria for minimal formation of THMs but was eliminated in favor of chloramines due to its greater cost and operational complexity. Free chlorine was effective, but because of its trihalomethane formation potential, conversion to chloramination was the recommended alternative.

Control of Tastes and Odors

As in the case of free chlorine, the applicability of chloramines for control of tastes and odors tends to be site specific. A number of utilities have found that formation of chlorinous tastes and odors can be avoided by replacing free chlorine with chloramines. These tastes and odors have been associated with reactions that take place between free chlorine and certain types of phenolic compounds, leading to the formation of chlorinated phenols (4). In some cases, only seasonal application of chloramines is necessary, depending on the time of occurrence of the phenolic compounds in the raw water.

Another example of chloramine use to avoid a specific taste and odor problem relates to control of household odors that have occurred in a number of the utilities that use chlorine dioxide. These odors are frequently observed to occur sporadically throughout service areas, with certain homes and businesses reporting odor features that range from "kerosene" to "cat urine." It has been reported that this phenomenon appears to occur when residual chlorine dioxide is vaporized from tap water and reacts in the air with compounds emitted by new carpeting. Free chlorine appeared to result in some regeneration of chlorine dioxide residual in distribution piping. Use of chloramines as a secondary disinfectant in place of free chlorine was observed to resolve the problem for some utilities (27).

Taste and odor problems are site specific, and it is important to note that chloramines may not resolve such problems in many situations. Therefore, an understanding of the nature of the problem is important in selecting the appropriate approach. Chloramines basically provide a strategy to avoid undesirable reactions such as those that occur between free chlorine and phenols. They are less likely to be effective in cases where previously formed taste and odor substances must be removed by oxidation reactions.

As discussed above, where oxidation is required, it is sometimes possible to provide a limited period of contact with free chlorine in the treatment plant flow prior to the conversion to chloramines by subsequent ammonia addition. This has been a common method for applying chloramines where oxidation is required for taste and odor control. However, chlorine doses necessary for oxidizing tastes and odors can sometimes be relatively high (e.g., 5 to 10 mg/l), and problems with disinfection by-product formation may still be encountered in spite of subsequent addition of ammonia to convert to chloramines.

The effects that can be encountered in selecting the sequence of chlorine and ammonia for taste and odor removal was demonstrated at plants of the Metropolitan Water District of Southern California. Taste and odor events were frequently correlated with the occurrence of certain organosulfur compounds that were thought to result from bacterial degradation of algae or other biological phenomena. Organic amine compounds were thought to be another possible source. However, these were not evaluated because of the lack of high pressure liquid chromatography equipment required for analysis of these compounds. In some cases, events corresponded with anaerobic conditions in finished water reservoirs. Other events were associated with in-plant recycle of wastewater (28).

For control of most of these events, a period of contact with free chlorine was necessary in order to remove the taste and odor compounds. While this practice was effective for control of tastes and odors, it resulted in significant trihalomethane formation as compared to a sequence in which free chlorine contact was minimized by an alternative approach that involved simultaneous addition of chlorine and ammonia. As an example of the differences between these approaches, one plant produced a finished water with THM concentrations of 2 to 11 μg/l with no prechlorine contact period as contrasted with concentrations of 60 to 90 μg/l when a prechlorine contact period was provided. However, control of taste and odor compounds was not effective without prechlorination, and other taste and odor control methods would be required if prechlorination were eliminated. At the time of this evaluation, prevailing standards did not require this change to meet more restrictive THM requirements. However, this result is one indication of the type of problems that might result from THM standards that are more restrictive than 0.10 mg/l.

Another study yielded further insight into complexities associated with eliminating the prechlorine mode of chloramination (29). These investigations indicated that potassium permanganate, a commonly available substitute oxidant that might be used in the absence of prechlorination, did not yield an effective oxidation pathway for five common taste and odor compounds: geosmin, 2,3,6-trichloroanisole, 2-isopropyl-3-methoxy pyrazine, 2-isobutyl-3 methoxy pyrazine, and 2-methylisoborneol. In contrast, more complete oxidation by other disinfecting alternatives, such as ozone and chlorine dioxide, was found to be effective for these particular compounds. These findings suggest some caution before selecting potassium permanganate as a substitute oxidant for taste and odor control in conjunction with chloramines, although several utilities have reported its successful use (30, 31). Application of chlorine dioxide and ozone are discussed in Chapters 6 and 7.

Other possible alternatives for taste and odor control in conjunction with chloramines include powdered activated carbon, aeration, and raw water management to minimize tastes and odors at the source (49). However, as in the case of alternative oxidants, the success of these methods varies and depends on site-specific conditions. Therefore, the availability of workable alternative methods for taste and odor control may be important considerations if the prechlorine approach for taste and odor removal must be abandoned.

BASIC CHLORAMINE FORMATION CONDITIONS

Significant differences in the effects of the chloramination process can occur depending on the conditions selected for reacting chlorine and ammonia. Two of the most important features are the sequence of chlorine and ammonia addition and selection of chlorine-to-ammonia ratio. Another significant factor to consider is pH. A near neutral pH is desirable, at least during the formation reaction. Lower pH levels will result in formation of higher levels of di- and trichloramines.

Sequence of Addition

One of the most basic decisions in chloramination process design is the selection of the sequence in which chlorine and ammonia are added.

Prechlorination

Under this method, free chlorine is added and allowed a period of contact with the process stream before ammonia is added to form chloramines. This sequence can provide a higher level of disinfection due to the contact time with free chlorine and, in some cases, may allow CT criteria for free chlorine to be met prior to conversion to chloramines. It can also retain the capability for oxidation-related process capabilities associated with free chlorine. These can include removals of iron, manganese, sulfides, color, and certain taste and odor compounds.

The major disadvantage of prechlorination is that it creates a period of chlorine contact that can increase the likelihood for forming THMs and other chlorinated organic byproducts. The magnitude of this effect is variable and depends on both the precursor content and the rates of formation. In some cases, formation of byproducts is rapid, a situation that could limit available contact time in the presence of a high precursor content. Therefore, this method of addition may not be applicable when the rapid formation situation exists or where the extent of byproduct formation must be minimized.

Preammoniation

This method involves the addition of ammonia prior to chlorine addition. The basic intent of preammoniation is to make ammonia immediately available for reaction when chlorine is added, thereby reducing the time of contact between free chlorine and the main process stream. This method can reduce the formation of chlorinated byproducts and may be particularly appropriate where it is necessary to limit formation of these byproducts. It may also be appropriate where formation of chlorinated taste and odor compounds can occur in the presence of free chlorine.

A major disadvantage of the preammoniation approach is reduced primary disinfection capability compared to free chlorine, especially for viruses and protozoan pathogens such as *Giardia* (as reflected in EPA CT criteria for viruses; these criteria credit only a prechlorination approach). In addition, the oxidation-related process capabilities of free chlorine are not available for removal of iron, manganese, sulfides, color, and certain tastes and odors. As has been discussed, these capabilities may have to be replaced through alternative treatment methods including other forms of disinfectants and oxidants.

Concurrent Addition

Under this method, chlorine and ammonia are added at the same location. As in the case of preammoniation, the intent of this method is to reduce the contact period of free chlorine with the main process stream. However, the chlorine contact period may be somewhat increased with this method as compared with preammoniation because of the need to disperse both chlorine and ammonia before chloramines can be formed. Although mixing may take place in a matter of seconds, some differences from the preammoniation approach have been observed. For example, one study showed that concurrent addition resulted in substantially greater levels of coliform disinfection as compared with preammoniation, while still achieving existing goals for reducing formation of THMs as compared with a prechlorination approach (32). More restrictive THM requirements, however, may favor preammoniation approaches. Also, although the study indicated that acceptable bacterial reductions were achieved with concurrent addition, it still may not be capable of achieving adequate disinfection for viruses and protozoan pathogens. Inactivation of protozoa and viruses usually requires a longer period of contact with free chlorine to meet CT criteria.

As in the case of preammoniation, oxidation-related capabilities associated with free chlorine are not available with the concurrent addition approach. Where such oxidation capability is required, it would have to be achieved through the addition of other oxidizing chemicals or other treatment methods.

Preformed Chloramines

Contact of a process stream with free chlorine can be virtually eliminated by using a strategy in which chlorine and ammonia feed are combined to form chloramines prior to addition to the main process stream. Under some conditions, this approach can yield very low levels of THMs and other chlorinated organic compounds. As was the case for concurrent addition and preammoniation, this approach may not be effective for disinfection of viral and protozoan pathogens. Also, full-scale operational experience with this approach is limited; most background experience has been gained in laboratory evaluations.

The effects of alternative chloramination methods on THM formation have been observed at several locations. As previously discussed, for one treatment plant serving the Metropolitan Water District of Southern California (28), THM levels of 2 to 11 μg/l were reported when preammoniation was applied as compared with 60 to 90 μg/l with the prechlorination approach.

In another case involving a pilot investigation in Thornton, Colorado (20), the prechlorination approach was compared with the preformed chloramine approach. The initial THM concentration for the preformed chloramine approach averaged 15 μg/l over an extended testing period compared to 25 μg/l for the prechlorination approach. These differences persisted and increased when the samples were incubated for a period of 5 days. In the case of prechlorination, the THMs increased from an average initial concentration of 25 μg/l to an average concentration of 40 μg/l over the 5 days of storage. Some of the 5-day prechlorination samples approached a maximum concentration level of 80 μg/l. Significantly, these increases occurred following the addition of ammonia, which was intended to eliminate further THM formation, thereby suggesting an aftergrowth phenomena in which a reaction sequence is initiated by prechlorine contact and continues in spite of the subsequent addition of ammonia. As a consequence, it would be good to minimize the contact of the main process stream with free chlorine in situations where there is a need to achieve very low levels of THMs and other chlorinated byproducts. This type of delayed-reaction phenomenon would have a significant effect on the sequence of ammonia/chlorine addition and could require elimination of prechlorination and, in extreme conditions, may require consideration of the use of preformed chloramines. Although these phenomena have not been factors for most utilities in meeting THM criteria of 100 μg/l, they could become significant for meeting more restrictive criteria.

Evidence that a delayed reaction phenomenon can lead to subsequent THM formation has been provided by laboratory evaluations using selected model organic precursor compounds. For example, in one experiment, a reaction sequence indicated initial formation of intermediate compounds, which subsequently degraded to form chloroform (33). Results indicated that while the chloroform formation reaction could be suppressed as long as an acid or neutral pH was maintained, a subsequent increase in pH caused conversion of the initial intermediates to chloroform. This pH-related phenomenon was observed even in samples dechlorinated following the initial reaction with chlorine. As a consequence, it was hypothesized that chloroform formation can be greatly affected by alkaline reactions that lead to its formation from intermediate products. Even under more neutral pH conditions, initial formation of intermediate products could result in delayed chloroform formation over time.

Additional evidence of subsequent byproduct formation has been provided by several air stripping evaluations of THM removal. As an example, an air stripping pilot study in Norfolk, Virginia (34), showed confounding results to be associated with continuing THM formation in effluent samples that were dechlorinated with sodium thiosulfate. Even after chlorine was removed from solution by the addition of sodium thiosulfate, chloroform levels continued to increase. In this case, chloroform was observed to increase from a level of 14 μg/l in a sample injected into a gas chromatograph 15 minutes following dechlorination to a level of 32 to 35 μg/l for a sample injected 24 hours after dechlorination. Not until this subsequent formation phenomenon was taken into account could reasonable modeling results be obtained. Although the byproduct increase was not as great, adjustments to counteract this effect were also required for an air stripping pilot plant in Riviera Beach, Florida (35).

Even if the intermediate forms generated by prechlorination do not convert to chloroform, they may still represent a concern. For example, in one laboratory study (36), the formation of several other byproducts of interest—pentachloroacetone, chloral hydrate, and trichloracetic acid—was observed in acidic and neutral laboratory solutions. Other studies have identified a larger number of alternative compounds that tend to be favored under different conditions. As discussed in Chapter 4, observations indicate that compounds such as trichloracetic acid tend to be favored under lower pH conditions, whereas conversion of byproducts to chloroform is favored under alkaline pH conditions. As a consequence of this possibility for either immediate formation of THMs or the formation of other byproducts of concern, some of which may have a potential for conversion to chloroform, restrictive standards for THMs and other byproducts may limit prechlorine contact times prior to ammonia addition at some locations. Primary disinfection of *Giardia* and viruses could be reduced in this case, placing greater emphasis on the need for chlorine dioxide, ozone, or other alternatives for achieving these primary disinfection goals. Alternative methods for achieving nondisinfection goals may also be needed.

Chlorine-to-Nitrogen Ratio

The chlorine-to-nitrogen ratio can have a significant effect on several phenomena. For example, concern for undesirable formation of dichloramines and nitrogen trichloride is a consideration that tends to favor lower chlorine-to-nitrogen ratios in the range of 3 : 1 to 4 : 1 (see Figure 5–2). Also, the results shown in Figure 5–4 indicate that the formation of both THMs and other halogenated organic compounds is increased as the breakpoint is approached, thereby providing an additional reason to favor lower ratios. However, it should be noted that problems with erratic biogrowths may increase when ratios become too low. These growths are associated with biological nitrification and can be caused by the presence of excess ammonia that can occur with chloramines, especially at low chlorine-to-nitrogen ratios.

Selection of the appropriate chlorine-to-nitrogen ratio involves a compromise between competing goals. Lower chlorine ratios reduce the tendency to form disinfection byproducts and also tend to minimize the taste and odor potential associated with the formation of dichloramine and nitrogen trichloride. However, problems with nitrification phenomena, and associated deterioration of microbial quality, can become a concern for ratios that are too low. Therefore, somewhat higher chlorine levels, approaching 5 : 1, may become more desirable for many utilities.

If unacceptable levels of byproducts are produced when higher ratios become necessary, consideration can be given to altering the sequence of chlorine and ammonia addition to minimize any contact with free chlorine. This may involve the use of preammoniation or concurrent addition approaches, and, in extreme cases, the preformed chloramine approach may be required. As has been discussed, these changes may introduce significant complexities at some water treatment plants if prechlorination functions must be replaced. Also, even when preformed chloramines are used, significant levels of TOX can still be formed (39) and lower ratios may be required, resulting in possible conflicts between objectives for simultaneously limiting both byproduct formation and nitrification. Resolution of these conflicts will become more difficult if standards for disinfection byproducts become more stringent.

There is also a need to control the chlorine-to-ammonia ratio throughout the distribution system as well as at the treatment plant. A degree of change in this ratio will occur as the chlorine component of chloramines degrades. A slightly higher chlorine-to-ammonia ratio may compensate for this effect. Problems may also be encountered in distribution piping that obtains water from several treatment plants with different chlorine-to-ammonia ratios. Shifting ratios can occur at points of intermixing between these sources, and these effects need to be considered. The most extreme shifts can occur when chloraminated water is mixed with water from a plant that applies free chlorine. This mix can cause the ratio to increase toward the breakpoint ratio resulting in an undesirable dissipation of the disinfecting residual in some cases and tastes and odors in others. Similar considerations apply when shifting from chloramine to free chlorine secondary disinfection modes from a single plant since two different waters will intermix under this condition as well.

AMMONIA HANDLING AND FEEDING

Formation of chloramines requires the addition of both chlorine and ammonia. Because chlorine handling and feed equipment are discussed in Chapter 4, the following discussions will focus primarily on ammonia. Alternative configurations for handling and feeding ammonia are discussed and information is presented that can serve as a basis for preliminary design and cost evaluations of alternatives. Additional information is available in the *Handbook of Chlorination* by George Clifford White (4), from manufacturers of ammonia feed equipment, and from suppliers of the various forms of ammonia.

The design of ammonia feed facilities needs to consider appropriate levels of both reliability and redundancy. These may be less stringent than requirements for chlorination, which is an essential process for providing continuous disinfecting capabilities. Regulatory and site-specific factors will dictate the extent to which reliability features are desirable for ammonia feed, since a free chlorination option would still be available if an ammonia system needed to be removed from service for a short period of time. Some care should be exercised when selecting a design dosage for chlorine since significant oxidation demand for free chlorine may occur within a system that is normally in contact with chloramines. This can cause a more rapid dissipation of chlorine residual that needs to be compensated for by a higher chlorine dose. This higher demand should be considered in systems where a free chlorine burnout is anticipated for control of nitrification, where seasonal switchover from free chlorination to chloramination is anticipated, or where water from several treatment facilities is being mixed.

As in the case of chlorine, ammonia is a potentially hazardous material that requires appropriate provisions for safety. The two predominant alternatives are the anhydrous and aqua ammonia forms. Dry forms, such as ammonium sulfate and ammonium chloride, may also be applicable, especially for smaller systems. In each case, state and local requirements should be reviewed for the selected form to assure proper adherence to codes and regulations, especially as they relate to required purity.

Anhydrous Ammonia

Anhydrous ammonia systems are similar to those used for gaseous chlorine. Molecular ammonia, NH_3, is compressed and stored in a predominantly compressed gas-liquid form in pressurized cylinders or tanks. Like chlorine, the liquid form vaporizes to a gas as it leaves the pressurized container, and ammonia feed can be sustained by this natural vaporization up to a certain level. For feed rates in excess of the maximum rate of vaporization, external assistance from a heated evaporator is required. Custom tanks often can be made large enough to provide an appropriate natural maximum rate of evaporation to eliminate the need for evaporator units. In systems in which rate of natural evaporation is inadequate, the evaporators can be connected directly to the storage tank. In some cases, ammonia is recirculated through the evaporator, thereby raising the temperature of the tank contents. In this type of system, tank pressure can be controlled to allow direct withdrawal of gas from the tank.

As in the case of gaseous chlorine systems, the main function of ammonia feed equipment is to control the rate of gas feed from an initial compressed gas-liquid form to the feed location. This is accomplished through a system of valving and by use of pressure and flow control devices. Equipment used for feed of anhydrous ammonia is similar to that used in gaseous chlorine systems. However, variations occur due to differences in the physical properties of the two chemicals. For example, the molecular weight of ammonia is 17 as compared to a molecular weight of 71 for chlorine. This results in a proportionate reduction in weight per unit volume of gas, thereby requiring a reduction in the rating of mass feeding capabilities of facilities when ammonia is used instead of chlorine. Appropriate adjustments and flow control are required to adapt to this difference. Changes are also required for rotameters and other metering devices to reflect this different density of ammonia.

In addition to differences in density, adjustments are required for differences in rates of vaporization. Ammonia has a vaporization rate approximately one-fifth that of chlorine. This affects the maximum rate of ammonia withdrawal as well as ratings for evaporation equipment, which must both be rated lower by approximately this amount for a given piece of equipment.

Unlike gaseous chlorine, which yields H^+ as an end product and acts as an acid, anhydrous ammonia yields OH^- as an end product and acts as a base when dissolved in water. This is illustrated by the following two reactions that occur when these chemicals are added to water:

$$Cl_2 + H_2O = HOCl + H^+ + Cl^- \qquad (5\text{–}23)$$

$$NH_3 + H_2O = NH_4^+ + OH^- \qquad (5\text{–}24)$$

As a result of this basicity, scaling problems due to formation of calcium carbonate and other precipitates can occur if dilution water has enough hardness, typically greater than 30 mg/l as $CaCO_3$. This often requires softening of the ammonia dilution water to avoid scaling of injectors and ammonia solution piping. The addition of phosphate chelates may also reduce scaling. As an alternative, direct feed systems that feed ammonia as a gas are often favored over vacuum-type solution feed systems.

Like chlorine, ammonia is a hazardous material that requires safety precautions. The predominant concern is for irritation and damage to the mucous membranes of the eyes, nose, throat, and lungs (4). It is also good practice to minimize the opportunity for contact between other reactive chemicals, such as chlorine. As such, AWWA Manual No. M3, *Safety Practice for Water Utilities* (40), recommends that ammonia not be stored near chlorine or in the same room with chlorine cylinders.

Systems for handling and feeding anhydrous ammonia consist of the following basic elements:

- Containment tankage
- Storage and weighing facilities
- Piping between containment tankage and feeders
- Evaporators (if required to achieve a high rate of ammonia vaporization)
- Feeders (and injectors where solution feed systems are used)

Containment Tankage and Storage and Weighing Facilities

Containment tankage for anhydrous ammonia, as well as associated storage and weighing facilities, can be similar to that used for gaseous chlorine. For example, an 800-pound container of anhydrous ammonia is the same size as a ton container of free chlorine and is provided with similar connections to allow either gas or liquid withdrawal. As in the case of chlorine, the liquid withdrawal connection would be used when a liquid stream was being withdrawn directly from the container for feed to an evaporator. Such a system would be required to accelerate the rate of ammonia vaporization when the ambient rate of vaporization within a container is less than the design feed rate. Where the ambient rate of vaporization does not limit feed capability, there is no need for an evaporator, and the connection for gas withdrawal can be used.

Smaller facilities can be supplied with cylinders in the 50-, 100-, and 150-pound range, while larger tanks can be used for larger facilities. These can include the standard 800-pound container, as well as 1,730-pound portable tanks and vendor-supplied 4,600-pound tanks available in some areas (5). Permanent on-site storage tanks of varying size can also be used. This approach should be strongly considered since it can provide significant economies in cases that involve either lease or purchase from bulk ammonia suppliers. These on-site storage tank systems also have more flexibility for design to yield a configuration in which the natural rate of vaporization is sufficient to eliminate the need for an evaporator. As in the case of gaseous chlorine, systems for handling anhydrous ammonia are equipped with safety valves and other features to protect against leaks.

Piping Between Tankage and Feeders

Configurations and valving for piping between containment tankage and feeders are similar to those used for gaseous chlorine systems. When moist, ammonia is corrosive to many piping materials, and potential for corrosion is a consideration. While there are many similarities between equipment used for chlorine and for ammonia, material compatibilities are somewhat different. In particular, copper and copper-containing alloys should be avoided with ammonia, while they can be acceptable for use with chlorine. For example, rubber hoses are normally used for connecting ammonia cylinders instead of the copper pigtails that are used for chlorine cylinders.

Schedule 80 high-temperature seamless carbon steel is commonly recommended for piping of dry gas, with fittings of forged carbon steel rated for 2,000-pound cold working pressure (42). It is good practice to consult suppliers for more detailed information on materials for piping and other components such as valves, traps, gas strainers, pressure gauges, and pressure switches.

Evaporators

Evaporators are required whenever the ambient rate of evaporation from a storage container cannot sustain the design maximum ammonia feed rate. The higher heat of vaporization for ammonia needs to be taken into consideration when applying evaporating equipment. For example, an ammonia evaporator must be derated by a factor of approximately one-fifth that used for chlorine evaporation.

As has been discussed, the need for external evaporation can be avoided in many cases through design of containment tankage that provides an adequate volume and surface area over which vaporization can occur, thereby compensating for limitations of vaporization rates in more confined tanks. When custom storage tanks are used, this approach should be considered in design in order to avoid need for evaporation equipment.

Feeders

Potential for scale formation in solution lines has become a major consideration in selecting the type of feed system for anhydrous ammonia.

While concerns for the extreme dangers of even small chlorine leaks has caused vacuum feed chlorine systems to be favored over pressurized, direct gas chlorine feed systems, concerns for anhydrous ammonia are not as extreme. Ammonia is also much more soluble than chlorine and is therefore more amenable to direct gaseous feed. However, the main factor that favors consideration of direct gas feed for anhydrous ammonia is the elimination of the potential for scaling problems that can occur in the ammonia solution lines required for vacuum feed systems. This is not a problem encountered with vacuum-feed chlorine systems, because chlorinated solutions are acidic and do not cause precipitation of hardness.

Commercial direct feed ammoniators are available in sizes up to a feed rate of 1,000 lb/day (41). Such feed units typically involve the use of pressure-regulating devices to develop a transition from high pressures in storage containers to a regulated pressure that allows for stable flow rates across a metering device in the ammoniator. Ammonia gas from these feeders is directly sparged into the main process stream, often through relatively simple diffusers. While these diffusers are much less prone to scaling than piping found in dilution water systems, some provision should be made for cleaning.

In spite of possible scaling problems, vacuum solution feed ammoniation systems are still widely used, especially where scaling is not a significant problem. Such arrangements are similar to those used for chlorine feed. These systems involve the use of pressure-regulating valves that provide for a controlled transition from the pressurized condition in the storage containers to a defined vacuum across the metering device in the ammoniator. Solution water is fed through an eductor to cause a venturi effect that creates the vacuum within the system, thereby drawing ammonia into solution at the eductor device. Solution feed often can be applied directly in soft waters (generally hardness less than 30 mg/l as $CaCO_3$) without severe problems of scaling in piping, but in some cases there have been problems even under these conditions. Where scaling is a problem, a softening system may be required to treat the dilution water before it comes into contact with ammonia. In many cases, an ion exchange system can be used for this purpose. However, problems may be encountered in disposing of the waste brine from this process, since it may not always be possible to dispose of this waste stream via the sanitary sewer because of local sewer regulations. The addition of a phosphate chelate to the dilution water may eliminate the need for softening, although experience with this approach is limited.

Provisions should be made for removing occasional scale buildup in solution pipes by cleaning with acid, even for systems with low hardness. This may affect pipe layout and material selection for compatibility with acid. Cleanouts should be provided in dilution water piping and some provisions for cleaning should also be made for direct feed systems since scale can form at the point where ammonia gas is introduced into the main process stream.

Choice of the type of feed system involves trade-offs. Direct feed systems offer significant operational advantages for minimizing scaling problems, but adequate submergence conditions are required for gas dissolution. Vacuum systems provide safety for controlling leaks and greater flexibility for addition points.

Another factor that affects the choice of system is the feed capacity. Vacuum feed systems become more favored at feed rates that exceed the size of commercially available direct feed equipment. Consideration can be given to a specialized direct feed system in these cases, although costs may become less favorable.

Direct feed systems also have a limited range of discharge pressure that should not exceed 15 psi. Excessive pressure at feed locations will limit the applicability of commercially available direct feed systems, particularly for pressurized piping. In vacuum feed systems pressure can be boosted simply by increasing the pump pressure of the dilution water. However, high pressures can be required for some of these types of applications, which could add to the complexity of these systems as well.

Aqua Ammonia

Aqua ammonia is commercially available as a solution of ammonium hydroxide (NH_4OH) that ranges in concentration from 29 to 30 percent. The standard commercial strength is a 26° Baume solution that equates to approximately 29 percent ammonium hydroxide by weight. However, some suppliers of aqua ammonia can provide lower solution strengths.

Aqua ammonia solutions can be quite corrosive to certain materials. In addition, ammonia can be vaporized from the solution as a gas and can be hazardous if not properly controlled. This vaporization can also create problems with vapor lock of feed piping, and some utilities have preferred to use more dilute aqua ammonia solutions as a means of minimizing these vapor-related problems, which are more prevalent under warm conditions and at high elevations (43).

Storage Tankage

Aqua ammonia can be stored in stainless steel, aluminum, carbon steel, or fiberglass tanks. On-site storage tanks should be enclosed because the evolution of ammonia gas at temperatures above 80°F can result in losses that reduce solution concentration and create a hazardous off-gas (44). Two basic storage alternatives have been used:

- *Vented tanks allow excess pressure to be released as temperature increases.* The off-gases in these tanks are commonly piped through an ammonia scrubber or through a container of water that serves as a trap to remove ammonia vapors prior to venting to atmosphere. One problem to consider is that periodic cooling of tank contents can cause a reduction in gas pressure within the tank, a condition that can result in a negative pressure that could collapse some tanks unless the pressure is equalized. With a water trap, air inflow through the trap is inhibited and negative pressure can be created unless some source of inflow or other method of vacuum relief is provided. Alternately, direct venting of the ammonia off-gases to the atmosphere can be considered if site conditions permit. This approach was used in Oceanside, California, under conditions where the vent could be strategically located to allow satisfactory dispersion of ammonia into the atmosphere above (43). Unlike chlorine, ammonia is lighter than air and can be dispersed upward into the atmosphere by this method. However, air quality standards are likely to limit this approach except for specific cases.
- *Low-pressure tanks that are designed to contain off-gas in the tank over a pressure range of 15 to 25 psi.* These tanks will also require a pressure relief valve that would vent under an excess pressure condition. An ammonia scrubber or a water trap should be considered for this vent line. Because the tank is allowed to operate under a slightly pressurized condition, negative pressure problems are reduced although provisions for vacuum relief might be considered as an added precaution (43).

Feed Pumps and Piping

The basic piping system includes fill piping into the storage tank and feed piping to the point of application. A feed pump is commonly required to transfer the solution to the point of application. However, in some cases the tank elevation may allow gravity feed, thereby eliminating pumping.

Both chemical metering pumps and progressive cavity pumps have been used for feeding. Piping systems should incorporate pressure relief and pulsation dampening as appropriate for the type of pump selected. Flow metering of the feed stream is required for either manual or automated control, and piping should include isolation valves to allow equipment to be removed from service. Care should be exercised in selecting equipment and piping components since aqua ammonia can be incompatible with a number of materials. For example, many standard elastomers found in valves and rotameter seals are damaged by ammonia. These include butyl rubber and neoprene. The synthetic rubber EPDM is one possible replacement material (43). Selection of metallic materials is also affected. Specifically, copper-containing materials need to be avoided as in the case of anhydrous ammonia.

Capability for control of solution feed rates can be a significant consideration when using aqua ammonia (4). Standard commercial ammonia at a solution strength of 29 percent equates to a concentration of 290,000 mg/l. Assuming a 5 : 1 chlorine-to-ammonia ratio at a chlorine dose of 5 mg/l, an ammonia feed rate of 8.34 lb/day would be required for a 1 million gallons per day (mgd) facility. This would equate to a volumetric feed rate for aqua ammonia of 0.14 gal/hr, a low feed rate for accurate control with many chemical metering pumps. Addition of water to increase the volumetric flow rate to a more accurate range could create scaling conditions unless a soft water is available for dilution purposes. However, this would negate a major advantage of aqua ammonia for limiting scaling problems.

These limitations for achieving accurate feed conditions would need to be addressed, especially at lower dosages for small plants. Pumps that can accurately feed in the low range should be selected. Note that low volumetric feed rates are not as significant for anhydrous ammonia, which is typically added to dilution water to produce an ammonia concentration of approximately 10,000 mg/l or less.

Where diffusers are used for injecting aqua ammonia, a localized region of elevated pH can cause scale formation. At a minimum, provision should be made for cleaning the diffuser to remove these deposits. White (4) further suggests the installation of duplicate diffusers, with one serving as a standby when the other is removed from service for cleaning.

Granular Ammonia Salts

Ammonia salts used in water treatment include ammonium sulfate and ammonium chloride. These are typically not cost effective for larger facilities and are normally not considered in plants where aqua ammonia or anhydrous ammonia can be used efficiently. However, for small facilities, the greater simplicity and safety afforded by these salts may offer significant advantages. Of the available ammonia salts, ammonium sulfate is the most widely used, primarily due to cost.

Two basic feed systems can be considered:

1. Dry chemical feeders can be used to control the chemical dosing rate to dilution water, which then transports the feed stream to the point of application. Operational problems can be associated with moisture absorption that causes caking in these systems. Several additives can be provided by chemical suppliers to minimize these problems. Use of detergent compounds for this purpose may create problems with water quality and other additives should be considered (44).
2. Ammonium sulfate can be dissolved in a solution tank and subse-

quently fed with a chemical metering pump. Ammonium sulfate solutions tend to be acidic and can be corrosive to some metals. Materials that are resistant to sulfuric acid should be used (45). Care must be taken not to increase the pH of these solutions since alkaline conditions cause a conversion to molecular ammonia that can be emitted as a hazardous gas.

Care should be taken in the storage of ammonium sulfate to avoid incidental wetting, since ammonia gas can be emitted under these conditions. Caking can also result, creating problems with feeding. Storage in confined areas should be avoided because of the fume potential, and appropriate protective devices such as goggles and dust masks should be worn when handling open bags or containers. In addition, ammonium sulfate should not be stored near sources of heat, and contact with reactive chemicals such as chlorine or lime should be avoided (40).

Ammonia Dispersion and Contacting

Reactions to form chloramines can occur very rapidly, and the need for rapid dispersion when the two chemicals are brought into contact becomes critical for achieving the desired reactions between chlorine and ammonia. Slow dispersion can result in regions of localized high chlorine-to-ammonia ratio, driving the reactions in these portions of solution towards breakpoint. This can be wasteful of both ammonia and chlorine, leading to process inefficiencies. In addition, localized conditions of free chlorine availability can result in undesired formation of chlorine by-products.

In general, ammonia feed solutions can be dispersed and contacted in a similar manner as chlorine using the methods discussed in Chapter 4. However, additional provisions may be necessary for the scaling potential in the case of ammonia feed. In the case of direct feed systems for anhydrous ammonia, gas diffusers can be used for dispersion. Adequate submergence conditions should be available with these diffusers to assure effective dissolution. Off-gassing of ammonia has been a problem in some locations where submergence was inadequate.

References

1. Wolfe, R. L., N. R. Ward, and B. H. Olson. 1984. Inorganic chloramines as drinking water disinfectants: A review. *JAWWA* 76(5): 74–88.
2. Dice, J. C. 1985. Denver's seven decades of experience with chloramination. *JAWWA* 77(1): 34–7.
3. Hack, D. J. 1985. State regulation of chloramination. *JAWWA* 77(1): 40–4.

4. White, G. C. 1986. *Handbook of chlorination,* 2nd ed. New York: Von Nostrand Reinhold Company.
5. Montgomery, J. M. 1985. *Water treatment principles and design.* New York: John Wiley & Sons.
6. AWWA. 1986. *AWWA standard for ammonium sulfate, B-302–86.* Denver, CO: American Water Works Association.
7. Kreft, P., M. Umphres, J. M. Hand, L. Tate, M. J. McGuire, and R. R. Trussell. 1985. Converting from chlorine to chloramines: A case study. *JAWWA* 77(1): 38–45.
8. Saunier, B. M., and R. E. Selleck. 1979. The kinetics of breakpoint chlorination in continuous flow systems. *JAWWA* 71: 164–72.
9. Gray, E. T., P. W. Margerum, and R. P. Huffman. 1978. Chloramine equilibria and kinetics of disproportionation in aqueous solution. In *Organometals and organometalloids: Occurrence and fate in environment,* Brinkman, R. F., and Bellamy, J. M., eds. Washington, DC: American Chemical Society.
10. Sanguisin, J. S., and J. C. Morris. 1975. The chemistry of aqueous nitrogen trichloride. In *Disinfection of water and wastewater,* Johnson, J. D., ed. Ann Arbor, MI: Ann Arbor Science Publishers.
11. Morris, J. C., and I. Wei. 1969. Chlorine-ammonia breakpoint reactions: Model mechanisms and computer simulation. Paper presented at Annual Meeting of the American Chemical Society, Minneapolis, MN, 15 April, 1969.
12. Wolfe, R. L., and B. H. Olson. 1986. Chloramine disinfection: The implications of interference by nitrogenous organic compounds. *Waterworld News* 2(4): 12–14.
13. Wetzel, R. G. 1983. *Limnology,* 2nd ed. New York: Saunders College Publishing.
14. Feng, T. H. 1966. Behavior of organic chloramine in disinfection. *JWPCF* 38: 614.
15. Worley, S. D., D. E. Williams, S. B. Barnela, and L. J. Swango. 1989. New halamine water disinfectants. In *Biohazards of drinking water,* Larson, R. A., ed. Chelsea, MI: Lewis Publishers, Inc.
16. Scully, F. E. 1986. N-Chloro compounds: Occurrence and potential interference in residual analysis. In *AWWA Water Quality Technology Conference proceedings: Advances in water analysis and treatment,* pp. 611–22. Denver, CO: American Water Works Association.
17. Hrudey, S. E., A. Gac, and S. A. Daignault. 1988. Odorous aldehydes produced by disinfectant reaction with common amino acids. Paper prepared for poster presentation at 1988 AWWA Conference, Orlando, FL, June 1988.
18. Bousher, A., P. Brimblecembe, and D. Midgeley. 1989. Kinetics of reaction in solutions containing monochloramine and bromide. *Water Res.* 23(8): 1049–58.
19. Krasner, S. W., M. J. McGuire, J. G. Jacangelo, N. L. Patania, K. M. Reagan, and E. M. Aieta. 1989. The occurrence of disinfection by-products in U.S. drinking water. *JAWWA* 81(8): 41–53.

20. Speed, M. A., A. Barnard, R. P. Arber, G. C. Budd, and F. Johns. 1987. Treatment alternatives for controlling chlorinated organic contaminants in drinking water. U.S. EPA Contract CR-80933-01 (EPA/60012-87/011).
21. Johnson, J. D., and J. N. Jensen. 1986. THM and TOX formation: Routes, rates, and precursors. *JAWWA* 78(4): 156–62.
22. Noot, D. F., W. B. Anderson, S. A. Daignault, D. T. Williams, and P. M. Huck. 1989. Evaluating treatment process with Ames mutagenicity. *JAWWA* 81(9): 87–102.
23. Mitchum, R. P., M. W. Shelley, and C. M. Wheadon. 1983. Free chlorine versus ammonia-chlorine: Disinfection, trihalomethane formation, and zooplankton removal. *JAWWA* 75: 196–8.
24. Cameron, G. N., J. M. Symons, S. R. Spencer, and J. Y. Ma. 1989. Minimizing THM formation during control of the Asiatic clam: A comparison of biocide. *JAWWA* 81(10): 53–62.
25. Cameron, G. N., J. M. Symons, S. R. Spencer, and J. Y. Ma. 1989. Effect of temperature and pH on the toxicity of monochloramine to the Asiatic clam. *JAWWA* 81(10): 62–71.
26. Ficek, K. J., and J. E. Bell. 1970. Potassium permanganate: An alternative to prechlorination. *Aqua* (July): 153–6.
27. Hoehn, R. C., A. M. Dietrich, W. S. Farmer, R. G. Lee, E. M. Aieta, D. W. Wood, and G. Gordon. 1989. Household odors associated with the use of chlorine dioxide during drinking water treatment. Presented at AWWA Annual Conference, Los Angeles, CA, June 1989.
28. Krasner, S. W., S. E. Barrett, M. S. Dale, and C. J. Huang. 1989. Free chlorine versus monochloramine for controlling off-tastes and off-odors. *JAWWA* 81(2): 86–93.
29. Lalezary, S., M. Pirbazari, and M. J. McGuire. 1986. Oxidation of five earthy-musty taste and odor compounds. *JAWWA* 78(3): 62–9.
30. Bonacquisti, T. P., and E. Petrovitch. 1988. Preoxidation using potassium permanganate at the Fairfax County water authority. Presented at Annual Section Meeting, Virginia Section AWWA, Fairfax, VA, October 1988.
31. Middlemas, R. E., and K. J. Ficek. 1986. Controlling the potassium permanganate feed for taste and odor treatment. Presented at AWWA Annual Conference, Denver, CO, June 1986.
32. Means, E. G., T. S. Tanaka, D. J. Otsuka, and M. J. McGuire. 1986. Effects of chlorine and ammonia application points on bactericidal efficiency. *JAWWA* 78(1): 62–9.
33. Morris, J. C., and B. Baum. 1978. Precursors and mechanisms of haloform formation in the chlorination of water supplies. In *Water chlorination: Environmental impact and health effects,* Vol. 2, Jolley, R. L., Gorchev, H., and Hamilton, D. H., eds., pp. 29–48. Ann Arbor, MI: Ann Arbor Science Publishers.
34. Pirnie, M. 1986. *Chlorination system modifications and organics control.* Engineering Report prepared for City of Norfolk, VA, Department of Utilities, March 1986.
35. Cummins, M. D. 1985. Field evaluation of packed column air stripping: Rivi-

era Beach, Florida. Internal report of U.S. EPA Office of Drinking Water, Cincinnati, OH, May 1985.

36. Boyce, S. D., and J. F. Hornig. 1980. Formation of chloroform from the chlorination of diketones and polyhydroxybenzenes in dilute aqueous solution. In *Water chlorination: Environmental impacts and health effects,* Vol. 3, Jolley, R. L., Brungs, W. A., Cumming, R. B., and Jacobs, V. A., eds. Ann Arbor, MI: Ann Arbor Science Publishers.
37. Singer, P. C. 1986. THM control using alternative oxidant and disinfectant strategies: An evaluation. Paper presented at AWWA Annual Conference, Denver, CO, June 1986.
38. Wolfe, R. L., E. G. Means, M. K. Davis, and S. E. Barrett. 1988. Biological nitrification in covered reservoirs containing chlorinated water. *JAWWA* 80(9): 109–14.
39. Hazen and Sawyer. 1989. *Safe drinking water act evaluation,* prepared for Tamarac Utilities West, Tamarac, FL, January 1989.
40. Anonymous. 1983. *Safety practice for water utilities,* AWWA Manual No. M3. Denver, CO: American Water Works Association.
41. Trussell, R., and P. Kreft. 1984. Engineering considerations of chloramine application. Presented at AWWA Seminar, *Chloramination for THM Control: Principles and Practices,* Annual Conference, Dallas, TX.
42. Fischer and Porter. 1977. Technical information for handling chlorine, sulfur dioxide and ammonia from supply to point of application. Instruction Bulletin 70-9001, April 1977, Fischer and Porter Company, Warminster, PA.
43. Ainsworth, L. D., and M. McGrath. 1987. Simple aqua-ammonia feed system for a water plant. *Public Works* 118: 107–9.
44. American Water Works Association. 1971. *Water quality and treatment.* New York: McGraw-Hill.
45. Rice, R. G. 1988. Emerging technologies for compliance with disinfection and disinfection by-products regulations. Prepared for presentation at *EPA Workshops on Emerging Technologies for Drinking Water Treatment,* 28 March, 1988.
46. LeChevallier, M. W., C. D. Lowry, and R. G. Lee. 1990. Disinfecting biofilms in a model distribution system. *JAWWA* 82(7): 87–99.
47. Robinson, K., and R. Elefritz. 1990. Monitoring organic performance and disinfection of a surface water, ozonation-softening facility in south Florida. *AWWA WQTC Proceedings,* pp. 877–99. 1990 Annual WQTC, San Diego, CA, November 1990.
48. Topudurti, K. V., and C. N. Haas. 1991. THM formation by the transfer of active chlorine from monochloramine to phenoacetophenone. *JAWWA* 83(5): 62–6.
49. Bartels, J. H. M., et. al. 1989. *Taste and odor in drinking water supplies,* AWWARF Report. Denver, CO: American Water Works Association.
50. Dennis, J. P., et al. 1991. Practical aspects of implementing chloramines. Presented at 1991 AWWA Annual Conference, Philadelphia, PA, June 1991.

6

Chlorine Dioxide

with contributions by

W. J. Masschelein
Brussels Intercommunal Water Board, Belgium

Alex J. Varas
Hazen and Sawyer
on *Design Concepts*

Chlorine dioxide is an alternative disinfecting form of chlorine that is quite different in character from either free chlorine or chloramines. Unlike free chlorine and chloramines, in which chlorine occurs in the +1 oxidation state, chlorine in chlorine dioxide is in the +4 oxidation state. This is a significant difference that sets chlorine dioxide apart chemically, yielding different reaction pathways for both disinfection and the formation of byproducts. One advantageous consequence of this difference is a limited tendency for the formation of trihalomethanes. Furthermore, many other chlorinated byproducts of concern that occur with both free chlorine and chloramines are also not formed. Therefore, much of the recent interest in the use of chlorine dioxide is largely a result of its possible role for achieving disinfection while minimizing the formation of certain unwanted byproducts.

While use of chlorine dioxide can greatly reduce formation of many of the principal free chlorine byproducts of concern, other byproducts must be considered. These can include the inorganic degradation products of chlorine dioxide, chlorate (ClO_3^-), and chlorite (ClO_2^-), as well as nonchlorinated organic end products. A degree of chlorinated organic formation can also occur, partially as a result of the presence of free chlorine as an impurity in many chlorine dioxide feed solutions. As a consequence of these phenomena, it is more appropriate to characterize chlorine dioxide as a disinfectant that alters the types of byproducts formed, as opposed to considering it to be an alternative for reducing the formation of byproducts that occur with the use of free chlorine. In other words, the effects of the byproducts of chlorine dioxide must also be considered, although they may be of much less concern based on prevailing information.

Major concerns about the use of chlorine dioxide have been raised with respect to possible health consequences resulting from the ingestion of chlorine dioxide and its two inorganic reaction byproducts, chlorate and chlorite. Because of these concerns, it may become necessary to limit the maximum chlorine dioxide level in water distribution systems. This limitation could make it difficult to maintain an adequate residual at all locations in the distribution system and could restrict its role in secondary disinfection applications under approaches normally applied in the United States. Because of this potential limitation, much of the current U.S. interest in chlorine dioxide centers on its potential for use as a primary disinfectant that could replace free chlorine within a water treatment plant. Other disinfecting chemicals might then be required for meeting downstream or distribution system criteria for secondary disinfection. Chlorine dioxide is successfully used, however, for maintaining secondary disinfection in several European applications where stringent limitations have not been placed on maximum residual levels.

A key factor in the application of chlorine dioxide is that it normally occurs as a relatively unstable gas that cannot be compressed to a liquefied form without danger of explosion. Because of this inherent instability, chlorine dioxide cannot be conveniently delivered from off-site locations and, therefore, is normally generated on-site on an as-needed basis. Typically, for the quantities encountered in water treatment, such generation employs chlorine and sodium chlorite as reactant chemicals. A need to rigorously control this generation reaction occurs as a result of both the safety and the product quality considerations. This represents a significant change in the nature of operations as compared with free chlorine. Even in chloramination, in which chloramines are formed within the process stream by reaction between chlorine and ammonia, the need for such level of reaction control is much less.

HISTORY OF THE USE OF CHLORINE DIOXIDE

Chlorine dioxide was discovered in 1814 by Sir Humphrey Davy as a product of a reaction between potassium chlorate and sulfuric acid. However, it was not extensively commercialized until 1940. Much of its early application developed around use in pulp and paper manufacture, where it could serve as a bleaching agent that was not as susceptible as chlorine to loss by unproductive reactions (1).

Chlorine dioxide was initially used in water treatment because it serves as an effective oxidant for eliminating taste and odor problems that occur when free chlorine is contacted with a water that contains phenolic compounds. Free chlorine tends to react with these compounds to form chlorinated phenols, which produce an offensive chlorinous taste, whereas chlorine dioxide destroys these compounds.

While chlorine dioxide has been applied to a limited extent in the United States, it has been more commonly considered in Europe where industrial discharge of phenols has been a greater concern in contaminating surface water supplies (2). However, interest in chlorine dioxide has recently increased, both in the United States and internationally, as a result of its possible role as an alternative that can reduce the formation of trihalomethanes and other disinfection byproducts that are of concern with the use of free chlorine.

COMMERCIAL CHEMICALS USED TO FORM CHLORINE DIOXIDE

Generation of chlorine dioxide generally results from reactions involving either sodium chlorite ($NaClO_2$) or sodium chlorate ($NaClO_3$). Sodium chlorate is employed in a process that generates chlorine dioxide through reduction of the chlorate component by sulfur dioxide. This process has been extensively applied to produce the larger volumes of chlorine dioxide required in pulp and paper bleaching operations. However, most water treatment applications have used generation techniques that involve sodium chlorite. These techniques involve reactions with chlorine or pH adjustment with acids. A typical reaction sequence using chlorine can be represented by the following general expression:

$$2NaClO_2 + Cl_2 = 2ClO_2 + 2NaCl \qquad (6\text{–}1)$$

Commercial sources of chlorine have been discussed in Chapter 4. Discussions in this chapter will, therefore, focus on sodium chlorite.

Sodium chlorite solutions are normally made up to a concentration of approximately 25 percent. This concentration achieves the lowest freezing point and is therefore less susceptible to handling difficulties in cold weather. Chlorate can occur as an impurity in commercial sodium chlorite at levels of 2 to 3 percent by weight of chlorite. A degree of alkalinity is sometimes introduced to stabilize these solutions since sodium chlorite tends to degrade prematurely under acidic conditions. However, a low alkalinity solution (less than 10 mg/l as $CaCO_3$) is desirable for many of the generation methods used for water treatment (3). The equipment supplier should be consulted to determine the appropriate solution conditions for a given generation system.

Sodium chlorite solutions are highly corrosive, and consideration should be given to proper material selection for storage, pumping, and piping. Even at the optimum concentration of 25 percent, these solutions are still subject to freezing at temperatures of −15°C (5°F) (3), and the need for heated storage should be considered for facilities that are located outdoors. Upper limits also need to be placed on temperature in order to avoid explosion. With this in mind, temperatures should be maintained at less than 40°C (104°F), and conditions should not be allowed that could increase temperatures above 80°C (176°F).

In dry form, sodium chlorite occurs as a flaked salt at a concentration of approximately 80 percent. It is naturally white in color, although other coloration may occur with impurities. For example, partial formation of chlorine dioxide in the solid form can lead to an orange color, which can be dangerous.

Dry sodium chlorite can be highly reactive, having a capability for violent reaction (explosion) when it contacts with organic substances such as clothing, gloves, cotton waste, sawdust, mops, brooms, and oils. Physical factors such as heat, friction, or impact can also lead to reaction. For these reasons, the liquid form is normally preferred for water treatment. When a dry form is used, it should be dissolved into solution as soon as possible. Because of possible hazards, care should be taken to clean any spills of the liquid form before evaporation can lead to a deposit of dry salt. To avoid potential explosions, provisions for spill containment and cleanup are an important consideration for design and operation. Manufacturers of chlorine dioxide equipment and sodium chlorite suppliers should be consulted for more detailed information on the appropriate safety provisions.

CHEMISTRY OF CHLORINE DIOXIDE

Chlorine dioxide chemistry is often presented in terms of oxidation characteristics (30). These characteristics define the tendency to accept electrons to oxidize other chemical constituents. Its role as an oxidizing chemical in water involves two steps.

1. Chlorine dioxide gains one electron to form chlorite (ClO_2^-):

$$ClO_2 + 1e^- = ClO_2^- \qquad (6\text{–}2)$$

2. Chlorite gains four electrons to form chloride (Cl^-):

$$ClO_2^- + 2H_2O + 4e^- = Cl^- + 4OH \qquad (6\text{–}3)$$

The first step to form chlorite can usually proceed in the pH range normally encountered in water treatment practice. However, the chlorite form is less reactive for many constituents found in water, and the second step does not proceed as readily. The predominant oxidizing capability of chlorine dioxide for organic matter as well as many inorganic constituents is characterized by the oxidation potential of the one-electron transfer that occurs in the first reaction step. As a consequence, the overall five-electron total transfer capability for complete reaction through the two steps is often not available.

The oxidation potential of the first reaction step is 0.95 V at standard conditions and 25°C. This compares with a greater oxidation potential 1.49 V for the common free chlorine specie, hypochlorous acid, defined by the following reaction:

$$HOCl + H^+ + 2e^- = Cl^- + H_2O \qquad (6\text{–}4)$$

This simple numerical comparison would seem to indicate that free chlorine has a stronger oxidizing potential for organic compounds. However, other factors must be considered for chlorine dioxide reactions. In particular, the oxidation effectiveness depends on the availability of reaction pathways that allow the oxidation potential to be exerted under a given set of circumstances. Chlorine dioxide and free chlorine cannot, therefore, be compared on a simple oxidation potential basis for a given oxidation reaction. Observations indicate that free chlorine may be more efficient for general removal of total organic carbon due to a wider range of reaction pathways (4), while chlorine dioxide can be more effective for oxidizing specific organic groups as illustrated by a reactivity with phenols.

Although some features of reactions between chlorine dioxide and organic constituents are understood, many specific aspects are still uncertain. In general, it is known that chlorine dioxide has an unpaired electron in its molecular structure. This is a less stable and therefore more reactive chemical condition that is termed a *free radical condition*. This characteristic can affect the nature of disinfection reactions as well as reactions that produce the first oxidation step that results from a one-electron transfer to produce chlorite. Some research suggests, however, that mechanisms other than free radical reactions may be important for certain conditions (5). Other types of mechanisms are also involved if the second step of reaction occurs in which chlorite loses four electrons to form chloride.

Chlorine dioxide reactions with inorganic compounds can follow different reaction pathways than those encountered with organic compounds. For example, chlorine dioxide can react with some inorganic constituents through a complete five-electron transfer (5) that involves both oxidation steps (Equations 6–2 and 6–3). Specific inorganic constituents that can undergo such reactions include hydrogen sulfide and the +2 oxidation state of iron (i.e., the ferrous, or Fe^{+2}, form).

With respect to general reaction properties, the +4 oxidation state of chlorine found in chlorine dioxide does not readily substitute into other chemical structures to form compounds such as chlorinated organics or chloramines. Chlorine dioxide also does not readily oxidize ammonia. Therefore, ammonia, a constituent that can represent a significant demand for free chlorine, does not exert a demand for chlorine dioxide. Where other sources of chlorine dioxide demand are low, this factor may result in lower dose requirements relative to free chlorine, especially where significant levels of background ammonia are present in a raw water.

Chlorine dioxide is relatively stable in neutral and mildly acidic solutions. However, under alkaline conditions, chlorine dioxide can more readily degrade to form both chlorate (ClO_3^-) and chlorite (ClO_2^-) according to the following reaction (7):

$$2ClO_2 + 2OH^- = H_2O + ClO_2^- + ClO_3^- \qquad (6\text{–}5)$$

This reaction does not proceed to an appreciable extent at a pH less than 8. However, it can be a consideration where highly alkaline conditions are encountered, such as those where high pH softening processes are employed (6). The rate of degradation is also influenced by the chlorine dioxide concentration. Degradation proceeds at higher rates at higher concentrations of chlorine dioxide. Phosphate and carbonate ions reduce the rate of degradation.

In addition to these reactions, chlorine dioxide is susceptible to photochemical breakdown when exposed to light. These degradation reactions can lead to the formation of hydrogen peroxide, chlorite, chlorate, oxygen, and chlorine (9). To minimize this form of degradation, care should be taken to shield chlorine dioxide feed streams from light.

Another important degradation reaction involves the breakdown of chlorite, where chlorite degradation to chloride, shown in Equation 6–3, proceeds in the acid pH range. This reaction can ultimately lead to complete degradation to the inert chloride form. Chlorite can also undergo significant degradation in other ways if sufficient time is available. For example, studies by Noack and Doerr (10) suggested that, with adequate reaction time, chlorite could react with chlorine to form chlorate as an end product at pH 7. These findings were based on observed reactant ratios and the fact that little chlorine dioxide was observed in solution. This hypothesis was not confirmed by analyses of chlorate levels, although varying results for this type of reaction have been reported to be dependent on time of reaction, reactant concentrations, and pH (6).

The total effect of reactions involving chlorine dioxide is a composite of all of the reaction pathways. In one study involving fulvic acids extracted from natural water sources, approximately 70 percent of the reacted chlorine dioxide was converted to chlorite at pH 7 (11). In a study of reactions with phenol (12), approximately 50 percent of chlorine dioxide reacted was converted to chlorite.

A further indication of the variability of chlorite formation was encountered in a recent study at the Orange Water and Sewer Authority water treatment plant in Carrboro, North Carolina (13). It was observed in this study that conversion to chlorite shifted from a range of between 60 and 66 percent in raw water to 76 percent in settled water treated with potassium permanganate.

The ultimate effect of all of these reactions is varied and appears to result in a range of chlorite production of between 50 and 75 percent (6, 13). Chloride typically accounts for most of the remainder of the reacted chlorine dioxide in many laboratory solutions. However, chlorate can also be produced at significant levels under some field conditions.

DISINFECTION BYPRODUCT FORMATION

Significantly, the +4 oxidation state of chlorine that occurs in chlorine dioxide does not readily substitute into organic matter to form chlorinated byproducts such as trihalomethanes. Other halogenated organic compounds can be formed but much lower levels are observed than with chlorine (22). A number of nonhalogenated organic byproducts are formed, predominantly as a result of oxidation reactions. Some selectivity in reaction pathways appears to occur for these oxidation reactions. For example, it is reported that chlorine dioxide is most reactive with tertiary organic amines and phenols. Its reactivity with secondary amines is less, and it is relatively unreactive with primary amines. Chlorine dioxide is also reported to react with aldehydes and with alcohols under acid conditions. It is moderately reactive with alkenes that contain unsaturated or double bond configurations between carbon atoms, and unreactive with saturated aliphatic hydrocarbon groups, saturated carboxylic acids, and amino acids under conditions normally found in water treatment (7).

In spite of these observations of selectivity in reaction pathways, chlorine dioxide can engage in some reactions with the humic materials that naturally occur in drinking water. End products are predominantly nonchlorinated organics that are formed as a result of oxidation. Many of these reactions are thought to involve phenolic groups—i.e., groups that consist of a basic benzene ring–type structure to which hydroxyl groups (−OH) are attached (see Figure 3–2). Chlorine dioxide has been shown to react with these types of compounds in a manner that opens the benzene ring to yield products such as di- and tricarboxylic acids, glyoxalic acid, and aldehydes. Formation of quinones, a group of compounds that contains a benzene ring structure to which two oxygen groups (=O) are attached, is also observed with some phenolic reactions (7). The outcome of these reactions depends on the character of the phenolic compound, some being more susceptible to reaction than others. Reactions with humic acids at conventional doses have produced many similar byproducts, including carboxylic acids and glyoxal and other aldehydes. High doses can also produce monochloroacetic acid and traces of monochlorsuccinic acid and di- and trichloroacetic acids.

The extent to which ring opening occurs in reactions with phenolic compounds can depend on the ratio of chlorine dioxide to organic carbon. At low chlorine dioxide ratios, the ring structure may be retained and the reaction can lead to formation of quinones. Some chlorine substitution may also occur at lower ratios, leading to the formation of chlorinated phenols and chlorinated quinones (7), both halogenated organic byproducts. This substitution may actually result from alternative chlorine dioxide degradation pathways in which hypochlorous acid becomes an intermediate product. This type of reaction has been proposed for reaction with phenolic and other ring-type organics according to the following general reaction in which R represents a benzene ring–type compound:

$$R{-}H + ClO_2 \longrightarrow R{=}O + HOCl \qquad (6\text{–}6)$$

Other reaction sequences leading to the formation of free chlorine have been proposed. Free chlorine also frequently occurs as an impurity, especially in cases where it is used for the generation of chlorine dioxide. Therefore, there is a potential for free chlorine to be present in chlorine dioxide reactions, irrespective of mechanism. Consequently, some halogenated organic byproducts can be formed as a result of side reactions with chlorine. Because of this potential, consideration can be given to maintaining a background level of ammonia to convert any free chlorine to chloramines, thereby limiting the potential for these side reactions.

Another significant feature of chlorine dioxide chemistry is the fact that bromide is not readily oxidized to hypobromous acid in dark solution. This is not the case with ozone, where some formation of halogenated organic compounds is thought to occur as a result of hypobromous acid formation due to bromide oxidation in ozonated waters. As a consequence, formation of brominated byproducts may be reduced when chloride dioxide is used in place of ozone. However, it should be noted that photosensitized oxidation of bromide is possible with chlorine dioxide. Therefore, the extent to which bromide-related reactions can be minimized may depend on the exposure to light.

Some research has indicated that chlorine dioxide can react with trihalomethane precursors to reduce the formation of trihalomethanes. The percent of reduction in such trihalomethane formation potential increases as the ratio of chlorine dioxide to total organic carbon is increased (11). One study indicated that in the treatment of Ohio River water with 2 to 3 mg/l of chlorine dioxide, a 50 percent reduction in the formation potential for trihalomethane resulted (14). However, such extensive reduction in the potential for THM formation may not always be possible, and the actual extent of such reductions should be confirmed based on experimental evaluation. For example, in other research, chlorine dioxide was found to increase the chloroform formation potential of certain laboratory compounds, which were predominantly in the benzoic acid group (15). In other instances, where high levels of organic material are encountered, it may be difficult to achieve appreciable reductions in the formation potential without producing excessive residual levels of chlorine dioxide, chlorite, and chlorate.

Although it is clear from available research that chlorine dioxide can react to form some byproducts of potential health concern, the actual significance of these byproducts is not as apparent. Glyoxal and glyoxylic acid are among classes of compounds that have exhibited mutagenic properties. Quinones are also a class of compounds of possible health concern. However, other than chlorite and chlorate, the health effects of these byproducts have not, as yet, been specifically evaluated in detailed studies. Some indication of possible reduced health concern relative to products of free chlorine is offered in several studies that indicate no increase in mutagenic activity in solutions subsequent to chlorine dioxide application. However, these types of studies, as discussed in Chapter 3, are not conclusive in nature.

DISINFECTION

Chlorine dioxide is regarded as a strong primary disinfectant that is effective for bacterial, viral, and protozoan pathogens. This is reflected in the EPA CT criteria for *Giardia* and enteric viruses. To achieve credit for a specified log removal of *Giardia,* these criteria can be met by chlorine dioxide at CT levels that are usually less than half of the required free chlorine CT. Under most pH conditions, the reduction in required CT, as compared with that for free chlorine, is even greater. However, in the case of removal of virus, free chlorine is given a higher credit for disinfection, thereby reversing the situation for this category of pathogens. However, virus removal is still reasonably achieved with chlorine dioxide. Also, in most cases, CT criteria for *Giardia* will dictate the disinfecting dosage conditions.

Unlike free chlorine, the disinfecting effectiveness of chlorine dioxide for *Giardia* is not affected by pH over a range of 6 to 9 (8). Therefore, it can have a further disinfecting advantage over chlorine as pH is increased. Care may still have to be taken to avoid excessive alkalinity, since it can accelerate degradation of chlorine dioxide, as shown in Equation 6–5.

Chlorine dioxide does not readily react with ammonia. As a result, where ammonia is present, the demand for chlorine dioxide may be reduced as compared with chlorine, a disinfectant for which ammonia can exert an appreciable demand. However, many waters can exert a considerable chlorine dioxide demand through other pathways that result from the presence of background organic matter or inorganic substances such as iron, manganese, and sulfides. In some of these cases, chlorine dioxide residuals can be difficult to maintain, and disinfection results can become more erratic as a consequence. Furthermore, concerns for excess finished water residual levels of chlorine dioxide, chlorite, and chlorate may restrict the latitude for increasing the chlorine dioxide dose to more consistently achieve the desired disinfecting residual. As an example of the effects of certain types of demand, investigations in a water treatment plant in Lexington, Kentucky, disclosed a deterioration in certain aspects of the bacteriological quality of filtered water at functional pretreatment dosages of chlorine dioxide as compared with previous plant experience with free chlorine (16). While coliform criteria were maintained with chlorine dioxide, capability for broader disinfection was a concern. In this case, the observed deterioration was associated with high levels of background colonies of a noncoliform nature.

Two approaches may be considered to resolve problems that occur with chlorine dioxide demand. In the first, the point of chlorine dioxide application can be moved to a location in the treatment train that is downstream of the pretreatment process, allowing for maximum removal of organic and inorganic demand prior to chlorine dioxide addition. If necessary, alternative oxidants such as potassium permanganate can be considered to achieve both preoxidation and reduction of demand. Additional removal of demand-causing substances can be achieved in filtration so that consideration can be given to locating the chlorine dioxide addition to points downstream of this particulate removal process as well.

The second approach for achieving more consistent chlorine dioxide disinfection involves the addition of an adequate chlorine dioxide dose to achieve primary disinfection goals under all demand conditions. Following the period of contact necessary to meet primary disinfection objectives, consideration can be given to removal of any excess chlorine dioxide residuals in a manner similar to the dechlorination processes used in water and wastewater treatment. Under this approach, another disinfectant, such as free chlorine or chloramines, would subsequently be added at dosages appropriate for meeting downstream secondary disinfection criteria.

It is important to note that, while methods are available for removing chlorine dioxide and chlorite, chlorate is not easily removed once it is formed. Therefore, reaction conditions for chloride dioxide generation and within the process stream, prior to adding the reducing agent, must be such that little chlorate is formed. In general, chlorate formation is variable and may initially occur in limited quantities as long as the chlorine dioxide generation process is properly controlled to minimize such formation. Subsequently, chlorate can form as a degradation product over time, with formation being catalyzed in the presence of sunlight. It can also occur as a result of reactions between excess chlorine and chlorite in a pH range of 6 to 10 (32). As a consequence of these phenomena, steps need to be considered to (1) limit chlorate formation during chlorine dioxide generation and (2) select conditions for removing chlorine dioxide and chlorite that do not produce chlorate.

Granular activated carbon (GAC) and sulfur dioxide were originally thought to show promise as agents for removing chlorine dioxide and chlorite residuals. However, under some conditions, chlorate appears to be a major end product when activated carbon is used and potentially negates benefits from this approach unless appropriate contacting conditions are employed. In the case of sulfur dioxide, both chlorine dioxide and chlorite can be removed at a pH less than 6 (17). However, this process also has been found to lead to the formation of chlorate. Other reducing agents that have been evaluated include sodium metabisulfite, sodium thiosulfate, and ferrous iron (Fe^{2+}) salts. Like sulfur dioxide and GAC, sodium metabisulfite has produced chlorate as an undesirable byproduct. However, sodium thiosulfate does not produce appreciable levels of chlorate. This agent was particularly effective in a pH range of 4.5 to 6.5. Ferrous iron has been highly effective in achieving removals in a pH range of 6.0 to 7.0 without producing chlorate (33).

While there are some health concerns regarding chlorine dioxide residuals, chlorine dioxide has been effectively used to provide a disinfecting residual for meeting secondary disinfection goals in some water distribution systems; several applications of this type exist in Europe (6). In this type of application chlorine dioxide can often be more stable than free chlorine by virtue of the fact that it does not readily react with water, ammonia, bromide ions, or most organic nitrogen compounds (8). The extent of this advantage depends upon the presence of additional oxidant demanding constituents that might react with chlorine dioxide. Therefore, the relative stability of chlorine dioxide may be site specific. Where chlorine dioxide is applied as a secondary disinfectant, attempts should be made to remove these oxidant demanding substances prior to its addition.

As has been discussed, the use of chlorine dioxide in a secondary disinfection role may be limited by criteria that restrict residual levels of chlorine dioxide, chlorite, and chlorate due to health concerns. Such restrictions would constrain the allowable chlorine dioxide dosage. As a consequence, sufficient latitude for adding an adequate dosage might not exist for many water systems.

NONDISINFECTION USES OF CHLORINE DIOXIDE

Many of the nondisinfection uses of chlorine dioxide result from its oxidizing properties. This allows it to serve as a potential replacement for free chlorine in certain applications in which oxidative removal of target substances such as iron and manganese, sulfide, color, and some taste and odor compounds can be achieved. Chlorine dioxide can also be effective as a biocide for the control of biological growths in water treatment systems. This latter feature can result in improved filter performance and sludge dewaterability (18).

In some cases, goals for control of target substances can be more effectively achieved by using chlorine dioxide rather than free chlorine. However, some caution should be exercised before arriving at such a conclusion. For example, the demand exerted for free chlorine compared to that for a chlorine dioxide alternative may have a significant influence on the relative effectiveness of these two chemicals for meeting nondisinfection goals.

Control of Biological Growths

Chlorine dioxide has not been widely cited as a biocide for control of nuisance biological growths. However, it appears to have a potential role in this area. For example, chlorine dioxide has been used in some industrial applications for control of biofilms (6). Chlorine dioxide may also be effective as a biocide for the control of Asiatic clams in raw water pipelines (19). Another evaluation in Philadelphia reported chlorine dioxide to be an effective algicide for an open reservoir (20). Chlorite also has a degree of biocidal capability, although it is not as strong as required for acceptable levels of pathogenic reduction (31).

Control of Tastes and Odors

One of the early applications of chlorine dioxide in water treatment is related to its effectiveness for controlling certain types of tastes and odors. For instance, phenolic compounds can react with free chlorine to form odorous chlorinated phenols. This phenomenon has been avoided in some cases by using chlorine dioxide, which degrades both phenolic and chlorophenolic compounds by oxidation (2). Other common taste and odor compounds such as geosmin, 2,3,6-trichloroanisole, 2-isopropyl-3-methoxy pyrazine, and 2-methylisoborneol (MIB) have been effectively removed by chlorine dioxide (21). Geosmin and MIB are typically the most difficult of these compounds to remove.

Chlorine dioxide also appears to be useful in eliminating sulfide odors; sulfide is rapidly oxidized by chlorine dioxide (6). This reaction appears to take advantage of the full oxidizing capability of chlorine dioxide for a five-electron gain to form chloride. The total end product of this reaction is not entirely clear, although it appears that sulfate is predominant.

While these experiences indicate a role for chlorine dioxide for controlling many taste and odor problems, a number of water utilities have had the opposite experience in the actual creation of a significant odor problem associated with the use of chlorine dioxide. These particular odors have been observed to occur sporadically throughout service areas, with certain homes and businesses reporting odors that range from "kerosene" to "cat urine." It has been discovered that these odors can be produced by reactions between chlorine dioxide vapor escaping from water at taps and showers and organic vapors found in the atmosphere of some homes (23). Water temperature is probably a factor since the solubility of chlorine dioxide in water decreases as temperature is increased (30). A common source of reactive organic vapors is new carpeting. Research (23) has indicated that, even in systems in which the chlorine dioxide residual was very low in finished water leaving a water treatment plant, chlorine dioxide could be reformed to some extent in the distribution system by a reaction of its major degradation product, chlorite, and the free chlorine species, hypochlorous acid (HOCl). The level of formation produced by this reaction was found to be capable of yielding the extent of chlorine dioxide off-gassing necessary for producing odors.

Ammoniation to convert free chlorine to chloramines was recommended as one means for eliminating the reformation reaction. This approach was reported to be effective by one utility (16). However, while this may be effective where there is only a limited chlorine dioxide residual in the finished water, such an approach may not be effective where significantly larger chlorine dioxide residuals leave the plant. In such cases, removal of chlorine dioxide from finished water may be required.

Removal of Iron and Manganese

Chlorine dioxide has been demonstrated to be effective for the oxidation of soluble forms of iron (Fe^{2+}) and manganese (Mn^{2+}) to the higher oxidation states (Fe^{3+} and Mn^{4+}) that are readily precipitated as hydroxides or oxides and subsequently removed. Notably, the iron oxidation reactions can take advantage of the full oxidation capability of chlorine dioxide to gain five electrons and form chloride (see Equations 6–2 and 6–3). However, the manganese reaction appears to involve only a single electron transfer to form chlorite. These reactions result in theoretical dosages of 2.5 mg of chlorine dioxide per mg of manganese (25) and 0.24 mg of chlorine dioxide per mg of iron (assuming full five-electron transfer to form chloride). Higher doses will actually be required due to the presence of other demand-causing substances.

While generally improved manganese removal has often been reported when converting to preoxidation with chlorine dioxide (18), the actual effectiveness for manganese control may depend on several key factors. Chlorine dioxide can be extremely effective in achieving initial oxidation, although it may not achieve effective manganese control if its residual is subsequently dissipated in the treatment plant, a condition that allows manganese to return to its reduced form and redissolve. Capability for maintaining a residual varies depending on the presence of demand-causing substances. In particular, naturally occurring organic material can represent a significant competing demand (25).

Specifically, redissolution phenomena are most likely to occur both in sedimentation basins that do not continuously withdraw sludge as well as at the surface of filter media where the manganese precipitate can attach. These phenomena can also occur in supernatant recycle streams from sludge handling and dewatering processes and in sedimentation basins that practice mechanical cleaning, especially at low cleaning frequencies. Redissolution has proved to be a problem in some plants upon conversion to chlorine dioxide. Conversely, previous use of free chlorine achieved a more continuous level of oxidation throughout the treatment train (24). The problem might be alleviated either by the use of a higher chlorine dioxide dosage or by multiple points of addition. Care may need to be exercised, however, to avoid excess residuals of chlorine dioxide, chlorite, and chlorate that could exceed health-related criteria.

Water chemistry can significantly influence the effect of chlorine dioxide on both iron and manganese. Iron can be complexed with humic and fulvic acids to form organic compounds that retard its rate of oxidation. While manganese is not as readily complexed by the same humic and fulvic matter (25), competitive oxidant demand is exerted. It also has been reported that the chlorine dioxide oxidation rate of manganese is pH dependent (25); removal rates increase with increased pH, although a pH in excess of 4.5 is adequate for most situations.

Removal of Color

Chlorine dioxide is widely recognized for its decoloring capabilities in industrial applications such as pulp- and paper-bleaching operations. However, its effectiveness as a decoloring agent for drinking water has not been as widely cited (2). A major consideration for use of chlorine dioxide in this role is the dose requirement, especially in cases where health concerns for chlorine dioxide, chlorite, and chlorate residuals may limit the applied dosage to a certain level.

ALTERNATIVE METHODS FOR APPLYING CHLORINE DIOXIDE

As has been discussed, two major issues limit the acceptable levels of chlorine dioxide residuals that can be maintained in finished water:

- Health-related criteria that limit the exposure to chlorine dioxide and its degradation products, chlorate and chlorite.
- Odor problems related to chlorine dioxide off-gassing and subsequent reaction with organic compounds emitted by household sources such as carpets (discussed in the section Control of Tastes and Odors).

The major questions related to these concerns are where and how to best apply chlorine dioxide to achieve the maximum benefit within the associated limitations on residual levels. The predominant factor that characterizes the application of chlorine dioxide is the point of application. In general, chlorine dioxide can be used either for a pretreatment application to raw water or for a posttreatment application to settled or filtered water.

Each type of application has its particular advantages and limitations. In a pretreatment application, chlorine dioxide can be used for achieving goals such as improved coagulation, oxidation of iron, manganese, and sulfide, control of certain tastes and odors, control of biological growth, removal of color, and reduction of the trihalomethane formation potential. It might also be used for achieving disinfection goals in this type of application, depending on the residual level available after demand. However, a major disadvantage of using a pretreatment location for disinfection is that the raw water demand may be high, making it difficult to maintain a consistent disinfecting residual. Also, high demand conditions can create problems for maintaining a consistent oxidizing residual to prevent problems with downstream release of manganese. As discussed in the preceding section, previously oxidized manganese precipitates in sludge or on the surface of filter media can become exposed to periodic reducing conditions upon intermittent loss of a chlorine dioxide residual, resulting in a potential for resolubilization.

A posttreatment location for chlorine dioxide application can reduce problems associated with maintaining a disinfecting residual under high-demand raw water conditions. With this approach, upstream processes such as coagulation and sedimentation are used to reduce the demand. Other oxidants, such as potassium permanganate, might also be applied prior to sedimentation and filtration to achieve the removal of iron, manganese, sulfides, color, and taste- and odor-causing substances. Problems with manganese redissolution may occur, however, with these oxidants as well. Alternative biocides may also be necessary to control nuisance biogrowths in settling tanks and filters.

Selection of the type of application will depend on water quality factors such as the level of chlorine dioxide demand in raw water, capability for reducing demand by treatment, the amount of downstream contact time available at posttreatment locations for meeting primary disinfection criteria, the possible need for pretreatment oxidation for iron and manganese control, and the availability of alternative oxidants for pretreatment when required. These features will vary with location, and the best combination of approaches will necessarily be specific for a given set of water quality conditions and treatment goals.

In addition to the location of the chlorine dioxide feedpoint, compatibility with other water treatment conditions is another consideration in selecting a feedpoint. Powdered and granular activated carbon can remove chlorine dioxide residuals and may, therefore, be incompatible. Both chlorine and potassium permanganate can also react with chlorine dioxide so that simultaneous addition may need to be avoided. Excessive air stripping and other gas transfer operations such as recarbonation can cause reduction in chlorine dioxide levels due to its volatility. Alkaline pH levels greater than 8 should be avoided due to a more rapid degradation to chlorite and chlorate as shown in Equation 6–5. Therefore, high pH processes such as lime softening may present a problem for chlorine dioxide application unless the pH can be adjusted downward prior to its addition.

Processes for removing chlorine dioxide after the necessary nondisinfection and primary disinfection goals have been achieved may become more significant if restrictions on residual levels excessively limit the permissable dosage range. These methods have been discussed in the section Disinfection.

GENERATION OF CHLORINE DIOXIDE

For the quantities usually required in water treatment, chlorine dioxide generation systems have typically relied on one of several reactions involving sodium chlorite ($NaClO_2$). Alternative methods involving sodium chlorate in place of sodium chlorite are more commonly used for the larger quantities of chlorine dioxide that are applied in pulp and paper manufacture.

Chlorine dioxide formation from sodium chlorite typically occurs as a result of one of the following general reactions: (1) reaction with chlorine,

$$Cl_2 + 2NaClO_2 = 2ClO_2 + 2NaCl \qquad (6\text{–}7)$$

or (2) an acidification reaction,

$$5NaClO_2 + 4HCl = 4ClO_2 + 5NaCl + 2H_2O \qquad (6\text{–}8)$$

The reaction with chlorine gives a 1-to-1 yield of chlorine dioxide from sodium chlorite compared to the 4-to-5 yield with acidification. Therefore, the chlorine reaction methodologies have the advantage of more complete utilization of sodium chlorite. This advantage has favored the use of chlorine reaction–based methodologies, and there are few plants where acid is used in water treatment.

Although extreme acidity is not desirable, a moderate level of acidity (pH 2 to 3) enhances the chlorine reaction and is commonly used (6). This enhancement results from two phenomena that occur with acidification (17, 26):

1. Conversion of free chlorine from hypochlorous acid (HOCl) to molecular chlorine (Cl_2):

$$2H^+ + 2HOCl = Cl_2 + 2H_2O \qquad (6\text{–}9)$$

This reaction can begin to occur in the pH 2 to 3 range and can be important for the formation of chlorine dioxide since molecular chlorine reacts more rapidly with chlorite to form chlorine dioxide.

2. Conversion of chlorite ion (ClO_2^-) to chlorous acid ($HClO_2$).

$$H^+ + ClO_2^- = HClO_2 \tag{6-10}$$

This reaction also begins to occur in the region of pH 2 to 3. Chlorous acid is more reactive with hypochlorous acid (HOCl), which may still be present in this region.

Some older-generation systems do not apply the appropriate acid conditions to fully form chlorine dioxide so that partial conversions occur as a result. Under partial conversion, an undesirable excess of hypochlorite and chlorite can persist. These conditions can also lead to formation of chlorate as an undesirable byproduct (17).

Relatively precise control of pH is important since extremely low pH levels can cause the onset of the less efficient acidification reaction (Equation 6–8). Conversely, inadequate acidity does not allow sufficiently rapid formation of chlorine dioxide. Reactant ratios must also be controlled to provide nearly complete conversion of chlorite while avoiding undesirable excess levels of chlorine.

Procedures used for the generation of chlorine dioxide include control of reactant ratios and other conditions such as pH. Direct monitoring of reaction products as a control measure, however, has been complicated by the cumbersome techniques used for analyzing chlorine dioxide, chlorite, and chlorate. Methods for analyzing chlorate have been particularly difficult. These complications have inhibited development of convenient methods for direct field analysis and control. Reactant ratio and pH control are typically relied upon for process control and are confirmed by periodic laboratory results that use the more cumbersome methods available for analysis (27). Newer direct analysis techniques under development include a recent method for assessing chlorate and chlorite by ion chromatography (28) and a flow injection analysis method (17). While these may eventually simplify laboratory methods, improved methods for routine field analysis would still be helpful for process control decisions.

Generation Methods

Acid-generating systems that rely primarily on the acidification of sodium chlorite (Equation 6–8) have been used in the past and may still have a role. However, as has been discussed, these systems are generally less efficient than those that rely on reaction of chlorine with sodium chlorite (Equation 6–7) and are not widely used. Basic alternative generation methods using chlorine and sodium chlorite are shown in Figure 6–1 and are summarized below.

Chlorine/Chlorite System

This system involves the dissolution of chlorine into a feed water stream followed by subsequent contact with a sodium chlorite stream in a generator or reactor. The two streams are mixed for reaction either within the reactor or in the reactor influent pipeline, as shown in Figure 6–1. Acid can be added if necessary for controlling the reaction within the optimum pH range for chlorine dioxide generation. In some systems, the chlorine feed stream can provide much of the necessary acidity. Additional acid requirements will depend on the system provided and the pH achieved with chlorine addition. In general, the chlorine/chlorite systems tend to require proper pH control. A slight excess of chlorine is usually applied for complete conversion of sodium chlorite. However, the excess quantity should be limited to avoid unnecessary levels of free chlorine in the feed stream and to minimize undesirable side reactions in which chlorine reacts to form chlorate (29) or where excess chlorine may form THMs at downstream points of application.

Chlorine Recycle System

With this approach, chlorine is applied to a recycle loop, allowing chlorine levels to build up to higher levels than can be achieved with single pass systems. These high chlorine concentrations have flexibility to provide a pH down to less than 2 by virtue of the acid properties of chlorine. A feed stream is drawn off of this recycle loop to mix with sodium chlorite in the generation reaction and a feed water stream is added to the recycle loop to make up the volume difference. As in the case of the chlorine/chlorite system, the chlorine feed must be maintained in a proper balance with the sodium chlorite feed to provide nearly complete conversion of sodium chlorite while avoiding excess chlorine levels. However, the problems that can occur in maintaining optimum chlorine/chlorite ratios in the absence of separate acid addition are reduced by the fact that the recycle loop is used for controlling pH. This allows the chlorine solution, at a proper pH, to be withdrawn to the chlorine dioxide generation system on an as-needed basis for achieving the optimum ratio.

Gaseous Chlorine System

The gaseous chlorine system involves direct addition of a gaseous chlorine stream to a liquid sodium chlorite stream, as shown in Figure 6–1.

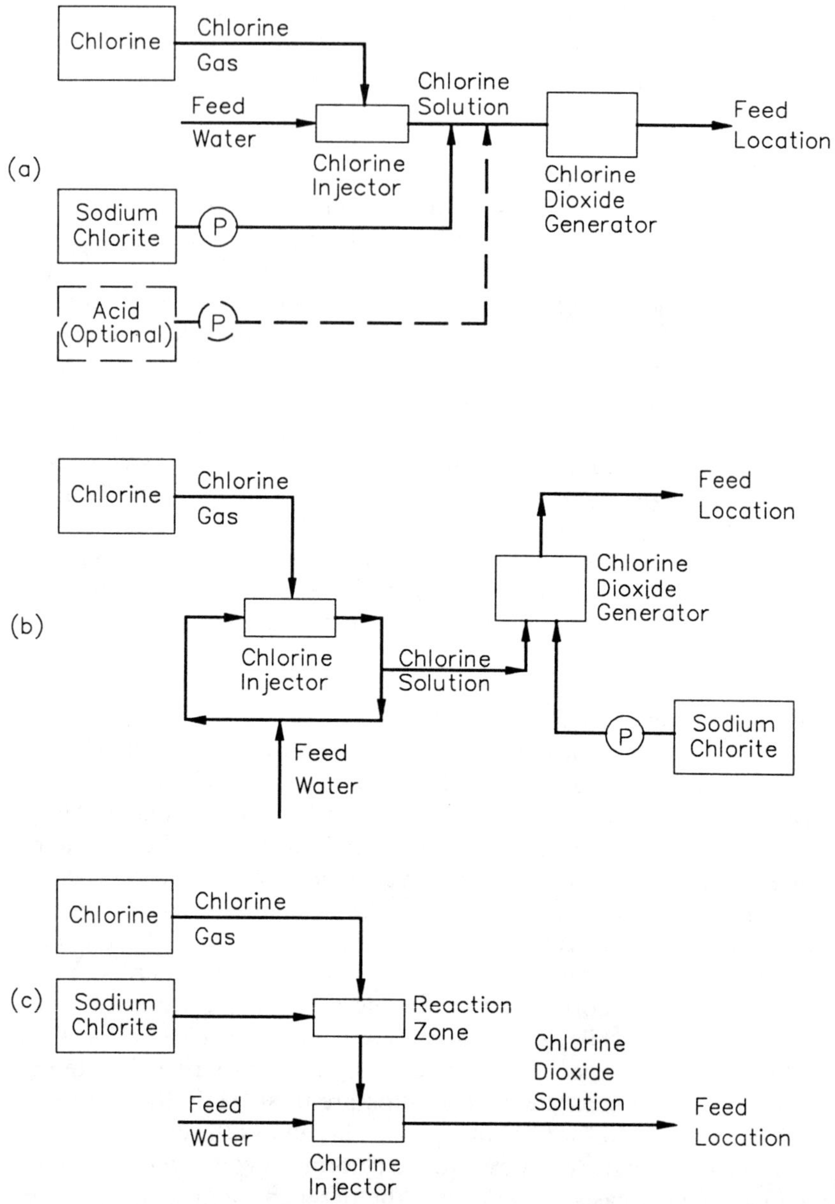

FIGURE 6–1. Basic chlorine dioxide systems using chlorine and sodium chlorite: (a) chlorine/chlorite system; (b) chlorine recycle system; (c) gaseous chlorine system.

Both streams are drawn by the vacuum created by the feed water flow through a chlorine injector. They are combined in the injector for mixing in a reaction zone. This method of contacting allows for a reaction between molecular chlorine, directly available from the gas stream, with chlorite in the liquid stream. A significant attribute of this system is a reduced need for rigorous pH control due to the fact that, as it is absorbed, molecular chlorine tends to react rapidly with the chlorite in solution before it can react with water to form hypochlorous acid (HOCl). However, chlorine feed must still be maintained in proper balance with sodium chlorite feed. It is claimed that this fast reaction method under a less acidic condition produces a high chlorine dioxide yield that minimizes contamination with chlorine and chlorate.

EQUIPMENT AND PIPING

Generation of chlorine dioxide requires handling of reactant and product streams that can include sodium chlorite, chlorine, acid, and chlorine dioxide. All of these chemicals are extremely corrosive and require appropriate material selection for equipment and piping. They are also hazardous, and appropriate safety measures need to be included in design. Containment barriers should be placed around all liquid storage tanks in the event of spill or rupture.

The basic components of chlorine dioxide generation systems are as follows:

- Sodium chlorite storage and feed system
- Acid storage and feed system (acid use depends on generation method)
- Chlorine storage and feed system (chlorine use depends on generation method)
- Chlorine dioxide generator
- Chlorine dioxide feed piping and dispersion equipment

Chlorine storage and feed equipment have already been described in Chapter 4. Acid and sodium chlorite storage and feed systems are basically liquid systems that consist of a storage tank(s) and solution feed pumps. In some cases, storage might be separated into bulk tanks and smaller operational or day tanks that are filled periodically. Fiberglass tanks are most often used for such storage. Diaphragm metering pumps are commonly used for control of liquid feed rate. The diaphragm compartment of the feed pumps is normally made of PVC, and corrosion-resistant diaphragms such as Teflon membranes are used. Sodium chlorite flows are frequently measured with magnetic flow meters or rotameters for precise control. Piping is of PVC, rubber, or Tygon materials. Provisions should always be made for back-flow prevention. Sodium chlorite is extremely reactive, especially in the dry form, and care should be taken to protect against potentially explosive conditions.

Chlorine dioxide generators are relatively simple mixing chambers that are constructed of Pyrex or PVC. The reactors are frequently filled with media such as Raschig rings or PVC rings in order to generate hydraulic turbulence for mixing. In many cases, glass is better than porcelain for Raschig rings since a small manganese content in dilution water can lead to a precipitate formation that clogs porcelain. A sample valve is desirable at the discharge end to allow for monitoring of the generation process.

Generation systems are available in sizes from 10 to more than 1,000 lb/day. In cases where a wide range of feed rates is encountered, it may be desirable to intermittently operate a chlorine dioxide generation system to fill an intermediate equalization tank as opposed to trying to maintain optimum generation for various reactant streams under varying conditions. Variable flows can then be withdrawn from the tank as required while allowing conditions in the generation system to remain constant. This type of system is described by Masschelein (29). Care must be taken in the design of these tanks to protect against the potential for toxic off-gases. The maximum acceptable concentration for chlorine dioxide in working areas is 1 ppm by volume in air; a gas phase containing more than 10 percent by volume is explosive. As in the case of chlorine, chlorine dioxide is denser than air.

Some suppliers of gaseous chlorine dioxide generation systems have developed equipment that can provide a high level of feed control of reactant feed streams under varying chlorine dioxide demand conditions. Such systems can eliminate the need for intermediate chlorine dioxide storage.

Basic System Design Considerations

The following basic features should be considered in the design of chlorine dioxide systems:

1. Inert material should be used in contact with the strong oxidizing and/or acid solutions involved in chlorine dioxide systems.
2. Separate containment should be provided for each liquid chemical.
3. Storage tanks should be provided with vents to outside.
4. Adequate ventilation and air monitoring should be ensured.
5. Gas masks and first aid kits should be provided outside of the chemical areas.

6. A washdown capability should be provided in chemical storage/mixing areas.
7. The reactor should be equipped with glass view ports if it is not made of transparent material.
8. Flow monitoring should be provided on all chemical feed lines, dilution water lines, and chlorine dioxide solution lines.
9. Dilution water should not be excessively hard in order to avoid calcium deposits and should be near neutral pH.
10. On-site and frequent testing of chemical solution strengths should be practiced to achieve efficient process control.
11. Air contact with chlorine dioxide solutions should be controlled to limit the potential for explosive concentrations. Chlorine dioxide concentrations in air higher than 8 to 10 percent volume must be avoided. Two methods can be applied: operation under vacuum or under higher positive pressure (45 to 75 psi) to prevent buildup of excess chlorine dioxide.

TYPICAL PLANT REQUIREMENTS

Commercially available sodium chlorite solution is usually 25 percent sodium chlorite by weight or 300 to 310 g/l (a tropical version of 400 g/l strength exists) and weighs 10.53 lb/gal. It takes 0.52 gallons of this solution and 0.5 pounds of chlorine to produce 1 pound of chlorine dioxide. A 10 mgd plant feeding 0.5 mg/l of chlorine dioxide would require about 20 gallons a day of sodium chlorite and 20 pounds of chlorine. Proportionate changes in feed quantities would be required for variations in plant size and dosage, respectively. For small capacity plants, sodium chlorite solution comes in many sizes of bulk packs and is pumped directly from these storage units. In larger plants, a 30-day storage tank should be installed with a transfer pump. Two chemical feed pumps would be required for each chemical for duplication of facilities as required by the EPA Surface Water Treatment Rule. It may be appropriate to install two chlorine dioxide generators or to provide the capability to substitute free chlorine for short periods of time.

Some small communities have arranged for the supplier to furnish and service the generator. The service could include regular testing for residuals of chlorite, chlorate, and chlorine dioxide in the treated water. This service could double or triple the cost of sodium chlorite but may be less expensive than arranging for the equipment, servicing, and testing separately. Since the chemicals for generating a pound of chlorine dioxide can be more expensive than per pound of chlorine, depending on local costs, local chemical suppliers' prices for various size deliveries should be used for estimating the operating costs.

References

1. CIFEC. 1978. Disinfection and protection of waters by pure chlorine dioxide, Notice 181A, Paris, France.
2. White, G. C. 1986. *Handbook of chlorination,* 2nd ed. New York: Van Nostrand Reinhold.
3. ASCE/AWWA. 1990. *Water treatment plant design,* 2nd ed. New York: McGraw-Hill.
4. Rav-Acha, C. 1984. The reactions of chlorine dioxide with aquatic organic materials and their health effects. *Water Res.* 18: 1329–41.
5. Chosen, E., R. Elits, and C. Rav-Acha. 1986. The formation of cation-radicals by the action of chlorine dioxide on p-substituted styrenes and other alkenes. *Tetrahedron Lett.* 27(49): 5989–92.
6. Aieta, E. M., and J. D. Berg. 1986. A review of chlorine dioxide in drinking water treatment. *JAWWA* 78(6): 62–72.
7. National Academy of Science. 1980. *Drinking water and health,* Vol. 2. Washington, DC: National Academy Press.
8. Rice, R. G. 1988. Emerging technologies for compliance with disinfection byproducts regulations. Presented at EPA Workshops on Emerging Technologies for Drinking Water Treatment, March 1988.
9. Gordon, G., R. G. Kieffer, and D. H. Rosenblatt. 1972. The chemistry of chlorine dioxide and chlorite. In *Progress in inorganic chemistry,* Vol. 15, Kippar, S. J., ed., pp. 201–86. New York: John Wiley & Sons.
10. Noack, M. G., and R. L. Doerr. 1981. Reaction of chlorine, chlorine dioxide and mixtures thereof with humic acid: An interim report. In *Water chlorination: Environmental impact and health,* Vol. 2, Jolley, R. L., Gorchev, H., and Hamilton, D. H., Jr., eds. Ann Arbor, MI: Ann Arbor Science Publishers.
11. Werdehoff, K. S., and P. C. Singer. 1985. Effects of chlorine dioxide on trihalomethane and total organic halide formation potentials. Presented at AWWA Annual Conference, Denver, CO.
12. Wajon, J. E., D. H. Rosenblatt, and E. P. Burrows. 1982. Oxidation of phenol and hydroquinone by chlorine dioxide. *Environ. Sci. & Tech.* 16: 396–402.
13. O'Neill, W. K. 1987. The applicability of chlorine dioxide as an alternative oxidant/disinfectant at the OWASA water treatment plant in Carrboro, NC. Masters paper, University of North Carolina, Chapel Hill, NC.
14. Miltner, R. 1976. The effect of chlorine dioxide on trihalomethanes in drinking water. Masters thesis, University of Cincinnati, Cincinnati, OH.
15. Lin, S., R. E. Liukkonene, J. G. Thom, M. T. Bastian, M. T. Lukasewycz, and R. M. Carlson. 1984. Increased chloroform production from model compounds of aquatic humus and mixtures of chlorine dioxide/chlorine. *Environ. Sci. & Tech.* 18: 932–5.
16. Routt, J. C. 1989. Chlorine dioxide trihalomethane control and distribution system odor problem: A utility's five-year experience. In AWWA Seminar Proceedings, *Impact of Changing Disinfectants,* pp. 17–48. Presented at AWWA Annual Conference, Los Angeles, CA.

17. Gordon, G., B. Slootmaeker, S. Tachiyashiki, and D. W. Wood. 1990. Minimizing chlorite ion and chlorate ion in water treated with chlorine dioxide. *JAWWA* 82(4): 160–5.
18. Hoehn, R. C., J. T. Novak, and W. E. Cumbie. 1987. Effects of storage and preoxidation on sludge and water quality. *JAWWA* 79(6): 67–75.
19. Cameron, G. N., J. M. Symons, S. R. Spencer, and J. Y. Ma. 1989. Minimizing THM formation during control of the Asiatic clam: A comparison of biocides. *JAWWA* 81(10): 53–62.
20. Ringer, W. C., and S. J. Campbell. 1955. Use of chlorine water for algae control in Philadelphia. *JAWWA* 47: 740.
21. Lalezary, S., M. Pirbazari, and M. J. McGuire. 1986. Oxidation of five earthy-must taste and odor compounds. *JAWWA* 78(3): 62–9.
22. Savoir, R., L. Romnee, and W. J. Masschelein. 1986. Incidence des centrales nucleaires sur l'eau de Meuse: Formation potentielle de derives organohalogenes du de past de l'eau de Meuse. *LeTribune du Ceebedeu* 59: 3–11.
23. Hoehn, R. C., A. M. Dietrich, W. S. Farmer, M. P. Orr, R. G. Ramon, E. M. Aieta, D. W. Wood, and G. Gordon. 1990. Household odors associated with the use of chlorine dioxide. *JAWWA* 82(4): 162–72.
24. Singer, P. C. 1986. THM control using alternative oxidant and disinfection strategies: An evaluation. Presented at AWWA Annual Conference, Denver, CO.
25. Knocke, W. R., J. E. Van Benschoten, M. Kearney, A. Soberski, and D. A. Reckhow. 1990. *Alternative oxidants for removal of soluble iron and manganese*. Report for AWWA Research Foundation, Denver, CO, March 1990.
26. Emmenegger, F., and G. Gordon. 1967. The rapid interaction between sodium chlorite and dissolved chlorine. *Inorganic Chem.* 6:633.
27. Lauer, W. C., S. R. Lohman, and S. E. Rogers. 1986. Experience with chlorine dioxide and Denver's reuse plant. *JAWWA* 78(6): 79–87.
28. Pfaff, J. D., and C. A. Brockhoff. 1990. Determining inorganic disinfection by-products by ion chromatography. *JAWWA* 82(4): 192–3.
29. Masschelein, W. J. 1984. Experience with chlorine dioxide in Brussels: Generation of chlorine dioxide. *JAWWA* 76(1): 70–6.
30. Masschelein, W. J. 1991. Unit processes in drinking water treatment. New York: Marcel Dekker.
31. Hansen N., M. Arnold, G. Fransolet, and W. J. Masschelein. 1990. Scope of use of chlorine dioxide in water disinfection role of residual chlorite ion. International Communication Laboratory of Brussels Intercommunal Waterboard, Brussels.
32. Gordon, G., and S. Tachiyashiki. 1991. Kinetics and mechanism of chlorite ion from the hypochlorous acid/chlorite ion reaction at pH 6–10. *Environ. Sci. & Tech.* 25: 408–75.
33. Griese, M. H., et al. 1991. Using reducing agents to eliminate chlorine dioxide and chlorite ion residuals in drinking water. *JAWWA* 83(5): 56–61.

7

Ozonation

with contributions by
David Nickols
and
Alex J. Varas
Hazen and Sawyer
on *Design Concepts*

Ozone, the strongest oxidant of the common disinfecting agents, was used as early as 1893 for disinfection of drinking water in Oudshoorn, Holland; Nice, France, has employed ozonation of drinking water since 1906. By 1916, there were 49 full-scale water treatment plants in Europe using ozone alone having a total capacity of 85 mgd (46, 77). Today, more than 2,000 water treatment plants throughout the world use ozonation for disinfection. Most of these plants, however, are in Europe, with more than 1,000 located in France alone.

Disinfection practice in the United States has developed principally around the use of chlorine. Partially because of concerns about byproduct formation, the alternative use of ozonation has generated considerable recent interest because of its ability to avoid the formation of halogenated organics inherent in chlorination of many water supplies. In many respects, the use of ozone in water treatment is still developing. While the use of ozone will avoid generating many known undesirable byproducts, there is some question about the possible formation of other undesirable constituents that cannot be determined because of limitations in both background knowledge and available analysis technology.

Still in the developing stage, understanding of the actual mechanisms of ozone reaction with raw water constituents is not complete. Scrutiny of earlier papers on research and operating experiences shows that some of the recognized influences of ozonation were associated with the oxidant demand exerted by the organic content of the source water as well as by a limited number of inorganics like iron and manganese. More recent research, however, has shown variations in reaction characteristics that can be influenced by pH, bicarbonate, carbonate, and other water quality characteristics that affect ozone degradation, but that do not directly assert demand. The chief lesson to be learned in the review of past research is the significance of raw water quality on ozonation reactions and results. It is important, therefore, that the influence of these raw water characteristics be considered both in the review of ozone research results and in the application of ozone in the treatment of specific water supplies.

CHEMISTRY OF OZONE

Ozone (O_3) is characterized by strong oxidizing properties. It is an unstable gas at ambient temperatures and pressures and decomposes rapidly to oxygen at temperatures above 35°C. For this reason, it cannot be manufactured and packaged at a central manufacturing plant, but must be generated on site.

Ozone has a characteristic odor, which can be detected by most humans at low concentrations (0.02 ppm by volume), far below the levels of acute toxicity. It is moderately soluble in water, with solubility depending on the temperature of the water and the ozone concentration in the feed gas. Typically, low feed gas concentrations (1 to 8 percent by weight) are produced by the corona discharge type generator that is commonly used in water treatment. Much more efficient contacting processes are necessary to transfer ozone into solution than those required for relatively undiluted chemicals such as chlorine and ammonia, which are also more soluble and more reactive in water.

Reactive Agents Formed from Ozone

While the ozone molecule is a strong oxidizing agent that can react directly with constituents found in a solution, it is also capable of forming highly reactive chemical agents that can contribute to additional oxidizing reactions. The most commonly cited of these reactive agents is the hydroxyl free radical ($OH^{\cdot}$), which is more reactive than ozone itself. (Note that a free radical configuration is one that contains an unpaired electron, a highly unstable chemical condition that promotes a high degree of reactivity.) Other reactive agents include the ozonide free radical anion (O_3^-), the superoxide free radical anion (O_2^-), the perhydroxyl free radical anion (HO_2^-), and hydrogen peroxide (H_2O_2) (39). Of these, hydrogen peroxide is much less reactive than the more highly reactive free radical species.

The formation of reactive agents can have a significant effect on the outcome of ozonation processes. Because conditions that contribute to the formation of such reactive agents can vary, however, their occurrence will not be the same for all water quality conditions. As a consequence, the effect of ozone addition can vary depending upon actual water quality conditions.

Decomposition Cycle

General phenomena associated with ozone reactions can be illustrated by ozone decomposition reactions as shown in the simplified representation, Figure 7–1. Several more detailed representations of this cycle have been developed (58), but this figure provides the general concepts. Degradation begins with the reaction between ozone and an initiating substance to form the superoxide anion (O_2^-). Once this process is started, the reactions enter into a cycle in which several intermediates are formed that lead to the ultimate production of oxygen as an external end product that leaves the cycle. Within this cycle, intermediates including the hydroxyl

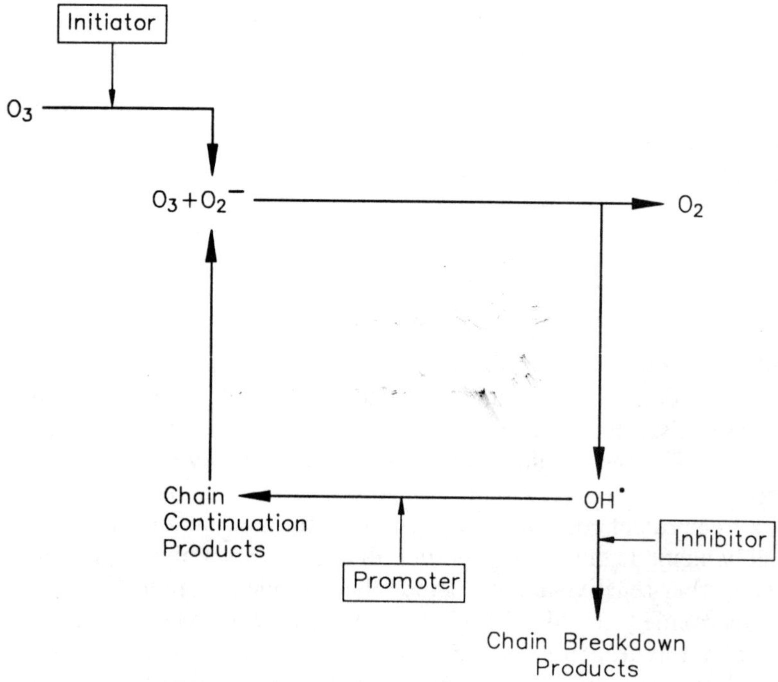

FIGURE 7–1. Ozone decomposition reactions.

radical ($OH^{\cdot}$) continue to react to produce superoxide anions that react with ozone to perpetuate the cycle.

A common initiating agent is the hydroxide ion, a constituent that increases in concentration as pH increases (45). Therefore, pH plays a key role in the ozone decomposition cycle. Increased rates of decomposition become significant at $pH > 8$, and ozone residual is particularly difficult to maintain at $pH > 9$. Elevated pH levels encourage the production of reactive agents by increasing the formation of hydroxyl radicals that occur as intermediates within the cycle. Several other initiating agents have been identified, which, when present, can accelerate the cycle to form increased levels of hydroxyl radicals. Some of these agents, such as hydrogen peroxide and ultraviolet radiation, have been used to promote this formation intentionally. Treatment processes have developed around the use of these agents to induce the formation of hydroxyl radicals; these processes take advantage of a greater reactivity for oxidizing many constituents that would otherwise be resistant to oxidation by molecular ozone alone.

Two types of external phenomena influence the cycle once it has begun: promotion and inhibition. Promoting agents continue the cycle through formation of the superoxide anion (O_2^-) (see Figure 7–1), whereas inhibiting agents derail the cycle by reacting with hydroxyl radicals to form other products (67). Ozone itself is a promoting agent and provides potential for continuing the cycle as long as it is present. Other promoting agents can further accelerate this portion of the cycle.

Commonly encountered inhibiting agents include carbonates and bicarbonates, which tend to scavenge hydroxyl radicals, slowing the rate of ozone degradation by interrupting the degradation cycle. For this reason, the presence of elevated levels of carbonate and bicarbonate can make ozone residuals more stable for longer periods (18). This can be advantageous for those disinfection applications where there is a need for maintaining a residual for the time needed for microbial inactivation.

For other ozone applications, formation of hydroxyl radicals may produce a desirable outcome by increasing reactivity for oxidizing certain contaminants. At significant levels, inhibiting agents have the undesirable impact of scavenging hydroxyl radicals upon formation, thereby reducing process effectiveness. Prominent scavengers, such as carbonates and bicarbonates, react with hydroxyl radicals to form other radical species, which do not produce the desired oxidation reactions (21). Of the two, carbonates are the dominant scavenger by a considerable factor (12), but the presence of either species is undesirable for these oxidation approaches.

As in the case of free chlorine, ozone can react to oxidize a number of inorganic compounds including iron, manganese, sulfides, nitrite, arsenic, bromide ion, and iodide ion (39). However, unlike chlorine, it does not have favorable pathways for oxidizing ammonia, except at a pH level greater than 9. Ammonia, therefore, does not exert a significant ozone demand under most water treatment conditions.

Reactions with organic compounds are somewhat varied. Molecular ozone is selective in its reaction pathways, whereas hydroxyl radicals are more indiscriminant. These reactions are discussed in more detail later in this chapter.

DISINFECTION WITH OZONE

Microorganism Inactivation

Ozone must be generated on site, and the gas stream (normally containing 1 to 8 percent ozone by weight) is applied to the water flow using appropriate gas/liquid contacting conditions. While ozone is highly reactive and will dissipate in a relatively brief time, ozone residuals still can be maintained for the short time required for disinfection. Dissolved ozone residuals of approximately 0.4 to 0.5 mg/l have been typical objectives for the disinfection process applied in past European practice. This was based on the observation that a 0.4 mg/l ozone residual could achieve a 99.9 percent inactivation of *Poliomyelitis* viruses in a period of 4 to 6 minutes (28). Contact times ranging from 4 to 12 minutes are now being considered. Criteria for future designs in the United States will be affected by EPA CT criteria that will require consideration of hydraulic distribution characteristics within a given contactor or configuration. These criteria are summarized in Appendix O of the U.S. EPA *Guidance Manual for Compliance with the Filtration and Disinfection Requirements for Public Water Systems Using Surface Water Sources* (47).

Ozone is thought to achieve disinfection largely through oxidation reactions that damage and destroy critical components of microorganisms, as described in Chapter 2. It has been recognized as an effective disinfectant for a wide range of pathogens and is applicable for achieving the primary disinfection goals for the pathogen categories regulated in the EPA Surface Water Treatment Rule (47).

Two types of primary disinfecting credit are considered for ozone under guidance criteria for the SWTR. The first type of credit is based on measured CT as with other disinfectants. However, ozone is also thought to achieve a very rapid initial kill that does not appear to be characterized by a CT relationship. In recognition of this phenomenon, EPA criteria provide a second type of credit for at least 1 log virus inactivation and 0.5 log *Giardia* inactivation within the first stage of a multistage contacting system as long as specified minimum ozone residuals are provided at the discharge from that stage. These credits are not specifically related to contact time and are available as long as the first stage is equal to or greater in volume than subsequent stages. Note that this credit can be extremely important for the widely used countercurrent porous gas diffusion type of contacting system discussed later in this chapter in the section, Ozone-Contacting Systems. In this type of contactor, ozone is not introduced until flow reaches the bottom of the first stage and the ozone concentration at the top is very low. As a consequence of this arrangement, much of the contactor volume of the first stage contains only a limited quantity of ozone. Credit available from CT calculations would, therefore, be extremely limited for this type of system.

pH Influence

pH can be an important factor in ozone disinfection. This may not be immediately apparent since the disinfecting properties at a given ozone solution concentration are not thought to vary significantly with pH, at least up to a pH of 9 (47). On the other hand, it is important to recognize that the actual ozone dosage required to achieve a target disinfecting concentration for ozone will vary since ozone decomposition rates increase with pH, especially above pH 8. For example, Figure 7–2 shows the effect of ozonating a water under two pH conditions: a range of 9.0 to 9.2 following lime softening and a range of 6.8 to 7.2 following recarbonation of the softened water with carbon dioxide to lower the pH. Note that no significant ozone residual concentration was achieved under the higher pH condition for any of the applied ozone dosages. It would, therefore, be a mistake to conclude that ozone disinfection under varying pH could be achieved with an equivalent level of ozone addition.

Disinfection may still be achieved under high pH conditions since the action of ozone is relatively rapid. Some supplemental site-specific testing of key pathogen indicators may be necessary to establish the relative disinfecting condition of ozonation under such conditions.

Influence of Particulates

While some laboratory studies have indicated that specific types of test particulates might not interfere with ozone disinfection (74), this might not be the case under some conditions encountered in full-scale water treatment applications. For example, a recent study has indicated decreased capability for inactivation of *Giardia* at elevated turbidity (greater than 1.1 NTU for this water) (70). Greater than 99 percent inactivation

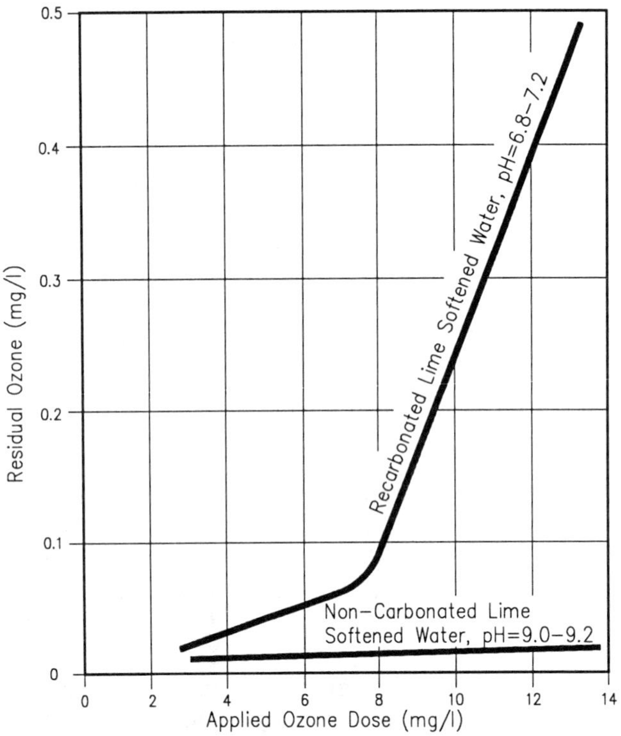

FIGURE 7–2. Effect of pH on ozone residual in lime-softened water.

was achieved in low-turbidity water, whereas more erratic results, with some removals at less than 90 percent, were reported in higher-turbidity waters. Possible protection of *Giardia* cysts by clumps of debris was suggested as one explanation of reduced efficiency under the higher-turbidity condition. This condition may have been further aggravated by autoflocculating phenomena that can occur under some conditions with ozone.

Secondary Disinfection Requirements

From the standpoint of secondary disinfection applications, ozone does not provide a lasting residual in distribution systems due to its short half-life, which eliminates it from consideration for this type of application. Therefore, a separate secondary disinfectant is typically added if ozone is used as the primary disinfectant. One effect of using ozone as the primary disinfectant or as a preoxidant is that the oxidant demand, and possibly the precursor content for formation of disinfection byproducts are frequently reduced, a condition that can reduce the required dosage of the secondary disinfectant and the associated formation of disinfection byproducts. Because the most likely secondary disinfecting agents in the United States are chlorine and chloramines, such dosage reductions can have beneficial implications insofar as reducing formation of halogenated byproducts.

Additional benefits are achieved if ozone is used with a biological activated carbon (BAC) process to provide removal of biologically degradable material. As discussed in Chapter 11, this ozone/BAC combination limits microbial regrowth in the distribution piping and results in more stable secondary disinfecting residuals. These benefits may justify use of ozone by some utilities regardless of disinfection byproduct considerations.

Point of Ozone Application

Selection of the location of ozone application for meeting disinfection goals depends on site-specific factors. In many pretreatment oxidation applications of ozone, particularly in waters with low ozone demand, it may be reasonable to provide an ozone residual over the contact time that also provides the CT required for primary disinfection requirements. However, where the ozone demand exerted in these pretreatment oxidation applications causes rapid depletion of the residual, ozone disinfection is often hampered. In such situations, ozone may have to be added at a second downstream location to accomplish disinfection. Such additional application points to consider are downstream of either the sedimentation or filtration processes, where both the oxidant demand and turbidity levels are much lower. When these alternatives are considered, caution should be exercised at locations downstream of the filters, since ozonating after filtration may generate other problems that are discussed in the subsequent section, Alternative Ozone Application Points.

When the location of an ozone disinfection step within a water treatment process sequence is selected, consideration should also be given to the pH level, especially in finished water where elevated pH levels might be used for corrosion control. This is because of the rapid depletion of ozone that may occur under excessively alkaline pH conditions.

BYPRODUCTS OF OZONATION

Ozone and its major reactive product, the hydroxyl free radical, are both strong oxidizing agents that are capable of a high degree of oxidation under appropriate doses and conditions. However, the natural organic matter found in most raw water typically is only partially oxidized under normal water treatment conditions: dosages of 1 to 5 mg/l and short contact times of 3 to 15 minutes. Some information has emerged on oxidized byproducts that result from these partial oxidation reactions with ozone. The extent of past research on many of these ozone byproducts, however, has been less than that for the halogenated byproducts that were the predominant concern in chlorine disinfection. In part, this apparent bias was the result of more readily available analytical methodologies for evaluating halogenated byproducts. Newer analytical methods are now being applied for evaluation of nonhalogenated oxidation byproducts of concern with ozone. Note that many of these byproducts may also be formed by chlorine to a certain degree and that the difference between chlorine, ozone, and other disinfecting agents may simply be the relative level of formation.

The public health significance of ozone byproducts relative to other disinfectants still remains to be fully determined. It is not possible to draw definitive conclusions based on compilations of the known byproducts of ozone and other alternative disinfectants, since many byproducts remain to be identified and much uncertainty remains about the health consequences of specific byproducts already identified. Ozone byproducts are generally of less concern than chlorination byproducts. In addition, there are preliminary indications, based largely on mutagenicity bioassays such as the Ames test, that the types and concentration of ozone byproducts may be of less concern than those produced by chlorine (33). However, caution must be exercised in interpreting these results, since ozonation tends to form compounds that are not as susceptible to extraction by the common methods used for preparing samples for mutagenicity assays. Many of these byproducts may escape evaluation under these procedures. Moreover, in spite of the value of mutagenic assays as screening tools, there are questions relative to test accuracy and the degree of correlation with carcinogenic effects (63). These tests, therefore, provide a glimpse at the comparative effects of disinfectants but cannot be taken as definitive.

Major Byproducts

Ozone exhibits selectivity in reaction despite its high reactivity. For example, the ozone molecule does not readily oxidize saturated aliphatic compounds (e.g., open chained organic compounds that contain only single carbon bonds such as C—C). However, it readily reacts with unsaturated bonds (organic compounds that contain a multiple bond such as C=C) to produce aldehydes, ketones, alcohols, and carboxylic acids as relatively stable byproducts (15, 19, 39, 42). Ozone also reacts with certain aromatic compounds (organic compounds that contain a benzene ring component), especially those that have attached —NH_2 and —OH groups (58). Reactions with these compounds may initially lead to formation of other aromatic oxidation byproducts such as quinones (aromatic compounds that contain two =O groups), followed by benzene ring rupture to form more linear byproducts upon further ozonation (39). It has also been demonstrated that relatively small doses of ozone can react with phenolic compounds to form aromatic polymers that can cause tastes and odors and which may also represent a possible health risk (35).

Hydrogen peroxide (H_2O_2) is an intermediate byproduct of nearly all organic oxidation reactions with ozone, especially at a pH of 6 or below. Under appropriate conditions, H_2O_2 can react with additional ozone to form hydroxyl radicals that are then eliminated by subsequent reactions with oxidizable materials (40). Other byproducts that might be anticipated include ozonides, epoxides, and organic peroxides (32). These tend to be more temporary in nature and ultimately convert to other byproducts, either in time or upon further ozonation. Although some of these intermediate byproducts are relatively reactive, they can be of health concern if they exist in a distribution system prior to their ultimate conversion. Surrogate measures for determining total oxidizing substances may be of some value to compensate for analytical complexities associated with specific compound quantification of many of these reactive compounds (48).

Within the major byproduct groups, several compounds are commonly observed. Oxalic acid (HOOC—COOH) is a carboxylic acid that occurs as a relatively stable oxidation product of many aliphatic, aromatic, and heterocyclic (ringed organic compounds that contain one atom different from the others in the ring) organic materials, because of its very slow rate of oxidation with molecular ozone once it has formed. Acetic acid (CH_3—COOH) is another carboxylic acid that is a relatively stable oxidation product and that is resistant to further oxidation by molecular ozone under water treatment conditions (40). However, note that both of these "final" byproducts of direct reaction with molecular ozone can potentially be further reacted with hydroxyl radicals through indirect pathways. Removal by biological degradation is also possible so that the ultimate outcome can vary.

A number of aldehyde byproducts have been found in ozonated drinking water. Although health effects of ingestion of drinking water are uncertain, these byproducts have become of interest in ozone applications because of a general tendency toward formation at higher levels than with other disinfection agents.

Greater aldehyde formation is associated with conditions that result in a slower rate of molecular ozone decomposition (i.e., conditions that enhance reactions with molecular ozone). For example, formation can be increased by the presence of free radical scavengers that reduce ozone degradation rates, as described in Figure 7–1 (15). Conversely, elevated pH levels increase ozone degradation due to the increased availability of hydroxide as an initiating substance (see Figure 7–1). This condition results in lower aldehyde formation as does the formation of hydroxyl radicals through the addition of hydrogen peroxide (49).

Low molecular weight aldehyde species, such as formaldehyde and acetaldehyde, have tended to be the focus of early studies of ozone byproducts. However, other higher molecular weight aldehyde species, such as heptanal, glyoxal, and methylglyoxal, also have been observed to be significant (15, 72). In fact, methylglyoxal may be found at higher levels than formaldehyde in many waters (71, 72). Although more information is needed, some of these other aldehydes are thought to be mutagenic and may be of health concern.

The level of ozone dose affects the formation of byproducts, but the relationship can be complex. For example, formation of low molecular weight aldehydes and carboxylic acids has been observed to initially increase with ozone dose (19). However, above an optimum ozone dose, the level of formation begins to decline (72). Formation also is decreased at downstream points of ozone application as succeeding processes reduce precursor content.

Other treatment process features also can affect aldehyde levels, the ultimate fate of which can vary. For example, some aldehydes have been observed to be much greater after ozonation where a chlorination step is provided ahead of filtration rather than downstream of filtration (23). In the absence of chlorine, biological degradation processes can develop in granular media to provide biological pathways for the removal of aldehydes (and other biodegradable byproducts). Studies have demonstrated this potential role for both filtration (19, 27) and biological activated carbon processes (59).

Understanding of biological removal processes is developing and may involve more than simply eliminating chlorination ahead of the filters. In this regard, contact time and total surface area of media are important features. These are affected by depth of media (i.e., contact time and surface area increase with increased depth) and size of filter media (i.e., surface area per unit volume of filter increases as size of filter media decreases). As expected, temperature also appears to be a significant parameter on biological removals, demonstrated by observation in one study of erratic aldehyde removals at temperatures below 10°C, in contrast to consistent removals observed at higher temperatures (62).

Formaldehyde removal has been reported to occur much more readily with biodegradation than removal of two other commonly encountered aldehydes, glyoxal and methylglyoxal (60, 71). Successful removal of methylglyoxal and glyoxal has been reported to occur in some biologically active filters (61, 70), while less success has been achieved in other situations that may have been influenced more by insufficient contact time and surface area (71). One study also reported removal of acetone, a low molecular weight ketone formed in an upstream ozonation process (61).

Halogenated Byproducts

Although much of the current concern for ozone byproducts is related to the nonhalogenated organic oxidation products discussed, halogenated products can be indirectly formed through a reaction sequence initiated by oxidation of the bromide ion (Br^-) to hypobromite ion (OBr^-) (65).

$$Br^- + O_3 = OBr^- + O_2 \qquad (7\text{–}1)$$

Subsequent conversion to hypobromous acid (HOBr) can occur by a reaction with H^+ that increases as pH is decreased.

$$(OBr)^- + H^+ = HOBr \qquad (7\text{–}2)$$

If the bromide ion is present in sufficient quantity and pH is sufficiently low to form HOBr, further reactions can occur to form measurable levels of halogenated byproducts, including bromoform, a trihalomethane species, and dibromoacetic acid (60). Other observed byproducts (in the presence of an appropriate nitrogen source) include bromopicrin and cyanogen bromide (30). From a regulatory standpoint, possible byproduct concerns are exacerbated by the fact that bromine is a much heavier molecular component than chlorine on the weight basis applied for regulation of these contaminants. In some situations, this indirect formation of halogenated byproducts could make it difficult to comply with extremely stringent criteria for trihalomethanes and other halogenated disinfection byproducts, especially if formation is in addition to levels generated by secondary disinfection processes.

Some research has indicated that ammonia can be added to react with HOBr to form bromamines, thereby reducing the level of halogenated organic formation (1, 9). In such addition, the fate of ammonia may need to be considered. For example, downstream free chlorine processes may require an added dosage to remove ammonia by breakpoint reactions. This added dosage will not only increase chemical costs, but will also increase the formation of chlorine byproducts.

Bromate and Iodate

In addition to brominated organic byproducts, significant concern has developed for further oxidation of the OBr^- species to form the bromate ion (BrO_3^-) (39, 65) which can be considered an inorganic byproduct. Although these oxidation reactions occur with other disinfectants as well, of particular concern is the use of ozone. Similar oxidation phenomena can also lead to formation of iodate ion when iodide is present. Both bromate and iodate are of possible health concern as carcinogens and are being considered for regulation (48).

Several factors exert an influence on the formation of bromate. In particular, pH has an important influence on the conversion of OBr^- to HOBr by the reaction with H^+ as shown in Equation 7–2. Occurrence of the OBr^- species that reacts to form bromate increases with pH, so that pH reduction during ozonation may represent one possible method for limiting bromate formation. However, as previously discussed, brominated organic formation can also increase with lower pH. Ozone dosage also affects these phenomena. For example, a somewhat higher ozone dose is required to achieve oxidation of HOBr to bromate, while lower dosages leave HOBr intact, resulting in a condition that may form brominated organics. As a result of these factors, process trade-offs may be necessary to accomplish desired conditions (76).

In some treatment situations, introduction of ammonia has been observed to decrease bromate formation, whereas the presence of hydroxyl radicals appears to increase the level of formation (1). These possible relationships should be considered when selecting operating conditions (significantly pH) that can affect the formation of hydroxyl radicals. The addition of initiating agents, such as hydrogen peroxide and ultraviolet radiation, to promote the formation of hydroxyl radicals should also be evaluated.

Mutagenic Potential

In some studies, mutagenic bioassays have been performed to assess the effects of different ozonation conditions. These studies indicate that low levels of oxidation increase mutagenicity, whereas mutagenicity is reduced by the increased oxidation that occurs at higher doses. These effects appear to vary depending on the ratio of ozone dose to the organic content to be oxidized. In one study, formation of mutagenicity was observed to occur at preozonation doses of 1 mg/l, whereas higher doses of 2 and 4 mg/l reduced the mutagenic activity (49). Similar results were observed in a subsequent study in which ozone doses of 10 mg/l or more were observed to either reduce or completely remove observable mutagenicity (25). Studies have also indicated that mutagenic activity formed by ozonation can be reduced by granular activated carbon (GAC) (39) and, in one case, by filtration (49). In the case of filtration, and perhaps in the case of GAC as well, biological activity is likely to have been a major factor in achieving such reduction.

Effect of Ozone on Precursors

Ozone can react with organic precursor compounds to change their potential for subsequent reaction with chlorine and other disinfectants. This effect, however, appears to be variable. At very low ozone-to-organic ratios, the THM-formation potential may increase as a result of a low level of oxidation that cleaves the organic material to make it more accessible to reactions with chlorine. As the ozone-to-organic ratio increases beyond a certain point, a greater level of oxidation may disrupt the basic structure of the organic material further, resulting in a decrease in the trihalomethane formation potential (41).

The ozone dosage–to–dissolved organic carbon (DOC) ratio is an important consideration when evaluating reaction phenomena. Normal ozone doses in high-DOC waters (greater than 10 mg/l) tend to result in a low ozone-to-precursor ratio, frequently causing increased trihalomethane-formation potential. This contrasts with conditions found at lower DOC levels, where higher ozone dose–to–DOC ratios are more typical and may be more likely to achieve reductions in formation potential. Conditions that affect THM-formation potential are subject to variation. Some research suggests that the generation of additional THM-formation potential may be associated with conditions that encourage hydroxyl radical–type reactions (e.g., low carbonate content and high pH), while reactions with molecular ozone are thought more likely to destroy precursor sites (58). For example, laboratory research using fulvic acid suggests that increased THM formation is more probable under alkaline ozonation conditions that are conducive to hydroxyl radical formation, whereas THM formation may be reduced by oxidation under neutral and acid conditions (75).

Other suggested phenomena that affect THM formation include a concept of ozone interaction based on two categories of precursor materials

(68). Type I precursors encompass a class that is characterized by a capability for formation of high levels of THM per unit of weight. The THM formation sites on these precursors are readily destroyed by ozone. Group II precursors are originally low in reactivity with chlorine to form THM. Ozone can react with these precursors to increase the level of THM formation. A maximum level of formation occurs at a given ozone-to-reactant ratio for compounds in this group. Beyond this ratio, THM formation from reactions with Group II precursors begins to decline as the ozone dose is further increased (68).

All of these observations imply that each treatment situation may be expected to be somewhat different depending on the composition of precursor materials and reaction conditions. These and other observations strongly indicate the need for site-specific testing. Note that because higher pH levels as well as other hydroxyl radical–related conditions appear to affect these phenomena, the effect of pH and other factors that influence hydroxyl radical formation should be considered in these evaluations.

Although the above effects of ozonation on trihalomethane formation are of interest, they do not indicate the complete picture for byproduct formation. For example, one study observed that while the potential for increased THM formation following ozonation occurred in some cases, there was a universal decrease in the amount of total organic halide formed in each of the four utilities under evaluation (23). Therefore, variations in trihalomethane formation may, in part, be an indicator of a shifting composition of byproducts but may not necessarily indicate total byproduct formation. This study also indicated shifts in the composition of the halogenated species based on several influencing factors. These included a tendency for greater formation of brominated species of trihalomethanes and haloacetic acid when ozone preceded chlorine as the final disinfectant. Note that this may represent a concern if brominated byproducts are more potent carcinogens and are regulated at lower levels as a consequence (see discussions in Chapter 3 in the section Direct Evaluations of Carcinogenicity). In some cases slight increases in chloropicrin formation were also observed with final disinfection using both chlorine and chloramine; a slight elevation of cyanogen chloride was observed where chloramine was used. Evaluation of ozonation using synthetic laboratory-created fulvic acid solutions has shown a greater destruction of formation potential for total organic halides, chloroform, trichloracetic acid, and dichloracetonitrile, while the formation potentials for dichloracetic acid and trichloracetone appeared to increase under test conditions (37, 73). The addition of bicarbonate appeared to increase the reduction in formation potential. Since bicarbonates scavenge hydroxyl radicals, this observation suggests that molecular ozone is a more efficient agent than hydroxyl free radicals under these test conditions.

Biodegradable Material

In addition to its other effects, ozone has been observed to alter the character of many organic constituents in water to make them more biodegradable, thereby increasing the opportunity for microbial growth in distribution piping and in components of plumbing systems. This can produce increased levels of coliforms and several opportunistic pathogens, resulting in new health concerns. The extent of this effect generally depends on the quantity of organic matter available for reaction with ozone. It is more likely that greater problems are encountered at higher DOC levels, which sometimes require processes such as downstream biological treatment methods to reduce the levels of biodegradable substances. These biological processes, which can be incorporated in activated carbon or filtration processes, allow the proliferation of a resident microbial population and can be effective in accomplishing the required reduction. The need and added cost for these processes may be significant factors in the selection of ozone as an alternative disinfectant, so these possible impacts should be considered in evaluating the use of ozone. Note that these same concerns may also need to be considered for other disinfecting alternatives as well. However, the level of conversion of organic matter is usually greater with ozone, thereby making the need for biological treatment processes more likely when ozone is used.

Some research indicates that biological processes can be induced simply by eliminating disinfecting residuals within conventional rapid sand media, thereby allowing a resident microbial population to become established. Other approaches can involve partial or complete replacement of conventional filter media with GAC to achieve a biological activated carbon modification of the filtration process. However, while these retrofit approaches may often be more economical than a biodegradation step that is separate from the filtration process, such retrofit may not achieve the required levels of removal. For this reason, some European plants apply a separate biological activated carbon process downstream of filtration.

Where prechlorination ahead of filters is eliminated to induce biodegradation, adjustments may be needed to improve filter wash efficiency in order to maintain the condition of the filter media for efficient solids removal. In addition, postdisinfection may be required downstream of any biological media to reduce the elevated bacterial levels that can appear in the effluent of a biologically active filter. Additional discussions of these phenomena and associated treatment methods are provided in Chapters 2 and 11.

NONDISINFECTION USES OF OZONATION

Nondisinfection uses of ozone can have a significant effect on its overall economic viability. For example, in cases where ozone can enhance coagulation processes, cost savings that result from lowered coagulant use can improve the cost-effectiveness of ozone in comparison with alternative disinfectants. Therefore, the full range of uses and benefits should be evaluated in making economic comparisons between ozone and other alternatives.

The principal nondisinfection uses of ozone are related to its strong oxidizing capabilities. These capabilities are advantageous for attaining immediate oxidation reactions. However, unlike chlorine, which has a residual that can be maintained for an extended period, the high reactivity of ozone results in a rapid depletion of residual, which may not be maintained throughout a treatment system. This inability to maintain a residual may be disadvantageous for some applications.

Ozone-Based and Hydroxyl Radical–Based Processes for Oxidation of Organic Material

Ozone is often considered as an oxidant for removing specific organic contaminants of concern. As discussed in the section Byproducts of Ozonation, molecular ozone can be quite selective in this regard. Process schemes that encourage the formation of highly reactive hydroxyl radicals have been developed as a means of increasing the range of oxidation to include a large number of organic contaminants. These processes involve exposing ozone to agents, such as ultraviolet light or hydrogen peroxide, that initiate the formation of hydroxyl radicals (see Figure 7–1). Elevated pH also increases the formation of hydroxyl radicals. An example of this effect is the treatment of the pesticide lindane where oxidation occurs only in an alkaline pH range (22).

Hydroxyl radical–based processes were originally developed for oxidation of synthetic organic compounds in waste treatment applications. Success has also been reported in the removal of organic contaminants in drinking water supplies (56). These processes have become commonly referred to as advanced oxidation processes (AOPs) due to the higher level of oxidation that can be achieved. This terminology is avoided here, however, because it is not always advantageous to convert ozone to hydroxyl radicals. Moreover, it is important to understand circumstances in which the presence of hydroxyl radicals will either enhance or diminish capability to achieve treatment goals. It is felt that these process characteristics are more clearly distinguished by use of the term hydroxyl radical–based processes.

One of the more prominent hydroxyl radical–based processes employs hydrogen peroxide and ozone. Termed PEROXONE, in recognition of the combination of hydrogen peroxide and ozone, this process has been evaluated for treating certain taste and odor compounds (specifically geosmin and MIB) that are resistant to other oxidants, including ozone by itself (29). As a consequence of the greater reactivity of hydroxyl free radicals, the PEROXONE process allows for removal of these compounds at a lower ozone dose, thereby increasing process efficiency.

A significant feature to consider when evaluating the use of hydroxyl radical processes in conjunction with drinking water disinfection is the rapid decomposition of ozone residual that occurs through the hydroxyl radical pathways, thereby reducing the available CT. Although initial studies indicated that the PEROXONE process was effective for control of coliforms (29), subsequent studies have confirmed a need to maintain some excess molecular ozone for effective disinfection of coliphage viruses, *Giardia muris* cysts, and heterotrophic plate count bacteria (13). This can be accomplished by maintaining a hydrogen peroxide feed level sufficiently low to limit reaction with ozone to a level that allows for some molecular ozone to remain. These studies developed an optimal ratio for oxidation of the target taste and odor constituents (i.e., taste and odor removal was not further improved by increasing the ratio), while still achieving disinfection goals.

Because of varying conditions, each situation needs to be evaluated individually. For example, hydroxyl radical–based processes are affected by the presence of free radical scavengers such as carbonates and bicarbonates. These scavengers, which occur under high carbonate alkalinity conditions, can result in increased dose requirements and perhaps reduced process effectiveness. Conversely, elevated pH can supplement initiating agents in the formation of hydroxyl radicals and may enhance the process (13). However, the effect of increased pH may be counterproductive in some cases where carbonate/bicarbonate species are present; increased pH results in a shift from bicarbonate to carbonate, which is a much stronger free radical scavenger.

When the applicability of both ozone and hydroxyl radical processes for oxidizing target organic species is considered, it is important to note that conventional ozone dosage levels in water treatment are not adequate to achieve complete oxidation of organic material. Under these conditions, the effect of ozonation processes is to partially oxidize target species, thereby achieving removal of a target compound by altering chemical structures. This partial effect should be taken into consideration when evaluating the applicability of ozone oxidation processes, since the outcome is the production of a new mixture of organic compounds whose properties should also be understood in order to judge process applicability. In a few cases, end products may be more toxic than the original compound. For example, ozonation of the pesticide heptachlor can produce a more toxic byproduct, heptachlor epoxide, which resists continued ozonation (20).

Some of the end products formed by oxidation can vary, depending on the conditions of reaction. For example, ozonation of parathion and malathion forms paraoxon and malaoxon, respectively, as undesirable initial oxidation products. However, the reactions continue with further ozonation and, providing the ozone dose and reaction time are adequate, innocuous final byproducts are ultimately produced (26).

Removal of Iron and Manganese

Oxidation Reactions

Soluble ferrous iron (Fe^{+2}) is oxidized rapidly by ozone to insoluble ferric ions (Fe^{+3}), at a theoretical dosage of about 0.4 mg of ozone per mg of ferrous iron (24).

$$2Fe^{+2} + O_3 + H_2O = 2Fe^{+3} + O_2 + 2(OH)^- \qquad (7\text{–}3)$$

Ferric ions can then precipitate as ferric hydroxide and be removed:

$$Fe^{+3} + 3H_2O = Fe(OH)_3 + 3H^+ \qquad (7\text{–}4)$$

Although ozone generally is effective for oxidizing iron, iron can be complexed in the presence of significant levels of humic materials, and under these conditions oxidation effectiveness can be significantly reduced (24).

Soluble manganous ions (Mn^{+2}) can be oxidized to manganic ions (Mn^{+4}); with a theoretical dose of about 0.9 mg of ozone per mg of manganese (24), Mn^{+4} can then react to form insoluble manganese hydroxides ($Mn(OH)_4$) and oxides (MnO_2).

$$Mn^{+2} + O_3 + H_2O = Mn^{+4} + O_2 + 2OH^- \qquad (7\text{–}5)$$

$$Mn^{+4} + 4(OH)^- = Mn(OH)_4 = MnO_2 + 2H_2O \qquad (7\text{–}6)$$

Oxidation reactions with manganese are affected by pH, with the oxidation rate decreasing as pH is decreased. With ozone, however, the rate of oxidation at lower pH levels is relatively rapid. Ozone, therefore, may offer some oxidation advantages at lower pH levels, where the effectiveness of other oxidants may be significantly reduced (58).

Another important fact to consider is that while ozone is effective for oxidizing manganese, the dose can be affected significantly by the presence of organic material. Manganese does not appear to be highly complexed by such organics; the organics represent more a competing source of demand that can divert ozone from the desired reaction (24).

Effect of Hydroxyl Radicals on Manganese Removals

Conversion of ozone to hydroxyl radicals generally diminishes the effectiveness for manganese oxidation apparently due to an increase in the potential for diversion into competing oxidation reactions. Therefore, chemical characteristics that retard ozone decomposition to form hydroxyl radicals tend to improve the efficiency of manganese oxidation. These can include higher concentrations of free radical scavengers such as carbonates and bicarbonates that may be found in high alkalinity waters (34). In contrast, PEROXONE processes, which lead to formation of hydroxyl radicals, are likely to reduce the efficiency of manganese oxidation.

Complexities of Manganese Removal

An important consideration in manganese removal is related to a tendency for an excess ozone dose to overoxidize manganese beyond the Mn^{+4} form that forms the precipitate shown in Equation 7–6. Overoxidation produces an undesirable permanganate ion (MnO_4^-), which is pink in color and remains in solution (28). Alternative steps necessary to limit such permanganate formation can be complex. Underdosing to avoid this situation is not feasible since an adequate oxidation level would not be provided for fully converting soluble manganous (Mn^{+2}) ions to insoluble manganic (Mn^{+4}) ions.

In some treatment situations, permanganate can be removed by reactions with organic material as long as an adequate retention time is available. A more specific process for achieving removal is the use of GAC (50) to reconvert the permanganate ion to insoluble manganic ions, which, as a precipitate, can be removed within the treatment plant. Some European applications use excess ozone to assure complete oxidation of Mn^{+2}, with subsequent removal of any undesired permanganate on GAC. Powdered activated carbon can also be used, although granular activated carbon is normally more effective. Moreover, required PAC doses can be quite high (e.g., 30 times the permanganate residual) (28).

Another feature to consider in the control of manganese with ozone is the inability of ozone to maintain an oxidizing residual throughout the entire treatment train. Problems may be encountered where sludges that are allowed to accumulate at the bottom of sedimentation basins can release manganese back into solution over time. This is likely to result from anaerobic conditions in the settled sludges. Recirculation and release of manganese can also occur where supernatant is recycled from sludge dewatering systems. Under such conditions, ozonation prior to sedimentation may not maintain the oxidizing condition necessary to reoxidize this subsequently released manganese. More effective or frequent sludge removal or additional manganese oxidation immediately prior to filtration may be required to resolve these problems.

While use of ozone prior to filtration may often appear to be the best approach for manganese removal, the filterability of the resulting precipitates needs to be considered. Oxidized manganese has a tendency to produce small, colloidal precipitates that can penetrate a filter (24). This may require a coagulation step to coalesce the colloids subsequent to the point of ozone addition.

As indicated by the above potential effects, manganese removal by ozone can be so complex that several manganese removal strategies should be evaluated within a plant to determine how best to apply ozone. It may also be advantageous to use other oxidants in a supplemental role. This was demonstrated in one treatment plant, where it was observed that manganese could not be maintained consistently below the target level of 0.05 mg/l after ozone addition to raw water. In this situation, chlorine was added as a supplmenetal oxidant to the filter influent to maintain an oxidizing condition across the filter media, resulting in a media coating of manganese dioxide that could adsorb the excess manganese in the manner described in Chapter 4 (51).

Basic Manganese Oxidation Approaches

Based on the observed characteristics, three principal ozone oxidation approaches to control manganese levels in drinking water can be summarized as follows:

1. Ozone can be added at dosages that are specifically optimized for manganese; i.e. an adequate dosage for conversion of manganese to Mn^{+4} while avoiding excess doses that may form soluble permanganate. This addition might be accomplished ahead of the sedimentation process if resolubilization of manganese can be limited in this process. Otherwise, the addition should occur prior to filtration, with consideration of a possible coagulant addition to improve the filterability of colloidal manganese. In optimizing the removal of manganese, some plants provide a prior recarbonation step that results in addition of carbonate and bicarbonate. The introduction of these inhibitors limits

ozone degradation to the hydroxyl radical that has a lower efficiency for removing manganese. In these situations, recarbonation is applied to react with lime to stabilize water for corrosion, and the effect on ozone oxidation of manganese is essentially a secondary benefit (58).

An important limitation of the optimized dosage approach can occur where the required ozone dose for manganese removal becomes difficult to control because of varying manganese concentrations. This optimized dose may also be inappropriate for disinfection and other oxidation goals of ozone, thereby requiring separate upstream or downstream ozonation steps for achieving these goals. If one of the points of ozone addition is located downstream of the filters, another process may then be required to remove increased levels of biodegradable material that can form at locations where ozone is added. This would eliminate the option for modifying the filtration process to remove biodegradable material.

2. Ozone can be added at excess dose rates for manganese removal, thereby resulting in permanganate formation but allowing ozone addition at levels that can meet disinfection and other oxidation goals. Removal of permanganate can subsequently be achieved by one of the following methods:
   a. Allowing adequate reaction time for permanganate to reconvert to Mn^{+4} prior to sedimentation or filtration.
   b. Addition of powdered activated carbon to catalyze the permanganate reducing reaction to form Mn^{+4}. The PAC dose requirement can be high for this approach.
   c. Use of downstream GAC systems to catalyze the permanganate reduction reaction to form Mn^{+4}. Other process goals, such as removal of the biodegradable organic carbon (BDOC) that is formed by ozone, may already dictate use of a GAC system. In this case, a GAC filter adsorber may allow a dual function both for removing biodegradable material and achieving catalyzed removal of permanganate.
3. Other oxidants can be used for supplemental manganese control. One example is the use of free chlorine to maintain an oxidized coating for manganese removal across the filters. This specific approach can overcome some of the limitations associated with the use of ozone for oxidation of manganese. Chlorine dosage may have to be controlled, however, to avoid the excess formation of chlorine byproducts.

Color Removal

Color in drinking water is commonly associated with naturally occurring humic materials and is frequently caused by the presence of specific carbon-to-carbon bonding patterns that consist of alternating double and single bonds (e.g., —C═C—C═C—). Color groups can also contain —OH and —NH_2 components, which are referred to as chromophores (66).

Ozone is particularly reactive with the carbon-carbon double bonds found in these configurations and is also reactive with some specific chromophoric groups, —NH_2 and —OH (66). Disruption of these color-causing configurations by oxidation will typically remove the color. This, however, does not necessarily mean that all of the original organic compound has been removed, but that the groups responsible for the original color have been altered. End products of these reactions can include ketones, aldehydes, and acids. Actual composition of such products depends on the nature of the color-causing compounds, the amount of ozone added, the reaction time, and other contacting conditions.

Dosage Requirements

While ozone is generally an effective decolorizing agent at relatively low dosages, the dosage requirement can be much higher in some specific cases. For example, high applied ozone dosages (e.g., 6.5 to 7 mg/l) were required for adequate color reduction of settled water from a lime-softening process in Fort Lauderdale, Florida. Adequate removal of the color found in raw water (11) could not be achieved with dosages greater than 13 mg/l. These waters generally contained high levels of DOC and color, both affecting the required ozone dose. In these high dose requirement situations, an alternative color reduction method may offer greater economy than pretreatment with ozone. However, these are unusual circumstances, and ozone is typically an excellent decolorizing agent for most applications.

The shapes of the color reduction curves shown in Figure 7–3 are typical. Note that these curves exhibit a relatively steep decline in color as the ozone dose is initially increased. However, the curves then begin to level off, leaving a refractory color component that is difficult to remove upon further ozonation. Because of this phenomenon, very high ozone dosages such as in the Fort Lauderdale example can be encountered in cases where extremely high levels of color removal are required. However, in recent studies for New York City the authors found that a large portion of the remaining refractory color could be removed by filtration, which is a possibility that should be considered.

In some cases, partial oxidation of the chromophoric groups may temporarily remove color, but unless oxidation of the original substance reaches an adequate level or the substance is removed by other means, the color may reform. This type of color reformation has been reported at

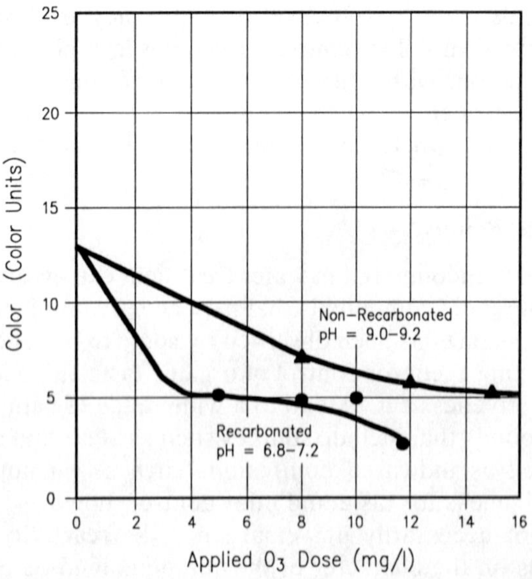

FIGURE 7–3. Effect of pH on color removal by ozone in a lime-softened water.

some locations. A two-stage ozonation process can allow flexibility for oxidation of any color that reforms (10). However, a one-stage process is normally adequate as long as the initial ozone dosage achieves the level of oxidation required to preclude reformation.

pH Influences

The effectiveness of ozone as a decolorizing agent has been observed to be affected strongly by pH in some locations, as demonstrated by the Tamarac, Florida, data (Figure 7–3). These data were obtained from studies in a lime-softening plant that was operated in the pH range of 9.0 to 9.2. Also shown in this figure are data obtained from a parallel evaluation of color removal by ozone following adjustment of pH to a lower level (6.8–7.2) by recarbonation. These data indicate that color was removed more effectively in the more neutral pH region that occurred upon recarbonation. Similar benefits of pH reduction of lime-softened water were observed in another study (6).

Similar pH effects have been reported in the treatment of lower hardness waters by the coagulation process (2). This suggests that reduced effectiveness may be associated with the rapid degradation of ozone to hydroxyl free radicals that can occur under the high-pH conditions. While hydroxyl radicals are very effective oxidants, they are less selective for reactions involved in color removal, resulting in a potential for greater diversion to reactions with other substances. As a consequence, the effect of pH and other phenomena that influence hydroxyl radical formation should be evaluated where color removal is to be achieved with ozone.

Taste and Odor Removal

Tastes and odors encountered in water treatment can involve a number of organic and inorganic compounds that may be susceptible to oxidation by ozone. In fact, ozone has been observed by some to be generally the most effective oxidizing agent for control of organic taste and odor compounds (31). This effectiveness can extend to a wide range of naturally occurring organic compounds that include sources such as algae and decaying plant matter, as well as industrial compounds such as phenols. Despite its general effectiveness for taste and odor control, however, the capability of ozone is not necessarily universal since the reactivity of molecular ozone depends on the character of the compounds to be oxidized.

Ozone can be a highly effective oxidant for removing many tastes and odors caused by plankton. Fishy odors are usually removed completely. However, some astringent and plastic tastes are not significantly removed, while fruity odors can actually be produced during oxidation of some of the taste- and odor-causing constituents. Production of these fruity odors has usually been associated with the formation of aldehydes (3). In treatment situations where oxidation may break the cell wall of the algae and actually release taste- and odor-causing substances, pretreatment by coagulation, settling, and filtration may be helpful to achieve a degree of algae removal prior to the addition of ozone.

Recent research has considered the capability of ozone for the removal of two taste- and odor-causing compounds that have been resistant to other oxidation methods: 2-methylisoborneol (MIB) and geosmin. Because of the resistance of these compounds, particularly of MIB, the Metropolitan Water District of Southern California has been evaluating the PEROXONE ozonation process. As discussed earlier, this process involves the addition of hydrogen peroxide to react with ozone to form highly reactive hydroxyl free radicals. This approach was observed to improve removal of MIB in comparison with the use of ozone alone (30). As would be expected, the process effectiveness is reduced in the presence of free radical scavengers such as carbonate and bicarbonate ions, thereby requiring higher ozone doses in water of greater alkalinity (13). The bromide ion also has been observed to decrease process effectiveness to varying degrees with both ozone and PEROXONE (1, 9).

In general, the effectiveness of ozone addition for removing these MIB- and geosmin-related tastes and odors may vary in other waters depending on the extent of hydroxyl radical formation under site-specific water quality conditions. The selection of process configuration will depend on the actual conditions encountered. In some situations, supplemental initiation of hydroxyl free radicals by processes such as the PEROXONE approach may be necessary. Other water quality situations, such as an alkaline pH, may be more conducive to hydroxyl radical formation without the need for a supplement.

Note that all of the hydroxyl radical approaches result in conversion of ozone to reactive forms. As a consequence, ozone disinfecting residuals may be only briefly available unless ozone is provided in excess of the quantity to be converted. Many other ozonation goals, such as color removal and iron and manganese oxidation, may also be adversely affected with the conversion to free radicals. Therefore, the PEROXONE process may require appropriate adaptations or adjustments. Evaluations by the Metropolitan Water District of Southern California have indicated that, with their supply, optimal hydrogen peroxide–to–ozone ratios range from 0.1 to 0.3 (13). This results in partial conversion of ozone to hydroxyl radicals, leaving some molecular ozone available for disinfection and other reactions. Some variations in the optimal ratio have been observed in different waters. It is essential, therefore, that adaptations required to meet multiple goals be confirmed for each PEROXONE application.

Enhanced Coagulation

Ozone oxidation of natural organic matter such as humic and fulvic materials can affect coagulation processes. With low applied ozone dosages, partial oxidation can occur that results in modification of certain structural components of organic matter without significantly breaking the molecular structure. Many of these partially oxidized organic materials appear to be capable of interactions that enhance the performance of coagulating agents. The application of ozone at low rates may also improve the neutralization and agglomeration of colloidal particulates through a microflocculation action.

When the ozone dose exceeds an optimum ratio for enhanced coagulation, excess oxidation can occur and cause molecular structures to be altered. This results in the formation of lower molecular weight compounds, which are not as easily flocculated with cationic flocculating agents, thereby reducing the coagulation benefits of ozone. In fact, excessive ozone doses have been reported to adversely affect coagulation processes in some instances (53). Figure 7–4 shows a relationship between ozone dosages and alum feed rates. This relationship results in an inverted bell curve characteristic, where more alum is required for ozone doses above and below the optimum.

As a consequence of the effect of dosage on the extent of oxidation, an optimum applied ozone dosage can occur for enhanced coagulation. In some situations, an important parameter is the ratio of ozone relative to dissolved organic carbon where an optimum ratio in the region of 0.1 sometimes is used as a rule of thumb (44). Other findings also agree with the importance of a ratio relationship (8). Reported optimum ozone doses for typical total organic carbon levels (3–6 mg/l) tend to be in the range of 0.5 to 1.0 mg/l. In Belle Glade, Florida, however, an effective ozone dose as high as 8.6 mg/l was reported for a high total organic carbon level (30 mg/l), a finding that supports the importance of using a ratio for control.

Although DOC content is an important consideration for ozone-enhanced coagulation, other factors appear to be involved as well. For example, in the treatment of certain waters, the presence of calcium ions has been identified in some research as an important factor that appears to contribute to ozone enhancement of coagulation (8). These results have indicated that such enhancement tends to be increased with an increased

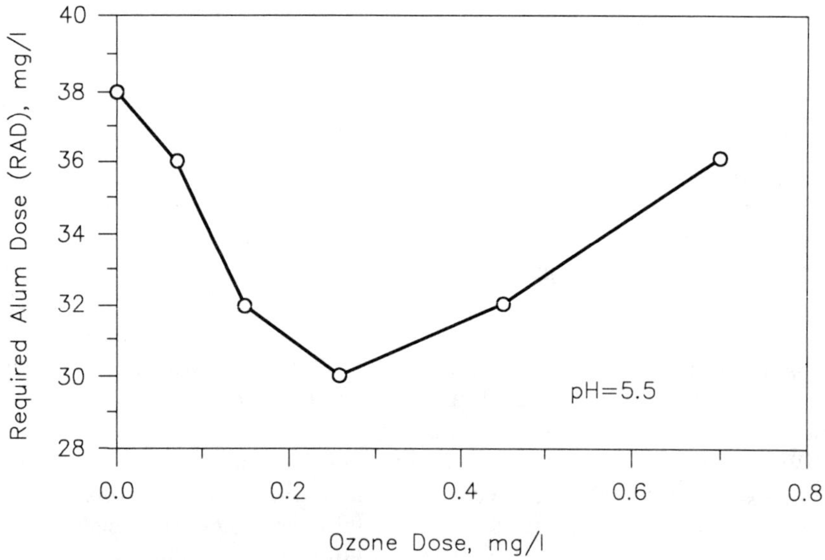

FIGURE 7–4. Ozone-induced coagulation effect on humic acids. (From Ref. 53. Reprinted by permission. Copyright © 1990, American Water Works Association.)

hardness–to–total organic carbon ratio and that enhancement is much less significant for any ozone dosage at low hardness ratios. The mechanism involved with this enhancement may be associated with a partial oxidation of some organic molecules to form carboxylic acid and other polar groups. Polarization refers to the extent to which positive and negative charge centers occur. Polar groups increase the potential for interaction with calcium and the small colloidal particles that are the target of coagulation processes (38).

Mechanisms other than those involving modified molecular characteristics have also been proposed to explain ozone enhancement of coagulation processes. For example, in some instances, addition of a strong oxidant such as ozone will change the nature or extent of charges on the surfaces of colloidal particles, thus making them more amenable to flocculation and removal by subsequent filtration. It is also possible that small colloidal particles may resist coagulation as a result of an adsorbed surface coating of natural occurring organic material. Under this circumstance, it is proposed that ozonation may improve coagulation by oxidizing the adsorbed material. Other proposed mechanisms include release of metal ions from organic material to serve as supplemental coagulants, reactions that result in polymerization of organic molecules, and oxidative attack and subsequent release of biopolymers from algae (38). Others have proposed that ozone enhancement of coagulation might result from the changes in pH that occur with ozone reactions (78).

In one novel application of enhanced coagulation, the Hackensack Water Company in New Jersey has modified the ozone-contacting system to use the rising gas bubbles to achieve a degree of solids removal through a flotation mechanism, thereby reducing the solids loading to downstream treatment processes. The process involves the addition of alum and polymer to the flow into the ozone contactor, which is then agitated by a submerged turbine type impeller system. Approximately 20 percent of the solids are removed by subsequent flotation in this approach, and the remainder of the turbidity removal occurs across what is predominantly a direct filtration process. This approach permitted an increase in filter rates to 6 gpm/sq ft with an overall increase in plant capacity from 50 mgd to 200 mgd. Flotation was facilitated by retrofit of former flocculation basins (14). Note that the flotation phenomena that occur in this plant may be associated with specific water quality characteristics, so testing should be performed to assess such applicability at other locations.

Other flotation applications have been reported for algae removal (28). In some locations, however, enhanced removal of algae also occurs due to ozonation without flotation. In some European plants, ozone is added in the initial flash mixing stages in conjunction with a hydrolyzed form of aluminum chloride called *polyaluminum chloride*. This is an alternate coagulation method that can yield enhanced flocculation, sedimentation, and clarification to result in further reduction in coagulant usage and associated reductions in sludge production as compared with alum coagulation.

ALTERNATIVE OZONE APPLICATION POINTS

As a strong oxidizing chemical, ozone can achieve a number of treatment goals. The desired goals will affect the selected points of ozone application and the dosages and contact times at each point. Several European systems use multiple points of ozone contacting within a plant, each application point focusing on a specific goal (28).

When an ozonation location is selected, it is important to consider the potential for interaction with other chemicals, since it is possible for ozone to react with hypochlorite ions, chlorine dioxide, and chloramines to result in a mutual destruction (39). These interactions can interfere with desired chemical reactions and complicate process control. Therefore, it may be necessary to dissipate the ozone residual as much as possible before these other chemicals are added. Dissipation can also be important for preventing uncontrolled ozone off-gassing in unwanted locations. In fact, without residual dissipation, it may be necessary to cover tankage and channels downstream of ozone-contacting systems just to prevent off-gas from contaminating the working atmosphere. Methods of residual dissipation are discussed later.

Pretreatment

Ozone has been used at pretreatment locations to achieve a full range of objectives that include primary disinfection, removal of tastes and odors, reduction in color levels, iron and manganese removal, enhanced coagulation, reduction in precursor level, and flotation for removal of algae and turbidity. Although best practiced at downstream locations in many plants that have a high ozone demand in raw water, primary disinfection may be an appropriate pretreatment goal at plants that practice direct filtration or in locations that have a low raw water ozone demand. In all likelihood, the goals for iron and manganese removal and enhanced coagulation are achieved as a matter of circumstance in many pretreatment disinfection applications since ozone doses may be dictated by disinfection, not oxidation, requirements. While effectiveness for these secondary goals may not be optimized by the use of disinfection dosages, they still may be achieved to a significant extent.

In many European applications, typical pretreatment doses for ozone are 0.1 to 0.2 mg of ozone per mg of DOC and are often intended to achieve limited oxidation of organic material for enhanced coagulation (28). Ozone pretreatment locations for this goal are generally prior to rapid mix. There are, however, exceptions to this practice, such as the previously cited plant in Hackensack, New Jersey, where ozone contact has been incorporated directly into the coagulation process in order to take advantage of the flotation effects produced.

For removal of iron and manganese, a pretreatment location may be favored at some plants since some of the precipitates formed by oxidation, especially those of manganese, can be of small size and require subsequent coagulation in order to be removed. In other situations, the presence of high levels of organic material at the pretreatment location may inhibit iron and manganese removal, thereby favoring a downstream location (7). It is also possible that manganese may redissolve in downstream sedimentation basins, thereby reversing the pretreatment removal initially achieved by ozone. This effect should not be overlooked in conventional water treatment facilities that employ sedimentation. An ozone addition point located downstream of sedimentation and just ahead of the filters may be more appropriate for some of these situations. Note, however, that these downstream locations may not provide for coagulation of colloidal manganese precipitates so that the need for adding this capability may have to be considered.

Dosage requirements for multiple goals may compete, requiring that priorities first be established to permit meaningful decisions. For instance, dose requirements for enhanced coagulation may differ from those for iron and manganese removal, and it may be necessary to provide supplemental methods for removing any remaining excess iron and manganese in situations where enhanced coagulation takes precedence.

Another concern that may be encountered in pretreatment applications of ozone is the tendency for formation of increased levels of mutagenicity. This occurs as a result of the higher concentration of organic materials at this location (40). A lower ozone dosage ratio relative to DOC usually prevails in this situation, resulting in a condition that can be more conducive to mutagen formation than at alternative addition points. Mutagen formation has been observed to reach a peak at lower ozone-to-organic ratios. It begins to decline as a result of greater levels of oxidation that prevail at higher ratios that occur in downstream treatment processes (i.e., ratio is reduced by removal of DOC in these processes). In cases where mutagen formation becomes a concern, capability for achieving a degree of removal of these substances by downstream processes such as biological filtration or further ozonation should be confirmed.

One phenomenon to consider when ozone is used at pretreatment locations to oxidize iron and manganese is that if the levels of iron and manganese are sufficiently high, copious amounts of a brown/black precipitate will be produced. These insoluble materials can interfere with the measurement of a dissolved ozone residual, even though a significant residual may be present. These complications need to be considered and can frequently be minimized by selection of an appropriate analytical technique (5).

Prefiltration

The addition of ozone at prefiltration locations provides an opportunity for removal of some demand-causing substances prior to ozone being applied, especially in conventional water treatment trains that employ coagulation and sedimentation processes. Such removal can reduce ozone demand significantly for many oxidation reactions and can reduce the dosage required to meet disinfection goals. As discussed in the section Removal of Iron and Manganese, a prefiltration application may be more appropriate in cases where manganese can be resolubilized from sedimentation basins. Depending on specific needs, use of prefiltration ozonation might also be considered with a pretreatment ozonation step to allow separate objectives to be optimized at both locations (40).

Ozone application at prefiltration and pretreatment locations can allow for biological activity in the downstream filters when other disinfecting residuals are absent. Such activity can be helpful in reducing the levels of many low molecular weight byproducts of ozonation such as aldehydes and organic acids (40). Biological processes may also be of value in reducing the levels of a larger group of biodegradable organic materials that can be formed by reactions between ozone and background (natural) organic matter. Removal of this material may be an important concern due to a capability to stimulate subsequent microbial growth in the distribution piping. In some cases, hydroxyl radical–based processes can be employed to further increase the biodegradability of organics, thereby increasing the capability for removal of organic material with biodegradation processes.

In a European adaptation of the prefiltration approach, ozone is added to partially oxidize organics ahead of slow sand filters, a filtration process that operates in a biological mode. Ozonation increases the biodegradability of organic material in the filter influent, making the slow sand filter biological process more effective (36). Enhanced removal of color by slow sand filters also is reported to occur as a result of preozonation (58).

The ease with which a prefiltration ozone application can be implemented varies from one plant to the next. Many plants have a system of interconnected piping, conduits, and channels on the influent side of filters, and it can be difficult to consolidate flow through a common point for transport to an ozone contactor. Also, there is a potential for air binding in the filter media, and provision should be made to dissipate gases prior to filtration.

Postfiltration

Postfiltration application of ozone typically allows opportunity for even greater removal of ozone demand–causing substances by upstream treatment processes. In addition, disinfection processes often are more effective at these locations since particulate matter that can shield pathogens from disinfecting agents has been substantially removed. In these respects, postfiltration would be an excellent location for achieving primary disinfection goals. Moreover, ozone contact facilities can often be installed much more readily at this location than at prefiltration locations.

Despite the advantage of a postfiltration application, this location eliminates the potential for using the filters to remove biodegradable material that may be formed by ozone, and a separate biodegradation process may be required as a consequence. In some situations, the ozonation of clear waters containing certain dissolved organic compounds can actually lead to increases in turbidity and color where microflocculation is generated. Because of such microflocculation, many European treatment plants follow ozonation with filtration. One plant follows ozonation with a second addition of ferrous iron compounds to increase the rate of microflocculation, which results in a very clear water after subsequent filtration (40).

Pre–Granular Activated Carbon

Granular activated carbon is often considered a complementary process for ozone systems, particularly in Europe, Canada, and Japan. In this configuration, ozone provides partial oxidation of organic material that makes it more susceptible to biodegradation on a granular activated carbon column or bed. This process configuration, termed biological activated carbon (BAC), combines the absorptive capabilities of activated carbon with the activity of an attached biogrowth to remove naturally occurring DOC as well as target organic substances that may not easily be removed by ozone alone. Also, chlorine demand can be reduced by BAC, providing for more stable residuals in the distribution system and a decrease in chlorine dosage. The removal of DOC, in conjunction with a reduced chlorine dose, results in a lower level of disinfection byproduct formation (69).

Biological processes are also being considered for removing the undesirable levels of biodegradable organic carbon (BDOC) that are formed in many ozonation systems. While conventional filters have some capability for biodegradation when disinfecting residuals are eliminated from the filtered water, GAC provides a much higher surface area for microbial attachment and may be more appropriate where the desired level of BDOC removal cannot be achieved with conventional filter media. GAC also can provide for removal of excess permanganate that can occur when ozone is used for manganese removal.

Granular activated carbon contact can be provided in separate contacting columns or beds located downstream of filtration. Alternatively, when criteria for contact time can be met, GAC can be incorporated into the filtration process at less overall cost than required for separate contactors. In this type of application, GAC is used as an alternative filter media to a sand or anthracite.

A significant problem in retrofitting existing filter plants with GAC media is the compatibility of existing filter boxes. Frequently this approach will require a deeper filter box in order to attain a sufficient empty bed contact time for the biodegradation process. In some cases, retrofit of new and more compact filter underdrain replacements will provide both added depth for GAC media as well as additional hydraulic gradient upstream of the filters. This type of retrofit may not be possible or may not be economical, so it may become necessary to construct a separate GAC contacting system to provide the empty bed contact time requirements. Alternatively, existing filters might be "derated" by reducing hydraulic loading to a level that achieves the desired contact time. Filtration capacity will be lost by this approach, requiring that new parallel filters be constructed to compensate for the derating. In addition, similar to prefiltration applications of ozone, the need to remove excess ozone prior to filtration will influence both filter replacement and postfilter GAC systems. All of these factors should be included in a complete evaluation of this approach.

OZONE SYSTEM DESIGN CONSIDERATIONS

The following sections give an overview of general considerations for evaluating and designing ozone systems. Major components of an ozone system include equipment for preparation of feed gas, ozone generation, ozone-contacting systems, and ozone destructors. Each major component requires specific evaluation.

Feed Gas Preparation

In the most commonly used corona discharge method, ozone is generated from an oxygen-containing feed gas stream (i.e., air or oxygen). Preparation of the feed gas for ozone generation is extremely critical because of the need for a clean, moisture-free gas that will protect equipment from damage. A designer is faced with a choice between air- and oxygen-based feed gas systems. In general, air systems, with a lower capital cost than many oxygen-generating systems, have been more common. However, since about 1980, there has been increasing interest in the use of oxygen generated on site. Purchase of liquid oxygen (LOX) from an outside source has received consideration as well. Relatively pure LOX has minimal equipment requirements, thereby reducing initial capital investment as compared with air preparation and on-site oxygen-generation systems.

Oxygen Systems

Oxygen gas has about five times as many oxygen molecules as the same volume of ambient air. This allows higher concentrations of ozone to be produced from this feed gas source; about twice the concentration is produced from oxygen as from air (Table 7–1). Significantly, use of oxygen feed systems generally reduces the overall ozone system power consumption. In the case of LOX systems, feed gas preparation equipment and its operation and maintenance is greatly simplified. As a consequence, LOX systems are being considered for small system applications in particular but may also have applicability for large systems as well.

LOX systems consist of insulated liquid storage tanks, evaporators, and flow metering. Although these systems are simple and maintenance is

TABLE 7–1. Ozone Concentrations[a]

Type of Ozone Generator	Air	Oxygen
Voltage controlled low- and medium-frequency generators	1.0–1.5	2.0–3.0
Frequency controlled high-frequency generators	2.5–3.0	5.0–10.0

[a] By % wt.

much less than with other gas feed systems, sufficient redundancy should be provided to permit regular maintenance. It is also essential that a reliable source of liquid oxygen supply be available. The cost of purchasing liquid oxygen is often such that the economics are more favorable because of the reduction in capital costs; capital costs often represent a large component of the total system cost, particularly for small systems. Care should be exercised in performing evaluations to assure that quoted LOX costs are not artificially depressed with a potential for substantial increase in the future as market conditions change.

On-site generation of oxygen is achieved by separating oxygen from air, using either cryogenic air separation or one of the pressure swing adsorption processes. Both types of processes are complex. Gas quality is important as for the air feed gas preparation systems described below, and although problems with particulates may not be as severe, filters should be used to provide protection of the ozone generators. Despite the complexity of these processes, economic analysis may demonstrate that the reduced cost for the ozone-generation step may justify on-site oxygen generation, especially for large-scale applications. Consideration must be given to costs associated with provision of appropriate levels of reliability. In some situations LOX can be used as an economical solution for either standby service or peaking service capabilities.

Recycling of the off-gas from a contactor can be considered a means for reducing the oxygen requirements in oxygen systems. However, this approach can result in a moisture-laden gas that can cause problems with equipment corrosion. As this may require systems for removing water vapor, single-pass systems have tended to be more common.

Air Preparation

When air is used for ozone generation, proper preparation is critical. Unless the ozone generator is supplied with dry, clean, and cool air, it will experience operating problems. If the air stream is too moist, water will condense on dielectrics within the generator and nitric acid will be formed, leading to reduced ozone yield and corrosive damage. Both particles and moisture can cause electrical arcing within a generator. This is an extremely undesirable condition that lowers generator efficiency and increases likelihood of equipment damage.

Air-preparation systems typically include compressors, air-cooling devices, air dryers, and particle filters. A critical design consideration is the target moisture content to be produced in the air stream at each location in the system. The present trend is towards very high levels of moisture reduction down to dewpoint levels of −65°C or lower. Somewhat higher

TABLE 7–2. Typical Drying Parameters

Location	Water Content (mg H_2O/kg air)	Moisture Removal (%)	Dew Point (°C)
Ambient air[a]	21,850	N/A	26
Compressor	13,790	37	19
Refrigerant dryer	2,737	87.5	5
Desiccant dryer			
Marginal	21.5	99.90	−51
Desirable	6.7	99.98	≤−65

[a] Assumes 80 percent relative humidity, 15 psig, and 30°C.

moisture levels might be tolerated in some cases. However, these begin to become marginal to unacceptable at dew point levels greater than −50°C.

Moisture removal is accomplished by various devices within an air-preparation process stream. Typical removals by these devices are summarized in Table 7–2. Several devices may be required at various points in the flow stream because of the potential for damage caused by improper moisture control.

Operating Pressure

Most air-preparation systems use compressors to provide the source of air. However, if the ozone contact tank is equipped with a vacuum-type turbine injector or other vacuum-creating devices, an air compressor at the head of the air-preparation system may be eliminated, although other air-preparation components will be required. A blower and aftercooler may still be required to supplement these systems during high-humidity periods.

The configuration of the air-preparation system can vary depending on a number of factors. Compressor/dryer air-preparation systems may be categorized according to operating pressure: low, medium, and high. Typical system configurations are shown in Figure 7–5. Under low- and medium-pressure conditions, more extensive drying is required to remove moisture from air, such as a two-stage drying system as shown in Figure 7–5. In higher-pressure systems, air is easier to dry and more options are available.

Basically the major difference in medium- and low-pressure system designs has been the type of compressor. Low-pressure systems can accommodate rotary lobe and other relatively simple, nonlubricated types of blowers. However, these blowers are typically limited to discharge

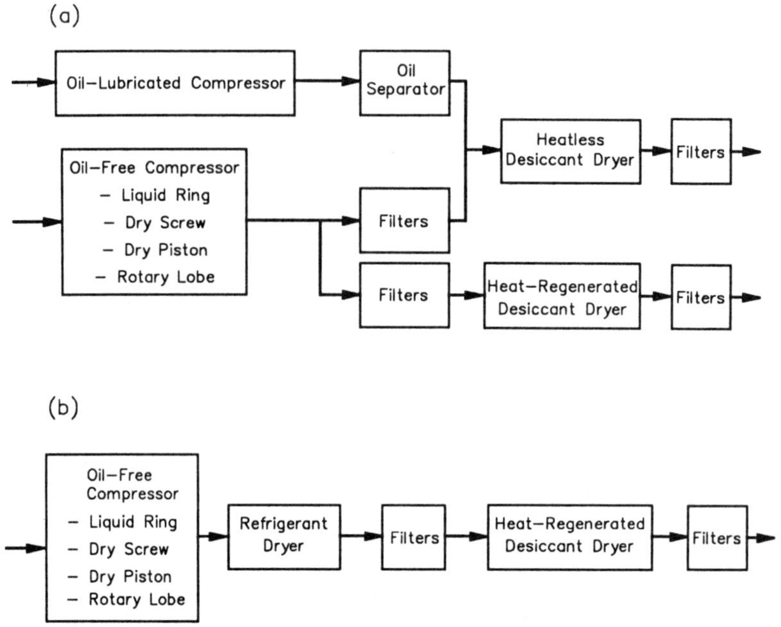

FIGURE 7–5. Typical air preparation systems: (a) high pressure; (b) medium and low pressure.

pressures of 15 psig. Medium-pressure systems typically employ compressors with a discharge capability of 25 to 30 psig or even higher. The liquid ring compressor is the more commonly used unit for this medium-pressure range, although it is also available for low-pressure applications as well. Other medium-pressure compressors include nonlubricated types such as the rotary screw design.

Typically a refrigerant dryer is used for achieving an initial or first-stage reduction in moisture level following the low- or medium-pressure compressors. These devices add to system complexity and may require specialty experience for maintenance. However, in spite of this disadvantage, they can have a significant effect on system economics by achieving an initial level moisture removal in an economic manner, thereby substantially reducing the sizing of heat regenerated dryers in a later stage. As an alternative to refrigerant dryers, other methods such as heat exchangers can be used to lower moisture content in the first drying step. Similar to the refrigerant dryer, moisture reduction occurs as a result of lowering the air temperature. Heat exchangers are generally more appropriate for larger systems.

The high-pressure system range begins at a compressor discharge pressure of approximately 100 psig. Moisture removal is easier to achieve in this higher range, often eliminating the need for refrigerant dryers, by allowing the use of heatless (pressure swing) dryers. These heatless dryers are also less prone to fouling and can accommodate the use of oil-lubricated compressors, which are not suitable with the heat regenerated dryers. In general, heatless dryers are less costly and have lower maintenance requirements than heat regenerated dryers. However, while these advantages may be achieved in the gas preparation components of high-pressure systems, the ozone generator shells need to be extra thick. Even where pressure-reducing valves are used, possible valve failure needs to be considered. The attendant higher pressure requirements for stainless steel ozone generator equipment can result in significant cost increase, especially for larger equipment sizes. The cost increase is less for smaller systems and can often be offset by savings that result with the use of heatless dryers. Therefore, high-pressure systems are more likely to be used for smaller systems, whereas low- to medium-pressure systems become more favored as system size increases.

Compressor/Cooler Alternatives

Selection of compressors requires consideration of a number of factors. Water-flooded compressors (liquid ring) have low efficiency but are reliable, durable, and need little maintenance. Dry compressors can be used over a wide pressure range, and multistage configurations (series) can often be used to obtain even higher pressures. Both oil-lubricated and dry compressors tend to produce a high-temperature air stream, which requires that these compressors be supplied with aftercoolers (usually an air- or water-cooled heat exchanger) to achieve temperatures suitable for downstream equipment that includes heat regenerated dryers and ozone generators. Supplemental downstream cooling can also be provided by additional refrigerant dryers. In contrast, water-flooded compressors tend to be cooled by the water that is used within the compressor to control exit air temperature. Aftercoolers are often not required for this type of equipment, although downstream cooling devices may still be necessary depending on site-specific temperature characteristics and other equipment needs. Thermocouple temperature elements should be installed in exit gas lines to monitor performance of this cooling equipment.

Air Dryers

Desiccant air dryers are critical components for achieving the extremely low moisture levels in air preparation. The heat regenerated dryers used for most low- and medium-pressure air preparation systems contain either alumina or silica as desiccant media. Each of these materials has good affinity for water, can be readily regenerated, and has a long life cycle. Molecular sieves are also used in heat regenerated systems, but are more commonly used as a bottom layer along with an upper alumina layer. Sole use of molecular sieves is more common in heatless dryer systems.

Heatless dryer systems that become applicable as alternatives for high-pressure systems require greater operating pressures to allow an adequate pressure swing that will achieve moisture removal during regeneration. It is this limitation that confines their use to high-pressure air preparation systems. Where they can be used, heatless systems have the advantage of extremely short downtime for regeneration as well as the tendency for less fouling, which often permits the use of oil-lubricated compressors. On the other hand, oil-lubricated compressors are not suitable for use with heat regenerated dryers.

Heat regenerated dryers fall into two general categories: internal and external regeneration. Internal heat regenerated systems that contain an imbedded heating element tend to result in a shorter desiccant life, whereas external systems that use an external air source can involve greater expense for piping and mechanical components. System size dictates the choice between these systems; external heat regenerated systems become increasingly favored as system size increases.

Run times for heat regenerated dryers are typically on the order of 8 to 16 hours. Such dryers are often cycled using timer control, although dew-point control can also be used. Regeneration typically consists of a heating period followed by a cool-down cycle, resulting in a total downtime on the order of 8 hours. Heating and cooling air for external regeneration systems should be filtered to 5 μm to help prevent particulate fouling of the desiccant.

Oversizing heat regenerated dryers adds slightly to the cost of the installation but can greatly increase reliability and the chance of success. Two rules of thumb are suggested: (1) desiccant weight should be 18 times that of the moisture to be removed in an 8-hour cycle, and (2) the residence time (with media in tank) should be greater than 5 seconds. The applicability of these criteria should be confirmed for actual humidity conditions in each location. Provisions should be made for the easy removal of desiccant media.

Air Filters

Filters are generally used at three locations within an air preparation system, as summarized in Table 7–3. The first set is normally installed where the air is introduced to the intake side of the compressors through filter/silencers that are intended to remove larger particles that could dam-

TABLE 7–3. Typical Filtering Parameters[a]

Location	Filter Size (μm)[b]
Before compressor—filter/silencer	5
Before dryer	
Particulate filter	3–5
Moisture filter	0.04 (coalescing)
Before generator—particulate	0.3 (acceptable)
	0.1 (desirable)

[a] Filters should be provided with differential pressure gauges and alarms.

[b] Actual sizes selected may vary and should be determined based on site-specific and equipment-specific considerations.

age the compressors. A second set of filters is typically located downstream of the compressors and refrigerant dryers before the inlet to the desiccant drying system. These usually consist of two groups of filters for removing particulates and moisture, respectively. An oil coalescer might be used for high-pressure systems that employ oil-lubricated compressors. A final set of filters is then placed at the inlet to the ozone generator that provides for removal of extremely small particles that may be associated with attrition of desiccant particles in the dryers. Filters should also be used on regenerant air intakes that supply hot air and cooling air for external heat regenerated dryers.

Filters should be positioned for easy access and rapid cleaning. A differential pressure gauge should be installed to indicate when the filters should be cleaned. For installations under vacuum, air filters should be installed before the air blowers.

General Gas Preparation Design Considerations

In all cases, design of feed gas preparation equipment should be reviewed carefully with ozone equipment manufacturers, taking into account the extremes of site-specific ambient air temperature and humidity. Standby systems should be provided for all major components with ample pressure and temperature indicators and alarms to monitor and control performance at various stages through the system. Dew-point monitors also should be supplied. Valves should be furnished as required to allow equipment to be removed from service, to allow air flow to be routed through bypasses and alternative equipment configurations installed for reliability and redundancy purposes, and to control pressures at required locations.

Ozone Generators

Although ozone can be generated by other energy sources such as ultraviolet radiation, electric corona discharge is the most common method employed in water treatment. Electric corona discharge generators are available in a variety of configurations. Most of those used have been the horizontal water-cooled tube configuration (Figure 7–6). However, alternative vertical tube and plate dielectric and air-cooled configurations are also available.

Ozone is formed in a corona discharge by the interaction between an electric discharge and oxygen molecules in a gas stream that is passed through the generator (see Figure 7–6). The electric discharge is induced by an alternating current which creates a voltage cycle across a gap between two electrodes. One of the electrodes is coated with glass or ceramic dielectric material that provides a smooth surface to distribute the electric discharge evenly along the surface. Otherwise, imperfections on the surface of an electrode could create hot spots, which tend to disrupt the electric discharge and result in undesirable and wasteful arcing at voltages below the level at which ozone formation can occur.

Within an applied voltage cycle, an electric discharge occurs only at voltage levels that exceed the ionization potential. If the ionization potential is exceeded at only the peak voltage along a cycle, then discharge will be confined to the time at which the peak voltage occurs. An increase in the applied voltage beyond this level will increase the period and the total quantity of discharge within a cycle. Therefore, the applied voltage has a significant effect on the extent of electric discharge and the associated ozone production and can be used as a means for controlling ozone output.

The frequency of the voltage cycle also affects the level of discharge by influencing the voltage patterns. The percent of time over which the ion-

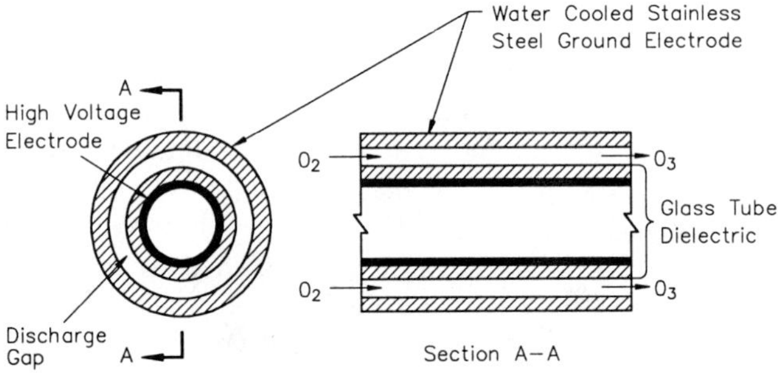

FIGURE 7–6. Schematic of ozone-generation tube. (Adapted from Ref. 52.)

ization potential is exceeded in a voltage cycle increases with voltage pattern changes that occur with increased frequency, thereby increasing the overall electric discharge. As a consequence of these relationships, frequency variation offers another method for controlling ozone output.

Before discussing generators in further detail, it is important to emphasize two major considerations that can affect performance as discussed before:

1. There is a need to protect and maintain the integrity of the generator dielectrics by providing the appropriate level of air preparation that will sustain efficient ozone generation and avoid damage to equipment. Excess moisture or particulate matter can cause hot spots that reduce efficiency and result in dielectric cracking. Moisture can also cause formation of nitrous oxides that can lead to corrosion and result in interferences in ozone production. A clean and dry gas stream is, therefore, essential for efficient, continuous performance of ozone-generation equipment. Neglect of these particular needs has been responsible for a number of ozone system failures.
2. The other significant consideration for ozone generation is effective control over temperature. Excess temperature can damage dielectrics. High temperatures also create conditions where ozone rapidly reverts to oxygen, thereby reducing efficiency. Therefore, temperature within the ozone generator needs to be limited by control of both the inlet air stream and the cooling of the internal elements. Inadequate generator cooling is another deficiency that has been responsible for a number of ozone system failures.

With the above performance features in mind, it is possible to review ozone generator design in more specific terms. Ozone generators are generally characterized by the frequency range of the applied voltage, as shown in Table 7–4. Low-frequency generators are operated using frequencies of 50 to 60 Hz, which are typically available from electric utilities. Medium- and high-frequency generators require conversion to higher frequency levels. This tends to result in more complex generators that

TABLE 7–4. Ozone Generator Characteristics

Type	Frequency (Hz)	Voltage (kV)	Power Factor
Low frequency	60	10–20	≥0.4
Medium frequency	700–800	8–14	≥0.8
High frequency	2,000–3,000	8–10	Unity

have a higher capital cost. Use of these increased frequencies, however, can increase the efficiency of generating an electric discharge with a possible savings in power costs. Also, the medium- and high-frequency generator designs are typically more compact, thereby requiring less installation space. These benefits tend to become more significant as ozone-generation capacity increases.

Other important attributes of increased frequency (medium and high) generators are as follows:

- *Capability for Both Voltage and Frequency Control.* When the operating frequency is increased, the opportunity exists for varying ozone output by imposing either frequency or voltage variations. However, this option is not always exercised, so many medium-frequency generators are still controlled using only changes in voltage.
- *Capability for Turndown.* Increased frequency generators generally tend to have higher turndown capabilities than low-frequency generators. This can be a significant advantage in cases where wide variations in desired ozone production create conditions that may require combinations of generators to match the full range of conditions. Under these conditions, the greater turndown afforded by increased frequency generators may allow a wider range of ozone production to be met with fewer generators.
- *Ozone Concentration in Gas Stream.* Increased frequency generators can generally produce higher concentrations of ozone within the gas stream. This can reduce the volume of the gas feed stream, resulting in significant savings for gas preparation equipment. However, the lower gas feed stream flow can reduce the gas-to-liquid ratio within porous gas diffusion contactors so that the consequent distribution of ozone within the contactor may be adversely affected. These influences need to be considered in design.
- *Power Factor.* Both medium- and high-frequency generators have much higher power factors (KW/KVA), thereby requiring much less, if any, need for adjustment. Low-frequency generators tend to have extremely low power factors, as shown in Table 7–4. This can require added expense to provide power factor correction equipment. Alternatively, the power factor might be corrected by synchronizing operation of several generators simultaneously. However, this may increase the number of generators required. Another approach is to synchronize generator operation with other major electrical loads within a plant.
- *Generator Cooling Needs.* Generator cooling needs tend to increase as frequency is increased. In most cases, water cooling systems are used, although a few systems have used air. If the locally available water

temperatures are sufficiently low, low-frequency generators can be cooled using the water supply directly. Water chilling systems are likely to be necessary to provide suitable cooling water temperatures for medium-frequency systems, although it still may be possible to eliminate these systems in locations where the maximum annual temperatures of the locally available water supplies remain relatively low. However, the opportunity for avoiding chilling water systems is generally greater with low-frequency generators. Additional complexity is often encountered with high-frequency generators, which may require a dual cooling system, using water in combination with oil or freon.

Water chilling systems can be relatively complicated and can have a significant impact on system layout and cost. Both single-pass and recycle chilled water systems can be considered. Single-pass systems tend to be favored for smaller installations, whereas recycle cooling systems may become attractive for larger chilling water systems, especially in cases where energy requirements can be significantly reduced. Water treatment may be required in recycle systems to reduce the tendency for chemical scaling.

There are no hard rules for selecting generator types in that each application will have site-specific features to be considered. Alternatives should be compared based on complete systems, which include air preparation and cooling water components, as well as the gas-to-liquid ratio considerations in contacting systems. The trend has been to opt for the lower capital cost and reduced complexity of low-frequency generators for small installations, whereas the efficiencies and improved turndown of increased frequency generators become more significant for larger capacity installations.

Among the increased frequency generators, medium-frequency generators have been favored over high-frequency generators, due, in part, to the increase in design complexity that occurs at higher frequency levels. However, properly designed and operated high-frequency generators have afforded good service. A significant consideration for the future of high-frequency generators will be the demand and the availability of suppliers, which has been somewhat limited in the past.

An important feature in system design is the selection of an appropriate generator size. It is critical that a generator be capable of sustained operation without damage under maximum design conditions. Problems have occurred with damage of some generators that have been operated at the manufacturer's *stated* peak output for extended periods. This has led to the recommendation that generators be sized based on 75 percent of peak output capacity (57). However, this is a somewhat vague generalization, and the key is to obtain appropriate equipment guarantees for the maximum sustained level of ozone production.

Ozone-Contacting Systems

The design of contact systems is strongly influenced by the relatively low ozone solubility in water at feed gas concentrations that range from 1 to 10 percent. Chlorine and ammonia are more soluble gases that, in addition, are available in a nearly pure form. As a consequence, these gases are more readily dissolved in water, requiring a modest degree of care in the design of injection systems. Ozone systems require a much more rigorous approach for achieving efficient transfer. As a consequence, ozone-contacting systems need to be configured not only for achieving appropriate detention times for disinfection or oxidation, but for efficient gas transfer as well.

Another consideration in ozone-contactor design is the need for control and handling of off-gases to avoid exposure of personnel to ozone. Typically, the off-gas stream is collected in a vacuum piping system and transported to an ozone destruction system. In many cases, there may be a need for destroying the ozone residual in the water prior to downstream treatment with chemicals that are incompatible with ozone (e.g., chlorine and chlorine dioxide) or to avoid excess ozone off-gassing that may represent a hazard in uncovered downstream basins.

Failure to dissipate ozone residual also can represent a significant operational problem in prefilter ozonation systems by causing gas binding of filters. When adequate head is available, use of turbulence generated by flow over a weir is a common method of stimulating release of ozone. Under other circumstances, dissipation of residuals and gases may simply involve a quiescent holding zone at the end of an ozone contact system to permit ozone die-off. Chemical methods also can be used for ozone removal such as dosing a reducing agent (sulfur dioxide, sodium bisulfite, or sodium thiosulfate), adding hydrogen peroxide to convert ozone to unstable hydroxyl radicals, stripping ozone by aeration, or, where sufficient head is available, using a cascade aeration system.

Various contacting configurations are available. The most commonly used systems can be placed in the following general categories (not necessarily in order of frequency of use):

- Ozone injection into feed stream
- Porous gas diffuser system
- Turbine system
- Off-gas reinjection systems

Other less commonly used systems include packed towers and spray contact chambers.

Ozone Injection into Feed Stream

The Otto contactor, which falls into this category, is an early version of ozone contacting (4). Ozone is drawn into the process flow stream through an aspirator, which operates by a venturi-jet principle. The ozone-laden water is then directed downward into a vertical tube, which discharges at the bottom of a contacting basin. The depth of this discharge creates the pressure and time of vertical travel necessary to provide effective transfer of ozone. More recently, deep U-tube configurations have been developed as another modification of ozone feed stream injection. This type of contactor has been constructed to depths to 66 feet in order to achieve a high pressure for efficient transfer of ozone (64).

A potential problem in the vertical tube approach is that the flow turbulence and small ozone bubble size required for efficient transfer may not be achieved over a full range of plant-operating flows. Therefore, turndown requirements should be evaluated for these systems and methods for increasing transfer under low flow conditions may need to be considered. In many cases, this problem can be resolved by confining injection to a side feed stream that is maintained at an optimum flow rate. The side stream is then intermixed with the main stream after ozone has been added.

Another recent modification of the ozone injection method involves the use of in-line static mixing devices located immediately downstream of the point of ozone injection. Although these devices can be extremely efficient for many conditions, problems can be encountered under other conditions:

1. Depending on design, gas dispersion in large static mixers may not be efficient, particularly in static mixers mounted in the horizontal position.
2. The efficiency of most static mixers is flow sensitive. Since the mixers rely on velocity for obtaining the proper back flow or mixing patterns, they tend to become inefficient below flows of 60 to 75 percent of maximum flow.

Figure 7- 7 shows a side stream arrangement that can overcome these problems in static mixers to a certain extent. The side stream flows (typically 5 to 10 percent of maximum) are designed for the ideal rate of mix at the desired level of ozone addition. The larger mixer then can blend the two flow streams. The small mixer should be in a vertical position and, if

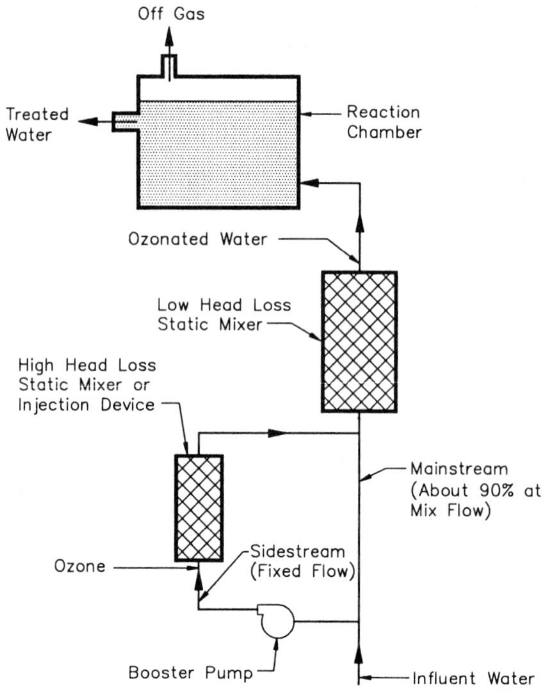

FIGURE 7–7. Static mixer system for ozone dispersion.

possible, the large mixer should also be in this orientation. Alternatively, the efficiency of static mixer systems can be improved through the use of multiple, parallel mixer units that are placed in service to match process flow requirements.

A major consideration in the case of each of the ozone feed stream injection systems is the amount of contact time available within the system itself. Where additional contact time is required for disinfection, some form of downstream detention may be necessary. This may involve detention in piping or a downstream chamber. Because of the strong oxidizing properties of ozone, consideration needs to be given to use of corrosion-resistant materials in downstream detention devices. There will also be a need to provide for withdrawing off-gas for conveyance to a destruct system.

Porous Gas Diffuser Systems

Porous gas diffuser systems can be arranged in either concurrent or countercurrent configurations. In a concurrent configuration, the process water flow stream is introduced at the bottom, where it comes into contact with the porous ozone gas diffusers and rises to the top in the same direction as the bubbles. This is contrasted with a countercurrent system in which the liquid flow is introduced at the top of a contactor and a downward flow is induced by flow withdrawal at the bottom of a contact chamber (Figure 7–8). The downward water flow is opposite in direction to the rising flow of gas bubbles. This countercurrent effect tends to retard the bubble rise rate to a certain extent, thereby increasing the opportunity for ozone transfer. In addition, the rising bubbles come into contact with water having a progressively increased demand for ozone reaction. Under this condition, ozone demand continually increases for bubbles as they near the surface. Conversely, bubbles in concurrent systems come into contact with solutions of decreasing ozone demand as they approach the surface. Under this condition, ozone levels can progressively increase, thereby reducing the ozone concentration driving force for mass transfer as the bubbles rise to the surface. As a consequence, the countercurrent configuration offers greater transfer efficiency, and its use has been favored in many designs.

While single-stage ozone-contacting systems can be used, many diffuser systems are multistaged, particularly when disinfection is the treatment objective. The concept of staging is illustrated in Figure 7–8 for a two-cell countercurrent contacting system. In compartment A, ozone can be added in a quantity sufficient to overcome the background demand and also provide a residual level that can subsequently be sustained for a few minutes of contact. Where disinfection is a predominant goal, a typical target residual has been 0.4 mg/l in the discharge from this contact chamber, although the residual levels should now be based on EPA's CT crite-

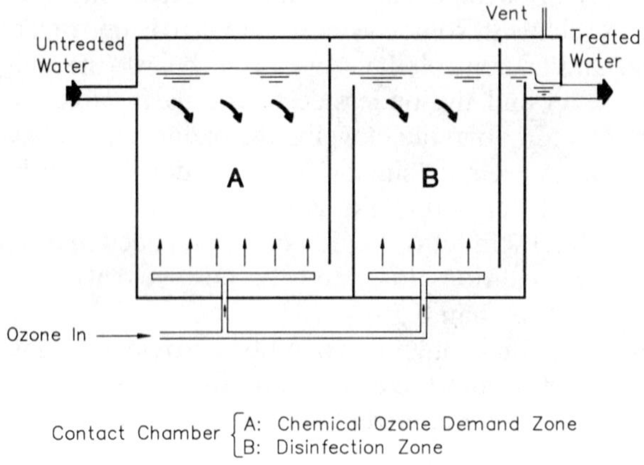

FIGURE 7–8. Two-stage countercurrent contacting system. (From Ref. 54. Reprinted by permission of International Ozone Association.)

ria. In stage B, additional ozone is added, thereby allowing the effective contact period to be extended. No limitation exists for the number of contacting cells, and it is possible to provide as many as desired. However, system complexity and costs increase with additional staging of the contacting system and associated increases in piping and flow-splitting devices for multiple points of ozone addition. A typical configuration involves a two-stage to four-stage countercurrent baffled concrete structure. Smaller installations can consider vertical tanks in series as an alternative.

Critical factors in design of gas diffusion contacting systems are depth of diffuser submergence and diffuser characteristics. Recommended minimum submergence depths for high ozone transfer efficiency are generally in a range of 16 to 18 feet, and greater depths may be preferred where they can be reasonably accommodated. However, the hydrostatic pressure at depths much greater than 18 feet can combine with piping losses to create back pressures that exceed the normal discharge pressure of many generators (approximately 15 psig).

Fine bubble, disc-type, or rod-type ceramic diffusers may be used for dispersing the gas, with the disc the more common. A bubble size between 2 and 3 mm is an objective, although good results can be obtained over a wider range (46). Typical ozone transfer efficiencies in diffuser systems exceed 80 percent and normally exceed 90 percent, but only if appropriate bubble sizes and depths of diffuser submergence are provided.

The overall depth of a contactor needs to be deeper than the diffuser submergence, since the diffusers are normally one to two feet off the bottom. An access and a drain should be provided to allow the unit to be removed from service to clean any accumulated solids. Foaming and scum can be problems in some systems, and provisions must be made for their removal and/or control. Increased free board (the height between normal water level and the underside of the basin cover) is frequently required in contactors to avoid clogging the ozone destruct system equipment with foam. A weir or similar overflow device may be needed to control the water level within the contactor. Also, gas–to–water flow ratios of 0.15 to 0.20 scfm/cfm should not be exceeded in order to provide proper hydraulic conditions (64), and the flow velocity between baffles should be kept to less than 0.5 fps.

When evaluating the contacting conditions provided by gas diffusion, it is important to understand the distribution of ozone residual throughout the contact basin. In countercurrent systems, it is common for most of the ozone transfer to occur at the bottom of the basin. As gas bubbles rise to the surface, they become depleted of ozone, and the quantity transferred in the upper portion of the first contact stage is frequently exceeded by the demand of the process flow stream at this location. Therefore, much of the cell volume at some distance above a diffuser in first-stage contactor volume can be relatively devoid of ozone. Variations in concentration also occur in downstream contactor cells. This can be an important consideration for assessing CT criteria for disinfection and for comparing the effects of disinfection contact times of different plants and different types of reactors. EPA criteria for these evaluations are described in Appendix O of the U.S. EPA *Guidance Manual for Compliance with the Filtration and Disinfection Requirements for Public Water Systems Using Surface Water Sources* (47).

In contrast with the contacting conditions in countercurrent contactors, ozone often is introduced at the influent of concurrent contactors, allowing residual to be more widely distributed in this type of contactor. Therefore, concurrent contactors may enjoy some advantage in this regard. However, the recent tendency has been to opt for the higher transfer efficiency available in countercurrent systems.

Turbine Systems

In these systems, a mechanically driven turbine mixing device is used to provide the agitation for contacting ozone with the process flow stream. Two general configurations of turbine mixing systems have been developed: a conventional turbine system (Figure 7–9) and an aspirating turbine modification (Figure 7–10).

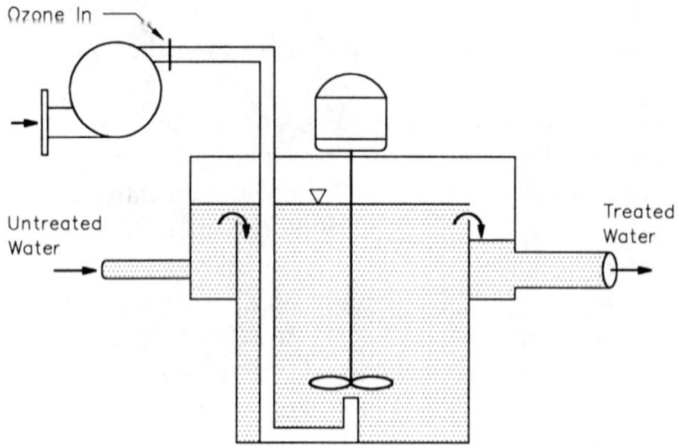

FIGURE 7–9. Turbine contactor. (From Ref. 55. Reprinted from *Waterworld News*, Vol. 3 (May/June 1987), by permission. Copyright © 1987, American Water Works Association.)

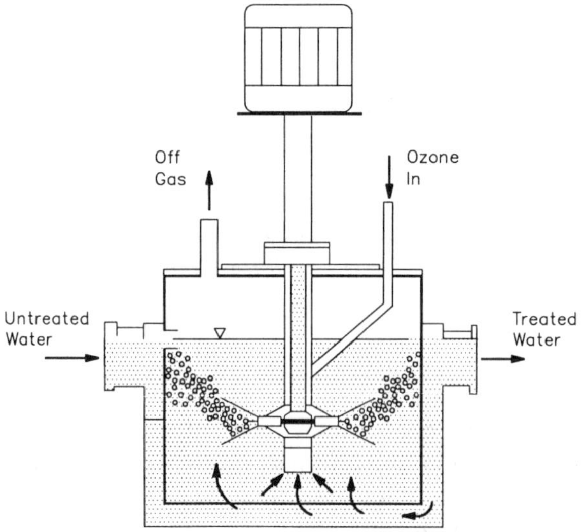

FIGURE 7–10. Aspirating turbine contactor. (From Ref. 55. Reprinted from *Water-world News,* Vol. 3 (May/June 1987), by permission. Copyright © 1987, American Water Works Association.)

In some cases, the mix chamber can discharge to another contacting chamber to achieve additional contact. However, ozone injection only occurs in the mix chambers, and this approach does not conveniently allow for multiple injection locations as can be applied in the case of multistage porous gas diffuser systems.

In the turbine contactor shown in Figure 7–9, the ozone gas stream is sparged under pressure into the main body of the contactor, and the bubbles are sheared and mixed by a mechanically driven turbine. In this type of contactor, the location for introducing the ozone gas stream is a key factor in maximizing transfer efficiency. Typically, gas is introduced below the turbine so that the rising bubbles can be sheared by the rotating vanes. However, modified versions using horizontally mounted turbines that entrain rising gas bubbles for mixing also have been used (28).

The aspirating turbine contactor (Figure 7–10) uses the internal pumping action of the turbine to induce a vacuum that draws ozone into the inner turbine column, thus eliminating the need for a gas preparation system compressor in some cases. The ozone then is entrained in a liquid stream that is injected back into the main body of the contactor, yielding a fine bubble stream that is mixed throughout the contactor volume.

Several alternative methods are available for mounting turbine motors. While vertical top entry mountings are most common, vertical bottom entry and horizontal side entry configurations also are possible in some systems, although potential problems with submerged shaft seals need to be considered. Submersible motors also can be used but can be more maintenance intensive.

Because of the dynamic mixing provided in turbine systems, the depth of turbine contactors can be much less than porous gas diffuser systems. This may reduce the cost for contactor construction. However, energy requirements often are significantly greater. Therefore, the trade-offs need to be considered.

Off-Gas Reinjection Recycle Systems

Off-gas recycle systems represent an effort to entrain some of the ozone that would otherwise exit the contactors in the off-gas. Several configurations of this type are shown in Figures 7–11, 7–12, and 7–13. The relative advantages of these systems will depend on site-specific economies associated with maximizing the use of ozone as well as associated benefits from reducing the requirements for ozone off-gas destruction.

Comparison of Contacting Systems

At present, gas diffusion systems are the most widely used method of contacting and provide the greatest level of experience. Internal baffling in these systems provides a high degree of retention for disinfection con-

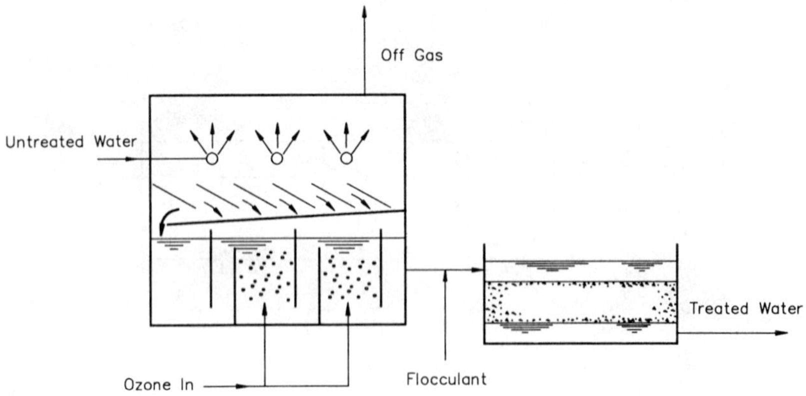

FIGURE 7–11. Off-gas recycle system A. (From Ref. 54. Reprinted by permission of International Ozone Association.)

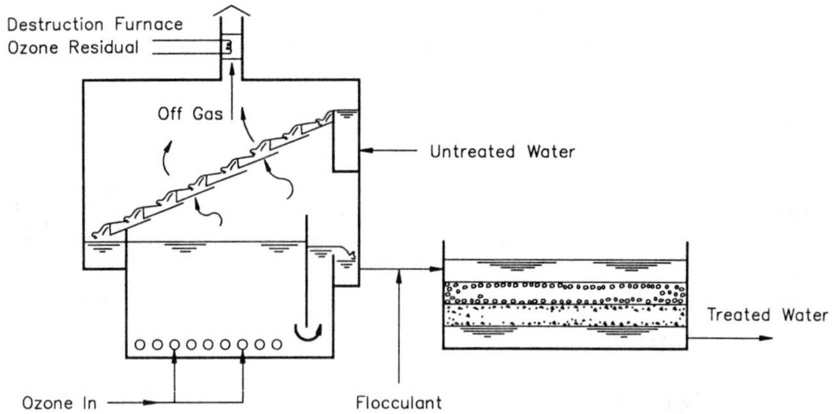

FIGURE 7–12. Off-gas recycle system B. (From Ref. 54. Reprinted by permission of International Ozone Association.)

tacting, in contrast to turbine systems that provide mixing without baffling.

Turbine systems are thought to achieve higher ozone transfer efficiencies and may be well suited to achieving oxidation goals, especially when disinfection contact times are not the primary consideration. Many of these reactions are quite rapid, thereby reducing the emphasis on contact time for these particular applications. Even in the case of disinfection applications, turbine mix systems may offer some advantages that could offset the added volume required for CT criteria. For example, porous

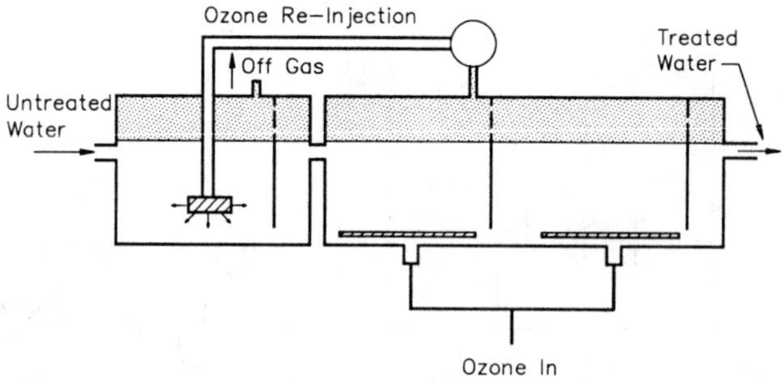

FIGURE 7–13. Three-stage ozone contactor with aspirating turbines and porous diffusion using off-gas recycle. (Reprinted from *Ozone System Design Manual,* by permission of Hankin Atlas Ozone Systems Inc.)

diffusers require a clean feed gas stream and are extremely prone to plugging, especially when used in pretreatment and in stop-start modes, or where encrustation by manganese, iron, carbonate, and other precipitates might occur. In addition, high pressure drops often can occur across plugged porous diffusers, exacerbating problems with air entrainment that can cause a slow degassing reminiscent of dissolved air flotation processes. Although this feature may be used to some advantage when ozonation systems are intentionally modified to achieve flotation for turbidity or algae removal, it can create problems with foam formation (28) and with possible air binding of filters (17).

Ozone injection contactors, including static mix and U-tube systems, are relatively new so that experiences are more limited. However, these systems may provide some advantages in terms of transfer efficiency and plug flow character where CT credit is desirable. Moreover, these systems are not subject to the clogging problems encountered with the use of diffusers (28). Problems may exist with some ozone injector systems where high water pressures (e.g., U-tubes) encountered at the bottom of deep contactors may exacerbate degassing conditions in downstream filters.

Ozone Destructors

Since contactor transfer efficiencies are always less than 100 percent and ozone usually cannot safely be vented to the atmosphere, an ozone destruction system is most often required. Standby equipment should be provided to ensure continuous protection. An exhaust stack may also be required to vent off gases at a safe elevation within the plant in the event that some ozone escapes the destruction system through faulty operation.

Destructors typically function either by using a thermal or a combined thermal/catalytic device to yield less than 0.1 percent ozone by volume in the discharge. The trend has been toward the use of newer thermal/catalytic destruct systems in the United States, although thermal systems have proved to be effective as well. Thermal systems alone have been favored in European applications where some chlorinated organic contaminants have been thought to poison catalysts in cases where the water supply contains significant VOCs.

The use of an exhaust fan allows the contactor to operate under a vacuum (1 to 3 inches of water column), which ensures that no ozone leaks out of the contactor into the building. If the fan is placed upstream of the destructor, it has to be constructed of ozone-resistant materials, listed in the following section.

Materials of Construction

Because ozone is corrosive and toxic and, as a gas, is prone to leakage, the selection of materials and joint/gasket systems is critical. Satisfactory materials for ozone gas systems are glass, 316L stainless steel, Hypalon, Viton, and Teflon. 304L stainless steel also can be considered for piping to convey a dry gas. Carbon steel and galvanized steel piping; rubber, nylon, and many elastomer gaskets; and aluminum are especially vulnerable to ozone attack. Experience has also shown that threaded joints are almost impossible to seal, even in stainless steel piping; therefore, all joints should be welded or flanged. It is also important to avoid the use of equipment components with rubber gaskets and threaded joints, especially where instruments are installed. Selection of materials is less critical for the air preparation system, although PVC piping is vulnerable to both vibration and the high-temperature conditions which occur.

Ozone is most corrosive in the presence of water or moisture, leading to special problems with destructor systems and contactors. High-density concrete and extra cover over reinforcing steel are measures that have been used in various installations in the United States. There seems to be less concern over the corrosion potential in Europe. A sealant for concrete joints should be chosen with care, since they may be subject to ozone attack especially at the top of contactors, where ozone gas is present. Some designers incorporate epoxy or PVC-coated reinforcing steel and Hypalon or stainless steel water stops in concrete construction. These measures can be costly and need to be evaluated for each case.

Ozone Measurement

Instrumentation should include an ambient monitor/alarm installed in the ozone generator room and any other enclosed areas with a potential for ozone leaks. On-line instruments can be considered for monitoring generator output. While these instruments, which measure ozone concentration in a gas phase, are generally effective and reliable, on-line instruments for measuring the ozone concentration in water have not been entirely satisfactory. A survey of analytical methods for residual measurements that pays special attention to interferences has been published (16). Although the accuracy and reliability of liquid phase ozone measurement instruments is still improving and may ultimately be satisfactory for process control, problems still persist with this method of monitoring. In fact, EPA criteria specify that compliance with the C component of CT criteria should be based on the Indigo Trisulfonate method, a wet chemical technique (47).

At present, instrument-based process control is usually achieved with gas phase monitors placed in the ozone supply stream and in the off-gas stream. Excessive or insufficient ozone concentration in the off-gas may be a general indicator of an excessive or insufficient ozone dose, respectively, assuming that the contactor transfer efficiency remains relatively constant. It also may be possible to correlate off-gas concentrations with liquid concentrations. However, note that where foam is generated in an ozone contactor, foam carried in the off-gas can interfere with the accuracy of measurements.

Electrical Requirements

Electrical requirements for operation of all equipment items associated with ozone generation is an extremely important aspect of system planning. Typical electrical requirements for air-based systems (including power required for gas preparation and operation of generators) are in the range of 10 to 12 kwh/lb of ozone generated at the rated system capacity. However, somewhat higher levels of use per pound (12 to 14 kwh/lb of ozone generated) may be encountered under average conditions where the generator is being operated at less than the rated capacity. Electrical requirements for oxygen-based systems will depend on the type of oxygen equipment. For example, generation from LOX might be accomplished at 5 to 8 kwh/lb of ozone, whereas a greater energy input will be required for systems that employ on-site generation of oxygen.

A major consideration in ozone system design is the need for electrical reliability in the event of a power failure. This will depend on overall plant reliability concepts and needs. In situations where finished water storage or availability of alternative finished water sources is limited, a high level of reliability may be necessary to ensure continuous supply. This will add somewhat to overall plant costs by requiring either a second electrical feed or standby electrical generation systems.

The time required to change over to a secondary electrical supply is a consideration in the design of operation protocols for ozone under standby electrical conditions. Unless the time required to convert to the secondary electrical supply can be very short, a restart of an ozone system may require a specified sequence of steps beginning with the gas preparation system. Therefore, some plant downtime may need to be considered for this type of occurrence.

One possible alternative to standby power capability for ozonation is the use of chlorine as a short-term emergency backup disinfection system. This may be an economical approach, since chlorine may already be available to meet secondary disinfection requirements with either free chlorine or chloramines. This alternative will require adequate tankage to meet chlorine-contacting requirements for primary disinfection along with possible permission for short-term exposure to chlorinated disinfection byproducts by regulatory authorities. Health concerns for chlorinated disinfection byproducts are generally related to chronic exposure, thereby providing a rationale that would allow short-term use.

TYPICAL PLANT REQUIREMENTS

The principal capital costs of ozonation installations include those for air preparation equipment, ozone generation, ozone contacting, ozone destruction, instrumentation and controls, housing/ventilation for equipment, equipment installation, and site requirements. To these costs must be added the cost for provision of an added electrical feed and costs for a cooling water system.

Specific monitoring needs will vary depending on the feed gas preparation system but will generally include temperature, pressure, and dew-point monitors as required for operation and maintenance decisions. As a minimum, monitoring equipment should also include the following:

1. Dew-point monitor of the air from the preparation equipment
2. Ozone output and gas flow rate from the generators
3. Ozone concentration in the plant ambient air
4. Ozone concentration in waste air after destructor

An ozone monitor/control capability might also be considered for the off-gas leaving the contactor. This type of system has potential applicability for control of oxidation reactions and as an indicator of ozone concentrations in the contactor. As discussed in the section Ozone Measurement, except where foam is a problem, equipment for off-gas monitoring of ozone is more reliable than equipment for monitoring ozone in the liquid stream.

The size and number of contactor stages can vary, as has been discussed. Ozone contact chambers are usually constructed of concrete or stainless steel. Some small installations use fiberglass-reinforced plastic or PVC contacting columns. Although these materials offer a low initial cost compared with stainless steel, more frequent replacement may be required. Therefore, the total life-cycle cost should be evaluated before making material selections.

Special and separate ventilation of the ozone area is important, with provisions for venting away from other HVAC intakes. In addition, some contacting systems may become slightly pressurized, requiring special pressure/vacuum relief valves.

Operating costs for ozonation systems vary and depend upon a number of factors such as these:

1. Whether air or oxygen is used as the feed gas source
2. Method of air preparation
3. Method of cooling the generator
4. Method for chilling of cooling water, if required
5. Method of contacting
6. Dosage of ozone required
7. Method of contactor off-gas destruction

Air preparation systems contain filters, which must be replaced regularly. Tube type ozone generators normally are shutdown once a year for cleaning and replacement of glass tubes, and for other general maintenance. The number of tubes to be replaced depends upon the quality of air supplied to the ozone generator and, most importantly, how they are handled to avoid breakage during cleaning and replacement.

Electrical energy is a major component of operating costs. When these cost evaluations are made, it should be noted that average efficiency is usually lower than the efficiency at the rated capacity for ozone generation. These effects need to be considered when operation costs for life-cycle evaluation are developed.

References

1. Aieta, E. M., B. M. Chow, A. Adamson, S. Liang, and D. Ferguson, 1990. The effects of ammonia, chloramines, and bromide on T&O oxidation and disinfection byproducts formation with ozone and PEROXONE. Presented at 1990 AWWA Conference, Cincinnati, OH, June 1990.
2. *Final report: In-Line ozone dissolution study: City of Long Beach, California.* Prepared by CH_2M-Hill, January 1990.
3. Anselme, C, I. H. Suffet, and J. Mallevialle. 1988. Effects of ozone on tastes and odors. *JAWWA* 80:(10) 45–51.
4. ASCE/AWWA. 1990. *Water treatment plant design,* 2nd ed. New York: McGraw-Hill.
5. Bader, H., and J. Hoigne. 1984. Determination of ozone in water by the indigo method: A submitted standard method. *Ozone Sci. Eng. 4: 169–176.*
6. Beaudet, B. A., and T. O. Mardam. 1988. Ozone pilot study at Palm Beach County water utilities department. Presented at Annual Meeting of Florida Section AWWA.
7. Bourbigot, M. M. 1990. Update on ozone applications in Europe. Presented at 1990 AWWA Conference, Cincinnati, OH, June 1990.

8. Chang, S. D., and P. C. Singer. 1988. The impact of ozone on the removal of particles, total organic carbon, and trihalomethane precursor. Presented at 1988 AWWA Conference, Orlando, FL, June 1988, pp. 1325–42.
9. Daniel, P., P. Meyerhofer, A. Lai, M. Lanier, J. March and Y. Board. 1990. Using ozone to meet conflicting water quality goals. Presented at 1990 AWWA Conference, Cincinnati, OH, June 1990.
10. Dimitriou, M. A., and E. Ivanco. 1989. The Myrtle Beach ozone system and water treatment plant. In *Ozone in water treatment,* Vol. 1: *Proceedings of Ninth Ozone World Congress,* Bollyky, L. J., ed. Norwalk, CT: International Ozone Association, Pan American Committee.
11. Environmental Science and Engineering Inc. 1981. Fort Lauderdale water quality and treatment study. Prepared for Malcolm Pirnie Engineers Inc., June 1981.
12. Farhataziz, and A. B. Ross. 1977. Selective specific rates of reaction of transients in water and aqueous solutions: Part 3—Hydroxyl radical and perhydroxyl radical and their radical ion. Washington, DC: National Bureau Reference Data Service, U.S. National Bureau of Standards.
13. Ferguson, D. W., M. J. McGuire, B. Koch, R. L. Wolfe, and E. M. Aieta. 1990. Comparing PEROXONE and ozone for controlling taste and odor compounds, disinfection by-products, and microorganisms. *JAWWA* 82:(4) 181–91.
14. Fung, L. C., R. A. Hensch, and B. J. Schwartz. 1989. Hackensack Water Company—Ozone: From pilot to design to operation. Presented at seminar *Impact of Changing Disinfectants,* 1989 AWWA Conference, Los Angeles, CA, June 1989.
15. Glaze, W. H., M. Koga, D. Cancilla, K. Wang, M. J. McGuire, S. Liang, J. K. Davis, C. H. Tate, and E. M. Aieta. 1989. Evaluation of ozonation by-products from 2 California surface waters. *JAWWA* 81:(8) 66–73.
16. Gordon, G., W. J. Cooper, R. G. Rice, and G. E. Pacey. 1987. *A survey of the current status of residual disinfectant measurement methods for all chlorine species and ozone*. Report for AWWA Research Foundation, Denver, CO, November 1987.
17. Gramith, J. T., D. W. Ferguson, M. J. McGuire, and C. H. Tate. 1990. Overview of Metropolitan's ozone/PEROXONE demonstration project. Presented at 1990 AWWA Conference, Cincinnati, OH, June 1990.
18. Grunwell, J., J. Benga, H. Cohen, and G. Gordon. 1983. A detailed comparison of analytical methods for residual ozone measurement. *Ozone Sci. Eng.* 5: 203–23.
19. van Hoof, F., J. G. Janssens, and H. van Dijck. 1986. Formation of oxidation byproducts in surface water preozonation and their behavior in water treatment. *Water Supply* 4: 93–102.
20. Hoffman, J, and D. Eichelsdorfer. 1971. On the action of ozone or pesticides with chlorinated hydrocarbon groups in water. *Wasser* 38: 197–206.
21. Hoigne, J., and H. Bader. 1976. Role of hydroxyl radical reactions in ozonation processes in aqueous solution. *Water Res.* 10: 377.
22. Ishizaki, K., R. A. Dobbs, and J. M. Cohen. 1978. Ozonation of hazardous and toxic organic compounds in aqueous solution. In *Ozone/Chlorine dioxide*

products of organic materials, Rice, R. G., and Coltruvo, J. A., eds. Norwalk, CT: International Ozone Association.

23. Jacangelo, J. G., N. L. Patania, K. M. Reagan, E. M. Aieta, S. N. Krasner, and M. J. McGuire. 1989. Ozonation: Assessing its role in the formation and control of disinfection by-products. *JAWWA* 81:(8) 74–84.
24. Knocke, W. R., E. Van Benschoten, M. Kearney, A. Soberski, and D. A. Reckhow. 1990. *Alternative oxidants for the removal of soluble iron and manganese*. Report for AWWA Research Foundation, Denver, CO, March 1990.
25. Kool, H. J., C. F. van Kreijl, and J. Hrubec. 1985. Mutagenic and carcinogenic properties of drinking water. In *Water chlorination: Chemistry, environmental impact and health effects,* Vol. 5, Jolley, R. L., et al., eds. Chelsea, MI: Lewis Publishers, Inc.
26. Laplanche, A., G. Martin, and F. Tonnard. 1983. Ozonation schemes of organophosphorus pesticides, application in drinking water treatment. Proceedings of the Sixth Ozone World Congress, International Ozone Association, Norwalk, CT, pp. 94–95.
27. Lykins, B. W., W. Koffskey, and R. G. Miller. 1986. Chemical products and toxicological effects of disinfection. *JAWWA* 78:(11) 66–75.
28. Masschelein, W. J. 1990. Overview of ozone installations in Europe. Presented at preconference seminar: *Practical experiences with ozone for organics control and disinfection,* 1990 AWWA Conference, Cincinnati, OH, June 1990.
29. McGuire, M. J., and M. K. Davis. 1988. Treating water with peroxone: A revolution in the making. *Water Eng. Manage.* 135: 42–9.
30. McGuire, M. J., D. W. Ferguson, and J. T. Gramith. 1990. Overview of ozone technology for organics control and disinfection. Presented at preconference seminar: *Practical experiences with ozone for organics control and disinfection,* 1990 AWWA Conference, Cincinnati, OH, June 1990.
31. McGuire, M. J., and J. M. Gaston. 1988. Overview of technology for controlling off-flavors in drinking water. *Waterworld News* 4(3): 18–21.
32. National Academy of Science. 1987. *Drinking water and health,* Vol. 7: *Disinfection and disinfectant by-products.* Washington, DC: National Academy Press.
33. Noot, D. K., W. B. Anderson, S. A. Diagnault, D. T. Williams, and P. M. Huck. 1989. Evaluating treatment processes with the Ames mutagenicity assay. *JAWWA* 81:(9) 81–102.
34. Paillard, H., B. Legube, M. M. Bourbigot, and E. Lefebvre. 1989. Iron and manganese removal with ozonation in the presence of humic substances. *Ozone Sci. Eng.* 11: 93.
35. Duguet, J. P., A. Bruchet, B. Dussert, and J. Mallevialle. 1989. Formation of aromatic polymers during the ozonation or enzymatic oxidation of waters containing phenolic compounds. In *Biohazards of drinking water treatment,* Larson, R. A., ed. Chelsea, MI: Lewis Publishers, Inc.
36. Rachwal, A. J., M. Bauer, and M. Chipps. 1987. Ozone's role in biological filtration processes. Presented at Second International Conference on Role of Ozone in Water and Wastewater Treatment, Edmonton, Alberta.

37. Reckhow, D.A., and P. C. Singer. 1985. Mechanisms of organic halide formation during fulvic acid chlorination and implications with respect to preozonation. In *Water chlorination: Chemistry, environmental impact and health effects,* Vol. 5, Jolley, R. L., et al., eds. Chelsea, MI: Lewis Publishers, Inc.
38. Reckhow, D. A., P. C. Singer, and R. R. Trussell. 1986. Ozone as a coagulant aid. Presented at conference seminar *Ozonation recent advances in research needs,* 1986 AWWA Conference, Denver, CO, 1986.
39. Rice, R. G. 1989. Ozone oxidation products—Implications for drinking water treatment. In *Biohazards of drinking water treatment,* Larson, R. A., ed. Chelsea, MI: Lewis Publishers, Inc.
40. Rice, R. G. 1987. Emerging technologies for compliance with disinfection and disinfection by-products regulations. Presented at EPA Workshops on Emerging Technologies for Drinking Water Treatment, 1987–1988.
41. Riley, T. L., K. H. Mancy, and E. A. Boettner. 1979. The effect of preozonation on chloroform production in the chlorine disinfection process. In *Water chlorination: environmental impact and health effects,* Vol. 2, Jolley, R. L., et al., eds. Ann Arbor, MI: Ann Arbor Science Publishers.
42. Schalekamp, M. 1978. Experience in Switzerland with ozone, particularly in connection with the change of undesirable elements present in water. Presented at Ozone Technology Symposium and Exposition of International Ozone Institute, Los Angeles, CA.
43. White, G. C. 1986. *Handbook of chlorination,* 2nd ed. New York: Van Nostrand Reinhold.
44. Sontheimer, H. 1985. Trends in ozonation roundtable discussion. *JAWWA* 77:(8) 30.
45. Staehlin, J., and J. Hoigne. 1987. Decomposition of ozone in water: Rate initiation by hydroxide ions and hydrogen peroxide. *Environ. Sci. & Tech.* 21: 229–30.
46. U.S. EPA. 1986. *Design manual, municipal wastewater disinfection.* EPA/625/1–86/021. Cincinnati, OH: U.S. EPA Office of Research and Development.
47. U.S. EPA. 1989. *Guidance manual for compliance with the filtration and disinfection requirements for public water systems using surface water sources.* EPA 68–01–6989. Washington, DC: U.S. Environmental Protection Agency, Office of Drinking Water.
48. U.S. EPA. 1989. Discussion of Strawman rule for disinfectants and disinfection by-products. Science Advisory Board Drinking Water Committee, meeting of October 11, 1989, Washington, DC.
49. van Hoof, F., J. G. Janssens, and H. van Dijck. 1985. Formation of mutagenic activity during surface water preozonation and its removal in drinking water treatment. *Chemosphere* 14: 501–10.
50. Weissenhorn, F. J. 1984. Removal of iron and manganese by ozone during drinking water treatment in Düsseldorf. In *Handbook of ozone technology and applications,* Vol II: *Ozone for drinking water treatment,* Rice, R. G., and Netzer, A., eds. Stoneham, MA: Butterworth Publishers.

51. Weng, C., D. L. Hoven, and B. J. Schwartz. 1986. Ozonation: An economic choice for water treatment. *JAWWA* 78:(11) 83–9.
52. White, G. C. 1986. *Handbook of chlorination,* 2nd ed., pp. 930–3. New York: Van Nostrand Reinhold.
53. Farvardin, M. R., and A. G. Collins. 1990. Mechanism(s) of ozone-induced coagulation of organic colloids. Presented at 1990 AWWA Conference, Cincinnati, OH, June 1990.
54. Richard, Y., and P. Blue. 1978. Ozone pretreatment of drinking water. International Ozone Institute, Ozone Technology Symposium, Los Angeles, May 1978.
55. Robson, C. M. 1987. Engineering aspects of ozonation. *Waterworld News* 3: 18–24.
56. Rulla, T. A. 1990. Demonstration project for groundwater VOC removal using ozone and hydrogen peroxide in North Hollywood, California. AWWA Seminar Proceedings: *Practical experiences with ozone for organic control and disinfection,* pp. 197–210, Cincinatti, OH.
57. Robson, C. M., E. G. Fujikawa, and B. T. Farver. 1990. Ozonation facility design: Consideration and experience. AWWA Seminar Proceedings: *Practical experiences with ozone for organic control and disinfection,* 1990 AWWA Conference, Cincinnati, OH.
58. Bablon, G., et al. 1991. Fundamental aspects. In *Ozone in water treatment: Application and engineering*, Langlais, B., et al., eds. Chelsea, MI: Lewis Publishers, Inc.
59. Huck, P. M., et al. 1990. Formation and removal of selected aldehydes in a biological drinking water process. *Aqua* 39(5).
60. McGuire, M. J., D. W. Ferguson, and J. T. Gramith. 1990. Overview of ozone technology for organics control and disinfection. Presented at seminar *Practical experiences with ozone for organics control and disinfection,* 1990 AWWA Conference, Cincinnati, OH, June 1990.
61. Miltner, R. V., E. W. Rice, and A. A. Stevens. 1990. Pilot-scale investigation of the formation and control of disinfection byproducts. Internal Report, U.S. EPA Drinking Water Research Division, Cincinnati, OH.
62. van Hoof, F., J. G. Janssens, and H. van Dijck. 1986. Formation of oxidation byproducts in surface water preozonation and their behavior in water treatment. *Water Supply* 4: 93–102.
63. Glaze, W. H. 1990. Overview of analytical methods for measuring disinfection byproducts. Presented at AWWA Water Quality Technology Conference, San Diego, CA, November 1990.
64. Bellamy, W. D., et al. 1991. Engineering aspects. In *Ozone in water treatment: Application and engineering,* Langlais, B., et al., eds. Chelsea, MI: Lewis Publishers, Inc.
65. Haag, W. R., and J. Hoigne. 1983. Ozonation of bromide-containing water: Kinetics of formation of hypobromous acid and bromate. *Environ. Sci. & Tech.* 17: 261–7.
66. Anderson, L. V., J. D. Johnson, R. F. Christman. 1986. Extent of ozone's reaction with isolated aquatic humic acid. *Environ. Sci. & Tech.* 20: 739–42.

67. Staehlin, J., and J. Hoigne. 1985. Decomposition of ozone in water in the presence of organic solutes acting as promoters and inhibitors of radical chain reactions. *Environ. Sci. & Tech.* 19: 1206–12.
68. Yamada, H., I. Somiya, and F. Inanami. 1986. The effect of preozonation on the control of trihalomethane formation. *Ozone Sci. Eng.* 8: 129–50.
69. Prevost, M. O., et al. 1990. Chlorine demand removal by biological activated carbon filtration in cold water. AWWA Water Quality Technology Conference Proceedings, pp. 407–28, San Diego, CA, November 1990.
70. Wallis, P., et al. 1990. Ozonation of *Giardia* cysts in high turbidity water. *AWWA,* Water Quality Technology Conference Proceedings, pp. 805–22, San Diego, CA, November 1990.
71. Sclimenti, M. J., S. W. Krasner, and W. H. Glaze. 1990. Ozone disinfection by-products: Optimization of PFBOA derivitization method for the analysis of aldehydes. AWWA Water Quality Technology Conference Proceedings, pp. 477–501, San Diego, CA, November 1990.
72. Glaze, W. H. et al. 1991. Trends in aldehyde formation and removal through plants using ozonation and biological activated carbon filters. Presented at 1991 AWWA Conference, Philadelphia, PA, June 1991.
73. Reckhow, D. A. et al. 1986. The ozonation of organic halide precursors: Effect of bicarbonate. *Water Res.* 20: 987.
74. Bablon, G., et al., 1991. Practical application of ozone. In *Ozone in water treatment: Application and engineering,* Langlais, et al., eds. Chelsea, MI: Lewis Publishers, Inc.
75. Reckhow, D. A., B. Legube, and P. C. Singer. 1986. The ozonation of organic halide precursors: Effect of bicarbonate. *Water Res.* 20: 987.
76. Amy, G. L., and M. S. Siddiqui. 1991. Bromide-oxidant interactions in water treatment. Presented at 1991 AWWA Conference, Philadelphia, PA, June 1991.
77. Rice, R. G., C. M. Robson, G. W. Miller, and A. G. Hill. 1981. Uses of ozone in drinking water. *JAWWA* 73: 44–56.
78. Edwards, M., and M. M. Benjamin. 1991. A mechanistic study of ozone-induced particle destabilization. *JAWWA* 83:(6) 96–105.

8

Potassium Permanganate

Kenneth J. Ficek
and
Arnold H. Reidies
Carus Chemical Co.

INTRODUCTION

Potassium permanganate is a widely used chemical oxidizing agent throughout the water industry. While it is generally not considered for a disinfecting role, it can still have an important effect on the development of a disinfecting strategy by serving as an alternative to chlorine or other disinfecting chemicals at locations in a plant where chemical oxidation is a primary goal. The purpose of this chapter is to review the theory and practice of using potassium permanganate in water treatment for oxidation-related removal of iron and manganese, elimination of tastes and odors, and control of disinfection byproducts (DBPs). A potential role for disinfection goals also is presented. Essential facts about potassium permanganate are discussed along with the primary and secondary uses for this chemical in current water treatment practice.

Potassium permanganate was originally introduced in Europe as a new disinfectant in 1862. It proved to be an immediate success, and by 1873, potassium permanganate had become a popular all-purpose disinfectant. Its effectiveness had been established in the control of epidemics of cholera in that early period of disinfection history. Not only was potassium permanganate used in hospitals and public comfort stations, but it was also accepted as a common household disinfectant (7). Potassium permanganate was gradually superseded as a general disinfectant by other chemical substances, notably chlorine. Its use was continued, however, for specific disinfection applications in both human and veterinary medicine.

Since that time, the use of potassium permanganate has increased in drinking water treatment but not for disinfection applications. As a strong oxidant, potassium permanganate is used in a primary role to control tastes and odors, to remove color, to control biological growth in treatment plants and to affect the reduction of iron and manganese content. In a secondary role, potassium permanganate may also be useful in controlling THM formation by the oxidation of precursors and in reducing demand for other disinfectants, thereby minimizing the formation of byproducts by other agents.

PROPERTIES OF POTASSIUM PERMANGANATE

Commercial Forms

Potassium permanganate is commercially available in crystalline form in a variety of grades and package sizes, as shown in Table 8–1. Because potassium permanganate is a strong oxidant, Department of Transportation regulations require that containers have warning labels marked *oxidizer*. A *corrosive* label is also recommended. Precautions for storage, handling, and use of potassium permanganate are printed on product labels and are also described in technical literature and in material safety data sheets prepared by manufacturers (6).

Physical Properties

Potassium permanganate ($KMnO_4$) occurs in the form of deep purple, almost black, crystals, which can have a blue metallic luster under re-

TABLE 8–1. Available Forms of Potassium Permanganate

Grade	Assay-Guaranteed % $KMnO_4$	Metal Container Package Sizes	Remarks
Technical	98	25 kg, 50 kg, 150 kg	
Free-flowing	97	As above plus bulk	Contains anticaking
Additives			
USP	99	50 kg	Available in different particle sizes
Reagent	99	50 kg	

TABLE 8–2. Solubility of Potassium Permanganate in Water

Temperature		Solubility	
°C	°F	%	g/l
0	31	2.8	28
20	68	6.5	65
40	104	12.5	125
60	140	23.0	230

flected light. Depending on the method of crystallization used in its manufacture, the crystals can either be needles (rhombic prisms) or somewhat irregularly shaped spheres. The density of potassium permanganate is 2.073 g/cm^3. Depending on the degree of compaction when delivered, the bulk density is about 100 lb/ft^3 or approximately 1,600 kg/m^3.

The solubility of $KMnO_4$ in water is strongly temperature dependent, as illustrated in Table 8–2. The dissolution rate depends not only on temperature but also on particle size, agitation, and the concentration of other salts already in solution. In the actual preparation of $KMnO_4$ solutions, elevated temperatures, small particle sizes, and vigorous agitation will reduce the time of dissolution.

Pure potassium permanganate is nonhygroscopic, but in technical and related grades individual crystals have a tendency to cake together, especially under high-humidity conditions. Therefore, the free-flowing grade (which contains an anticaking additive) should be used where flowability is important.

Chemical Properties

Potassium permanganate is highly reactive, particularly in the dissolved state, and nearly all of the chemical reactions are exothermic (release heat). Except under very acidic and very alkaline conditions, oxidations entail the reduction of heptavalent manganese (+7 oxidation state) found in potassium permanganate to a +4 oxidation state found in hydrous manganese dioxide (MnO_2), which forms a precipitate.

In the pH range of 4 to 9, permanganate oxidizes a wide variety of inorganic and organic substances. Under acidic conditions, the reaction is as follows:

$$MnO_4^- + 4H^+ + 3e^- = MnO_2 + 2H_2O \tag{8–1}$$

Under alkaline conditions, the reaction is as follows:

$$MnO_4^- + 2H_2O + 3e^- = MnO_2 + 4OH^- \quad (8\text{–}2)$$

Most oxidation reactions with organic materials occur faster under alkaline than under acid conditions because alkaline conditions favor formation of organic anions. Permanganate will oxidize many organic anions more readily than neutral molecules. Under normal raw water treatment conditions, which are most often only slightly acidic, most contaminants that cause tastes and odors, such as phenols and algae, are readily degraded by permanganate, and iron and manganese are oxidized and precipitated. If shorter reaction times are required because of specific plant design, raising the pH can increase the rate of the oxidation reaction and improve the coagulation of the manganese dioxide. Some of these reactions, for example, the oxidation of aldehydes, may consume alkalinity. This depletion should be taken into account when permanganate treatment is used with alum coagulation, which also requires alkalinity to form precipitates. More information on the reactive behavior, health, safety, and environmental aspects of potassium permanganate can be found in the *Encyclopedia of Chemical Technology* (37).

Biocidal Effects

The biocidal effects of potassium permanganate are largely attributed to direct oxidative degradation of cell material or specific enzyme destruction (32). In this fashion, the permanganate ion attacks a wide range of microorganisms: bacteria, fungi, viruses, and algae. The severity of the attack is determined by permanganate concentration, time, temperature, pH condition, the presence of other oxidizable matter, and the specific susceptibility of a particular microorganism to permanganate deactivation.

Although alkaline conditions generally enhance the capability of potassium permanganate to oxidize organic matter, the opposite holds true for its disinfecting power; $KMnO_4$ is generally a better biocide under acidic than under alkaline conditions (9, 31).

Manganese Dioxide as Coprecipitant for Microorganisms

As shown in Equations 8–1 and 8–2, the application of $KMnO_4$ results in the precipitation of manganese dioxide (MnO_2). MnO_2 contains chemically bound water and has a polymeric structure. In colloidal form, a hydrous MnO_2 particle has an outer layer of exposed OH groups capable of adsorbing charged species/particles as well as neutral molecules (25).

As MnO_2 colloids coagulate they can coprecipitate any adsorbed matter. This action can include microorganisms, so that coprecipitation by manganese dioxide represents an additional mechanism for the removal of microorganisms from water (9).

NONDISINFECTION USES OF POTASSIUM PERMANGANATE IN DRINKING WATER TREATMENT

Taste and Odor Control

One use of potassium permanganate is to oxidize contaminants that cause tastes and odors in surface water supplies. Most of these contaminants originate from algae—either from their metabolism or their decay. Other contaminants are the result of industrial and municipal waste discharges and decaying biological matter such as aquatic plants and fish. As with other methods, varying degrees of success have been reported depending on reactivity with specific taste and odor compounds. Even where direct oxidation does not occur, removal can sometimes be achieved by adsorption onto MnO_2 precipitates as they are formed (38). Applicability for specific tastes and odors needs to be confirmed based on testing.

In most cases, the destruction of organic contaminants requires reaction times ranging from a few minutes to several hours. Dosage rates can vary from less than 1 mg/l to about 5 mg/l. Customarily, the dosages range between 0.5 and 2.5 mg/l. Potassium permanganate is normally added at the intake to treatment plants to provide maximum time for oxidation. Where this is not possible, it is frequently added ahead of the rapid mix.

In the early 1960s, Cedar Rapids, Iowa, encountered a severe taste and odor problem caused by decaying algae and actinomycetes in the raw water (8). The problem was solved, first by the application of $KMnO_4$ at the intake at an average dose rate of 5 mg/l during the peak of the problem, and later at an average rate of 3.2 mg/l plus addition of an average dose of activated carbon of 5.3 mg/l before the secondary mixers.

To reduce the formation of chlorinated organics, chlorine is preferentially fed after $KMnO_4$ has been added. Hydrous manganese dioxide, generated in reaction, is removed by filtration (11). Examples of plants that have benefited from this practice are St. Joseph, Missouri; Davenport, Iowa; and Fairfax, Virginia, all discussed later in this chapter.

Removal of Iron and Manganese

The application of $KMnO_4$ for iron and manganese removal involves oxidation of the dissolved divalent species of iron (Fe^{2+}) and manganese (Mn^{2+}) to their tri- (Fe^{3+}) and tetravalent (Mn^{4+}) states, respectively. Precipitation of the oxide and hydroxide forms of iron and manganese enables removal by sedimentation and filtration. Theoretical doses for precipitation are 0.94 mg of potassium permanganate per mg of iron, and 1.92 mg of potassium permanganate per mg of manganese. Other demand-causing substances will result in somewhat higher doses than these theoretical ratios (39). Permanganate is also capable of oxidizing (and precipitating) organically bound iron. Manganese, not thought to be organically bound in this case, may involve competitive demand for oxidation between manganese and actual organic substances in source water (39).

In iron and manganese removal, the chemical condition at the point of introduction of permanganate is not as critical as in taste and odor control because at pH values above 7 the oxidation of Fe^{2+} and Mn^{2+} occurs almost instantly, and at pH 6 and 5 it takes about 5 and 15 minutes, respectively. However, selection of location and determination of applicability can be affected by variation in oxidation potential throughout a plant and possibility for resolubilization of manganese in particular. These features of manganese removal are discussed in Chapters 4 through 7.

In general, permanganate is added ahead of coagulation since the precipitate, MnO_2, can be colloidal and may need to be coagulated. At the normal coagulation pH ranges, MnO_2 particles are negatively charged and are capable of sorbing inorganics and organics (11). These particles may also aid in coagulation. Filtration systems employed for iron and manganese removal sometimes use greensand regenerated with a continuous feed of $KMnO_4$ (11).

Disinfection Byproducts

Pretreatment with potassium permanganate in combination with the relocation of the point of chlorination will generally result in lower DBP values than are obtained with traditional prechlorination (13, 28) for achieving oxidation (33). Under this approach, potassium permanganate serves as a substitute oxidant, allowing a reduction in chlorine use within the plant. $KMnO_4$ also can sometimes reduce the DBP precursor concentration to some extent. However, performance results have varied, thereby requiring site-specific testing. In most cases, DBP control is combined with iron and manganese removal or taste and odor control in a multipurpose application.

Algae Control in Raw Water Reservoirs and Filtration Basins

Currently, there is no EPA registration for potassium permanganate as an algicide, but $KMnO_4$ has been used to control problem algae that cause tastes and odors, as well as those that clog filters (14). Field applications of permanganate directly to raw water reservoirs and basins for the purpose of discouraging algae growth have been reported (12, 17). Potassium permanganate has also been successfully applied (as an alternative to treatment with chlorine) to control biofouling in an aqueduct (33).

BACTERIAL DISINFECTION CAPABILITY

A number of investigations of the relative capability of potassium permanganate as a disinfectant have been recorded. In four studies presented in this discussion, high dosage rates of potassium permanganate were required to accomplish nearly complete kill of bacteria.

Water from the Marne River in France was dosed with potassium permanganate at rates from 0 to 2.47 mg/l (18). After thorough mixing, the samples were kept for 2 hours at a constant temperature of 19.8°C in a darkened room. Results obtained were as shown in Table 8–3. No data were reported for the overall quality of the water involved in this investigation.

Banerjea (1) investigated the effect of $KMnO_4$ on several waterborne pathogenic microorganisms, including cholera, typhus, and dysentery bacilli. The objective in this investigation was to establish the conditions required for the treatment of bacterially contaminated drinking water with potassium permanganate. The experiments indicated that $KMnO_4$ dosages of 20 mg/l and contact times of 24 hours were required to deactivate pathogens; however, the complete absence of typhoid or dysentery bacteria was not assured with such conditions.

A study involving *Escherichia coli* bacteria was performed in the early 1960s (9). *E. coli* was selected as the test organism since it is generally regarded as a good indicator of fecal contamination and can be easily cultured under laboratory conditions. Results indicate that permanganate caused some bacterial kills over a range of pH values and temperatures at various concentrations and contact times. However, only in a few cases

TABLE 8–3. Effect of $KMnO_4$ on *Coli* Bacteria in River Water

$KMnO_4$ Dosage (mg/l)	*Coli* Bacteria per Liter
0	9,000
0.5	1,800
1.0	500
2.5	0

Source: Adapted from Ref. 18.

were nearly complete kills attained. Hydrogen ion concentration proved the most influential factor, with more effective bactericidal action occurring at lower pH values (see Figure 8–1). This finding is consistent with earlier observations concerning the effects of pH on the performance of commercial antiseptics (3). Higher temperatures somewhat enhanced the bactericidal action. This study also showed that the presence of oxidizable organics in the water reduces the bactericidal effectiveness of the $KMnO_4$ applied, as some of the permanganate will be consumed in oxidation of the organics.

The suitability of potassium permanganate as a substitute disinfectant was investigated in a laboratory study at the Las Vegas Valley Water District/Southern Nevada System (20). Agitated raw water samples from Lake Mead (pH 8.3) were treated with 1, 2, 3, 4, 5, and 6 mg/l of $KMnO_4$

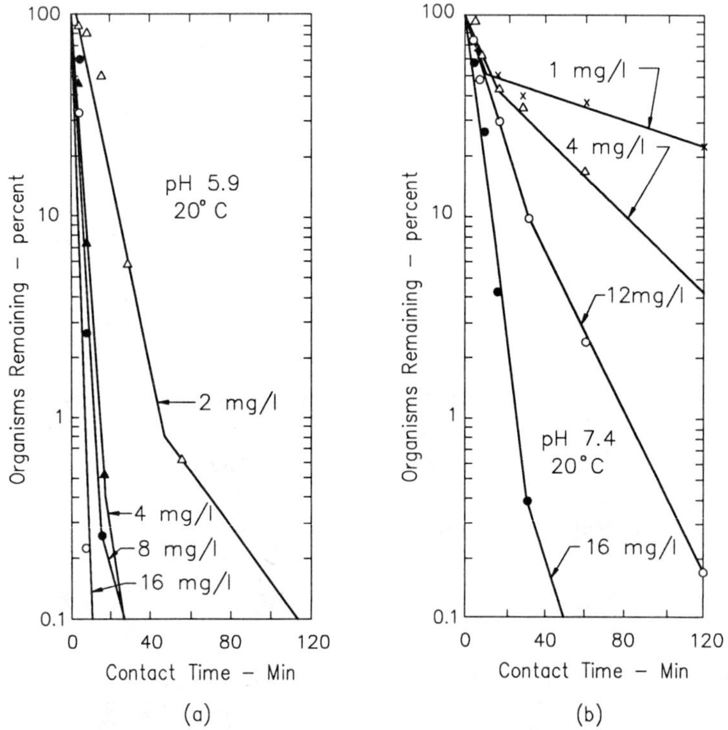

FIGURE 8–1. Influence of concentration on bactericidal effectiveness of potassium permanganate: (a) at pH 5.9; (b) at pH 7.4. (Reprinted from *Journal American Water Works*, Vol. 56 (April 1964), by permission. Copyright © 1964, American Water Works Association.)

at 15°C, using contact times of 30 minutes for dosages of 1 and 2 mg/l and 10 minutes for higher dosages. In all cases, complete kills of the coliforms were attained (raw water total coliform counts were reduced from 80–168/100 ml to less than detectable). Under the same conditions, noncoliforms showed survival rates of 0 to 1.1 percent. Based on this study, $KMnO_4$ at 4 mg/l is considered to be an effective disinfectant for coliforms and appears to be a satisfactory substitute disinfectant for Lake Mead water.

Legionella pneumophila is a bacterial pathogen responsible for Legionnaires' disease and Pontiac fever. A recent study at the University of Arizona indicates that potassium permanganate will inactivate *Legionella pneumophila* more rapidly at pH 6.0 than at pH 8.0. By exposure to 5 mg/l $KMnO_4$, more than 99 percent (2 log) reduction in bacterial numbers was achieved within 10 minutes at pH 6.0. Mean CT values for 99 percent reduction using $KMnO_4$ at pH 6.0 were 42.7 at 1.0 mg/l $KMnO_4$ and 41.9 at 5.0 mg/l $KMnO_4$ (35).

VIRAL DISINFECTION

Not all bactericides are necessarily active against viruses, but oxidizing agents are among the more effective virus deactivators (30). $KMnO_4$ is among a few substances that have proved at least partially effective against certain viruses (16).

Of interest are specific studies involving poliomyelitis virus (19, 23, 26) and influenza virus (2, 31). In one study, a large number of chemical agents with disinfecting properties were applied to a suspension of polio virus (strain MVA) at 37°C for 2 hours (26). The initial concentration of the disinfectant to be tested was adjusted in such a way that the viral suspension was exposed to 1 millimole of the agent. If deactivation occurred, the test was repeated with progressively lower concentrations. Of the 121 chemicals tested, 31 showed deactivation capabilities; but only 10 ($KMnO_4$ included) were effective at concentrations of 1000 mg/l or less. In the case of potassium permanganate, virus deactivation at pH 6.8 was found to occur at a concentration of 50 mg/l of $KMnO_4$.

Lund investigated the effects of temperature and pH on the deactivation process of polio virus (for types 1, 2, and 3) with potassium permanganate at concentration levels of 79 and 7.9 mg/l (19). He found that not only is oxidative deactivation enhanced by higher temperatures and lower pH, but spontaneous deactivation also takes place. This latter mechanism is favored at higher pH levels and higher temperatures, respectively. The investigation showed a definite functional relationship between inactivation rate and oxidation potential was found to exist at the test temperature of 37°C.

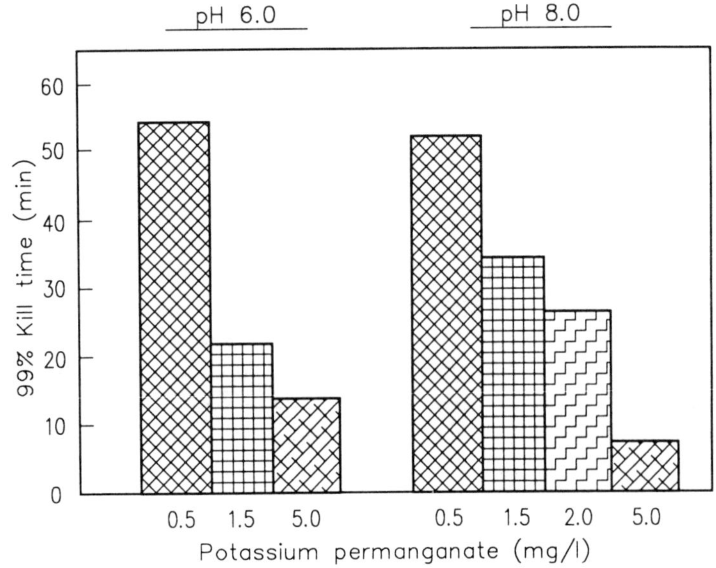

FIGURE 8–2. Inactivation of bacteriophage MS-2 by $KMnO_4$. (Reprinted from Ref. 34, pp. 979–89, by courtesy of Marcel Dekker, Inc.)

In tests conducted by Yahya et al. (36), 5 mg/l potassium permanganate was found to achieve a 1 log reduction (90 percent) of the type 1 poliovirus after 33 minutes of exposure. Further testing showed a significantly higher inactivation rate at 23°C than at 7°C, but showed no significant difference at pH 6.0 or pH 8.0.

Tests conducted at the University of Arizona verify that dosages of potassium permanganate from to 0.5 to 5 mg/l are capable of obtaining at least a 2 log inactivation of the surrogate virus, MS-2 bacteriophage with *E. coli* as the host bacterium (34). Concentrations of potassium permanganate (0.5, 1.5, 2.0, and 5.0 mg/l) were studied at two different pH levels, 6.0 and 8.0. Results showed that at pH 6.0 or 8.0, a 99 percent inactivation or reduction in the Plaque Forming Units of MS-2/ml occurred after at least 52 minutes with exposure to 0.5 mg/l $KMnO_4$. At a 5.0 mg/l $KMnO_4$ residual, a 2 log inactivation required 7.1 minutes at pH 8.0 and 12.8 minutes at pH 6.0 (see Figure 8–2).

TREATMENT OF FISH POND WATER

In fish farming and fishery management, potassium permanganate is quite widely used to treat pond water to counteract the acute effects of oxygen depletion, to remove organic contaminants, and to detoxify fish toxicants such as rotenone and antimycin. $KMnO_4$ is also effective in the control of certain fish diseases and parasites (10).

TYPICAL WATERWORKS EXPERIENCES

Potassium permanganate is used for multiple purposes in present-day waterworks operations. The more recent incentives for the consideration of potassium permanganate are principally the result of concerns for disinfection byproducts. When prechlorination of the raw water was stopped in water treatment in an effort to reduce the formation of THMs, new problems erupted in many treatment plants. Prechlorination had been effective in varying degrees in the control of algal and other biological growths in settling basins and filters. Prechlorination was also helpful in many locations in improving coagulation and flocculation through the oxidation of certain source water organic matter. Without prechlorination, there was a noticeable change in many plants in biological fouling of treatment units and in generally less effective treatment performances. The substitution of potassium permanganate for prechlorination has been helpful in restoring former treatment levels in many plants. This supplemental oxidation role of potassium permanganate can be an important consideration in developing a comprehensive alternative disinfecting strategy to meet a number of total disinfection and nondisinfection goals.

Water Treatment Plant Application

Observations reported for $KMnO_4$ use at the Crum and Pickering plants of the Philadelphia Suburban Water Company illustrate its effectiveness as a disinfectant (27). At these locations, taste and odor control was achieved by treatment with $KMnO_4$ at dose rates between 0.5 and 1.5 mg/l in conjunction with feeds of 30.8 mg/l alum and up to 10 mg/l powdered activated carbon. In addition, as illustrated in Table 8–4, when treated with 0.75 mg/l of potassium permanganate for a contact time of 60 minutes, raw water showed a MPN reduction from 3,678 to 180 coliforms/100 ml, corresponding to a 95 percent reduction.

From December 1966 to March 1967, a plant scale treatment study was conducted at the Kansas City, Missouri, water purification plant (24). One objective of this study was to determine the feasibility of chemical pretreatment of raw water drawn from the Missouri River. $KMnO_4$ dosages were applied in accordance with the actual permanganate demand of the water. The monthly averages were as follows: December, 1.0 mg/l; January, 1.1 mg/l; February, 1.3 mg/l, March, 2.7 mg/l. With a few exceptions,

TABLE 8–4. Effect of $KMnO_4$ as a Disinfectant

Jar No.	$KMnO_4$ (mg/l)	Contact Time (min)	Coliform Organisms (MPN/100 ml)
1	0.75	0	3,670
2	0.75	1	1,200
3	0.75	5	950
4	0.75	10	820
5	0.75	40	228
6	0.75	60	180

Source: From Ref. 27. Reprinted from *Journal American Water Works*, Vol. 54, No. 10 (October 1962), by permission.

the coliform content was reduced to less than detectable levels; fecal streptococci removal ranged from 48 to 96 percent. Actinomycetes removal was as high as 96 percent and as low as 27 percent.

In a disinfection byproduct reduction program conducted at the St. Joseph, Missouri, Water Company, prechlorination at that plant was replaced by potassium permanganate treatment (4). $KMnO_4$ was added to the discharge from the clarifier (see Figure 8–3) at a dosage from 1.0 to 1.1 mg/l. The bacteriological effects of the permanganate treatment, with retention time varying between 7.9 and 10.8 hours, are summarized in Table 8–5.

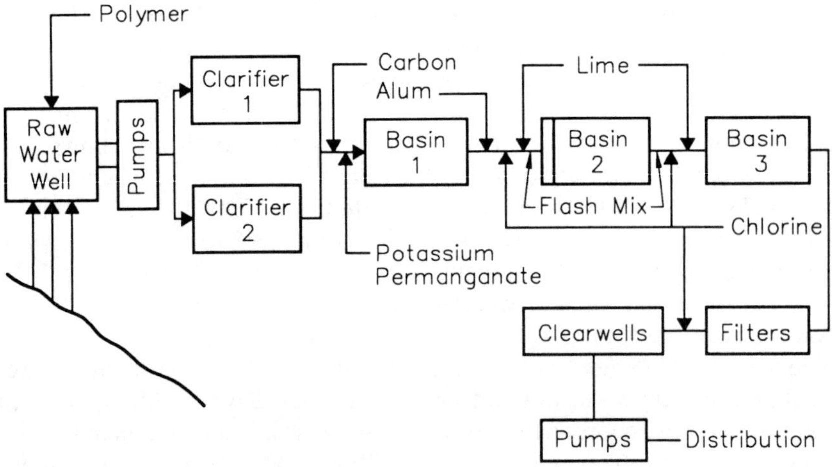

FIGURE 8–3. St. Joseph Water Co. water treatment process. (From Ref. 4. Reprinted by permission. Copyright © 1983, American Water Works Association.)

TABLE 8–5. The St. Joseph Water Company Membrane Bacteriological Data Test Run—1982

August	$KMnO_4$ (mg/l)	Retention Time (hr)	Total Coliforms: Missouri River Water (per 100 ml)	Total Coliforms: Basin No. 1 Exit (per 100 ml)
5	1.1	7.9	52,000	300
8	1.0	8.7	38,000	0
9	1.1	7.9	50,000	22
10	1.1	9.3	69,000	31
Potassium Permanganate Off				
15	0	10.8	87,000	35,700

Source: Adapted from Ref. 4.

The same reference reports use of $KMnO_4$ at the Davenport Water Company. This 30-mgd plant treats water from the Mississippi River by clarification, sedimentation, filtration (granular activated carbon media), and disinfection (see Figure 8–4). In August 1982, prechlorination was shifted from the raw water to the outlet of two parallel sedimentation basins. This measure was taken to control THM formation. However, the discontinuation of prechlorination resulted in odor problems in the flocculation basin areas caused by bacterial activity. Potassium permanganate at an average dosage rate of 0.63 mg/l and an average retention time of 38 minutes was then used to control the odor. In addition to achieving the desired odor control, there was a significant reduction in bacterial count.

While both of these plants added $KMnO_4$ later in the treatment process, most plants have found it advantageous to add it to the raw water. A test was conducted with potassium permanganate treatment from June 2 to August 31, 1987, at the James J. Corbalis Water Treatment Plant in Fairfax County, Virginia (5). Raw water for this plant is obtained from the Potomac River at an intake located 4.7 miles from the treatment plant. Potassium permanganate was applied at a typical dosage rate of 1.3 mg/l at the intake with a resulting contact time of 2 to 3 hours. Results show that potassium permanganate treatment significantly reduced total coliforms, heterotrophic plate count organisms, as well as the plankton count. In addition there was a reduction in the concentrations of manganese, total organic carbon, and threshold odor number.

Control of Rapid Sand Filter Media Growths

The city of Hamburg, Germany, prefers permanganate over chlorine for control of biological growths in filters such as are used in iron and manga-

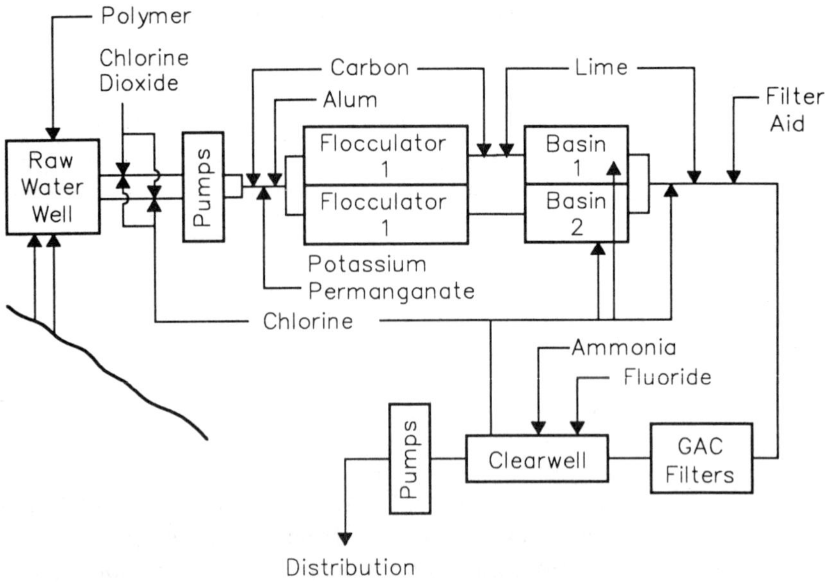

FIGURE 8–4. Davenport Water Co. water treatment process. (From Ref. 4. Reprinted by permission. Copyright © 1983, American Water Works Association.)

nese removal (15). In a "shock" treatment operation, $KMnO_4$ is applied either as a solid or in the form of a concentrated solution directly to the surface of the filter. Subsequently, enough water is added so that the effluent from the filter will show a distinctly pink-purple coloration, corresponding to a $KMnO_4$ concentration of 5 to 10 mg/l. This solution is then allowed to stay in contact with the filter for 24 hours, after which time samples for bacteriological analysis are taken. After the permanganate treatment, all residual $KMnO_4$ is removed by a thorough water rinse. If the filter contains excessive quantities of organic matter, it was found advisable to remove the organics after transferring the filter medium into another basin for treatment.

In a pilot study at the water treatment plant in Rantoul, Illinois, the parameters for controlling bacterial growth in sand filters were investigated (22). The entire filter was soaked for 3 hours in a 5,000 mg/l $KMnO_4$ solution, the pH of which had been adjusted with sodium carbonate to about 10.5. At the end of the contact period, the potassium permanganate solution was pumped into a holding tank and transferred—after replenishing the consumed potassium permanganate (about 30 percent)—to the next filter to be disinfected. Bacterial counts were performed before and after permanganate treatment on a suspension of organisms dislodged from the filter sand by vigorous shaking. The permanganate treatment reduced the number of bacteria on the filter medium by about one order of magnitude.

The dissolved oxygen in the filter effluent was also measured as an indicator of bacterial presence. This was based on earlier studies that had shown that the growth of nitrifying bacteria was accompanied by oxygen depletion. Permanganate treatment resulted in restoration of the normal dissolved oxygen level of about 7.5 mg/l from practically anaerobic conditions. Normal oxygen levels persisted for about 20 days, after which time regrowth of the bacteria with progressive deterioration of the dissolved oxygen level took place. A repeat of the $KMnO_4$ treatment would then be necessary.

Distribution Systems

Newly laid water mains or sections of existing distribution systems that have undergone major repairs must be disinfected before they can be put into service. The most frequently used disinfectant for this purpose is chlorine, but potassium permanganate—either alone or in combination with chlorine—has also been recommended and actually been used as an alternate agent. Sunnen recommends exposure of the pipes to be disinfected to a $KMnO_4$ concentration of 30 mg/l with a contact time between 2 and 24 hours or even longer (29).

Golda suggests use of permanganate for mains that are lined with cement mortar (15). Cement lining initially releases alkali, which can cause pH values to rise to 10 or even higher in the vicinity of the pipe wall. As discussed in Chapter 4, high pH conditions reduce the effectiveness of chlorine as a disinfectant. Golda recommends potassium permanganate doses at levels such that the concentration at exit from the pipe under disinfection is between 10 and 20 mg/l. Recommended contact time is from 12 to 24 hours, after which time the disinfectant solution is flushed out.

Permanganate has been used routinely in the disinfecting water supply mains in Mainz, Germany (21). Initial $KMnO_4$ concentration is 15 mg/l, and the retention time is 24 hours. Of particular interest in this operation is the use of ascorbic acid for the reduction of residual $KMnO_4$ in the spent disinfecting solution before its discharge into the Rhine River.

Principal objections against potassium permanganate for water main disinfection include a lower bactericidal efficiency than obtainable with chlorine, particularly with regard to heterotrophic plate count (HPC) data. The current AWWA standard for disinfection of water mains

(AWWA C-651-86) calls for the use of chlorine and specifies that the disinfected water must show the absence of coliform organisms.

TYPICAL PLANT ARRANGEMENTS

In the typical 5.0-mgd plant the addition of 2.0 mg/l of $KMnO_4$ will require a feeding system of about 150 lb/day, including standby capacity. For plants exceeding a capacity of 25 lb/day, dry volumetric feeders with hoppers and dust collectors would be appropriate. Injectors could be used for powering the flow to the feed point, drawing from a float-controlled solution tank under the feeder.

For plants utilizing fewer than 25 lb/day of potassium permanganate, the dry chemical is often dissolved in a solution tank prior to feed. The feeding facility would normally include two solution tanks with two chemical feed pumps. Each pump should be capable of meeting peak day needs with the tank having capacity for a 3-day supply. The potassium permanganate solution is normally prepared at a concentration of about one third of a lb/gallon.

Materials used for handling potassium permanganate can be steel, 316 stainless steel, PVC (Type 1), and fiber-reinforced plastic. The tanks should be supplied with mixers and covers. Care should be taken in storing dry potassium permanganate so that the material does not mix with other chemicals with which it reacts violently. The types of chemicals are listed on the material safety data sheet supplied by the manufacturer.

References

1. Banerjea, R. 1950. The use of potassium permanganate in the disinfection of water. *Ind. Med. Gaz.* 85: 214–9.
2. Barker, S. M., and L. Hoyle. 1972. Nature of the toxic reaction of influenza virus towards lung tissue. *J. Hygiene* 70(3): 425–37.
3. Bittenbender, W. A., E. F. Degering, P. A. Tetrault, C. F. Feasley, and B. H. Gwynn. 1940. Bactericidal properties of commercial antiseptics, a further study of the effect of pH. *Ind. Eng. Chem.* 32: 996–8.
4. Blanck, C. A. 1983. Total coliform reduction during treatment of Mississippi River water using potassium permanganate. *Proceedings of the AWWA Annual Conference* (1983): 961–70.
5. Bonacquisti, T. P., and E. Petrovitch. 1988. Preoxidation using potassium permanganate at the Fairfax County Water Authority. Paper presented at Virginia Section AWWA, Fairfax, VA, 20 October, 1988.
6. Carus Chemical Company. 1988. Material Safety Data Sheet. CAIROX® Potassium Permanganate. Ottawa, Illinois.
7. Cassebaum, H. 1979. Die Geschichte des "Mineralischen Chamäleons" (Permanganate). *Pharmazie* 34: 740–4.

8. Cherry, A. K. 1962. $KMnO_4$ improves water quality. *Water Sewage Works* 109: 266–7.
9. Cleasby, J. L., E. R. Baumann, and C. D. Black. 1964. Effectiveness of potassium permanganate for disinfection. *JAWWA* 56: 466–74.
10. Duncan, T. O. 1974. Review of literature on the use of potassium permanganate in fisheries. U.S. National Technical Information Service, Springfield, VA, PB Rep. No. 235453.
11. Ficek, K. 1978. Potassium permanganate for iron and manganese removal and taste and odor control. In *Water treatment plant design for the practicing engineer,* Sanks, R. L., ed. pp. 461–79. Ann Arbor, MI: Ann Arbor Science Publishers.
12. Ficek, K. J. 1983. Raw water reservoir treatment with potassium permanganate. Paper presented at the 74th Annual Meeting, Illinois Section American Water Works Association, Chicago, IL, 24 March, 1983.
13. Ficek, K. J., and J. E. Boll. 1980. Potassium permanganate: An alternative to pre-chlorination. *Aqua* (7): 153–6.
14. Fitzgerald, G. P. 1964. Laboratory evaluation of potassium permanganate as an algicide for water reservoirs. *Southwest Water Works J.* 45(10): 16–17.
15. Golda, W. 1973. Disinfektion von Rohrleitungen und Trinkwasser Aufbereitungsanlagen mit Kaliumpermanganat. *Goldschmidt Informiert* 6: 34–5. (A periodic technical publication of Th. Goldschmidt AG, Essen, FRG.)
16. Gönnert, R., and M. Bock. 1956. Zur Chemoresistenz der Viren. *Arzneimittel-Forsch.* 6: 522–7.
17. Kotter, K. 1979. Experience with potassium permanganate. Oxidation techniques in drinking water treatment—drinking water pilot project. Report II A: Advanced Treatment Technology Karlsruhe FRG. 1979. EPA-570/9–79–020.
18. Le Strat. 1944. Comparison des pouvoirs stérilisants du permanganate de potasse et de l'eau de javel a l'égard d'eaux contaminées. *Ann. Hygiene* (1944): 112–6.
19. Lund, E. 1963. Significance of oxidation in chemical interaction of poliovirus. *Arch. Ges. Virusforsch.* 12(5): 648–60.
20. Monscvitz, J. T., and D. J. Rexing. 1976. Disinfectant properties of potassium permanganate. Las Vegas Valley Water District Internal Report (unpublished).
21. Obst, U., and W. Kannenberg. 1988. Praktische Erfahrungen beim Einsatz und der Entsorgung von Kaliumpermanganat-Desinfektionslösung. GWF, *Gas-Wasserfach Wasser/Abwasser* 129(10): 656–7.
22. O'Connor, J. T., and K. Y. Baliga. 1970. Control of bacterial growths in rapid sand filters. *J. Environ. Div. ASCE.* 96(SA6): 1377–86.
23. Perrets, L. G., O. V. Bychkovskaya, A. M. Bazhedomova, N. S. Babina, and N. S. Semenova. 1960. Effect of potassium permanganate on poliomyelitis virus. *Vopr. Virusol.* 5(4): 407–11.
24. Popalisky, J. R., and F. Pogge. 1967. Studies on 3-phase water treatment at Kansas City, MO. Paper presented at the Missouri Section of AWWA, Columbia, MO, 4 April, 1967.

25. Posselt, H. S., F. J. Anderson, and W. J. Weber. 1967. The surface chemistry of hydrous manganese dioxide. Paper presented at meeting of Water, Air, and Waste Chemistry Division, American Chemical Society, Bar Harbor, FL, April 1967.
26. Schultz, E. W., and F. Robinson. 1943. The in-vitro resistance of poliomyelitis virus to chemical agents. *J. Inf. Dis.* 70(3): 193–200.
27. Shull, K. E. 1962. Operating experiences of Philadelphia suburban treatment plants. *JAWWA* 54(10): 1232–7.
28. Singer, P. C., J. H. Borchardt, and J. M. Colthurst. 1980. The effects of permanganate pretreatment on trihalomethane formation in drinking water. *JAWWA* 72: 573–6.
29. Sunnen, T. 1950. The disinfection of potable water pipeline systems before they are put into service. *Rev. Tech. Luxemb.* 42: 157–62.
30. Sykes, G. 1958. *Disinfection and sterilization.* Princeton, NJ: D. Van Nostrand Company, Inc.
31. Wagner, R. R. 1951. Studies on the inactivation of influenza virus. *Yale J. Biol. Med.* (1951): 288–98.
32. Posselt, H. S. 1972. Disinfection. In *Physicochemical processes in water quality control,* by Weber, W. J., Jr., pp. 413–56. New York: Wiley Interscience.
33. Whalen, P. J., V. D. Adams, and D. L. Sorenson. 1986. The use of potassium permanganate to reduce trihalomethane formation: The Deer Creek Reservoir example. *Chem. Environ. Proc. Int. Conf.* (1986): 162–70.
34. Yahya, M. T., N. R. Forsthoefel, K. Kujawa, and C. P. Gerba. 1989. Evaluation of potassium permanganate for the inactivation of bacteriophage MS-2 in water systems. *J. Environ. Sci. Health,* A24(8): 979–89. Marcel Dekker, Inc., N.Y.
35. Yahya, M. T., L. K. Landeen, and C. P. Gerba. 1990. Inactivation of *Legionella pneumophila* by potassium permanganate. *Environ. Technol.* 11: 657–62.
36. Yahya, M. T., T. M. Straub, and C. P. Gerba. 1990. Inactivation of poliovirus type 1 by potassium permanganate. University of Arizona Preliminary Research Report, Tucson, April 1990.
37. Reidies, A. H. Manganese compounds. 1981. In *Kirk-Othmer: Encyclopedia of chemical technology,* Grayson, M., and Eckroth, D., eds., pp. 844–95. New York: John Wiley & Sons, Inc.
38. Lalezary, S., M. Piribazari, and M. J. McGuire. 1986. Oxidation of five earthy-musty taste and odor compounds. *JAWWA* 78(3): 62–9.
39. Knocke, W.R., et al. 1990. Alternative oxidants for the removal of soluble iron and manganese. Report for AWWA Research Foundation, Denver, CO, March 1990.

9

Specialized Treatment Methods

with contributions by

Robert E. Fergen
Hazen and Sawyer
on *Air Stripping*

Ian Watson
Rostek Services, Inc.
on *Membranes*

INTRODUCTION

This chapter focuses on three processes that are somewhat specialized in application for either disinfection or the control of disinfection byproducts. By virtue of their characteristics, each of these processes has a specific treatment niche in which it might be applicable:

- *Ultraviolet radiation.* Ultraviolet radiation can inactivate bacteria and viruses; it is less effective for inactivation of *Giardia*. This process has potential for application to disinfection of groundwaters and other water sources where exposure to *Giardia lamblia* and other protozoan pathogens are not a concern.
- *Membrane processes.* Depending on water supply characteristics, membrane processes are sometimes capable of removing disinfection byproduct precursors as well as achieving treatment goals for removing undesired inorganic constituents found in many groundwater supplies. The potential for application to surface water treatment is also developing. Basically, these processes have multiple treatment potentials that include precursor removals as one of the principal objectives. Membrane filtration methods can also remove waterborne pathogens.
- *Air stripping.* Benefits of this process are limited to a capability for removing volatile disinfection byproducts such as THMs. Note that many of the byproducts formed in disinfection are nonvolatile in char-

acter, a condition that is likely to relegate air stripping to a relatively narrow role for controlling disinfection byproducts. Benefits may accrue, however, wherever air stripping can be justified for removal of additional volatile compounds that may contaminate partial water supplies.

DISINFECTION BY ULTRAVIOLET RADIATION

The disinfection capability of ultraviolet radiation has long been recognized in association with the purification properties afforded by sunlight. While this natural source is available, it is not generally adequate due to the limited water depth–penetrating properties of sunlight. Therefore, it has been necessary to develop more efficient methods of contact using artificial sources of ultraviolet radiation.

One of the keys to development of effective sources of ultraviolet radiation is efficient production of light at a wavelength in the range of 240 to 280 nm, an ultraviolet light range that is optimal for biocidal efficiency. This can be achieved with modern low-pressure mercury vapor lamps, whose origins actually extend back to 1835. This lamp is capable of efficiently converting electrical energy to light that is emitted at a characteristic wavelength of 253.7 nm. Low-pressure mercury arc lamps, a common source of ultraviolet light, are now capable of converting approximately 85 percent of the energy input into light at this wavelength (23). More recently, medium-pressure ultraviolet lamps have been developed that are capable of much higher intensity across a broader spectrum of the biocidal range. As a consequence, a much higher disinfecting capacity per lamp is possible.

Although ultraviolet disinfection was recognized as a method for achieving disinfection in the late nineteenth century, its application virtually disappeared with the evolution of chlorination technologies. In recent years, there has been a resurgence in its use in the wastewater field, largely as a consequence of concern for discharge of toxic chlorine residuals. In some wastewater applications, ultraviolet disinfection systems have been competitive with chlorination systems since the latter disinfection method frequently requires additional treatment for elimination of the chlorine residual prior to discharge. Such elimination is usually accomplished with reducing chemicals, such as sulfur dioxide.

Interest in ultraviolet disinfection for water treatment has not developed as rapidly as for waste treatment. Slow development has been partially influenced by initial findings of ineffective disinfection of the protozoan pathogen *Giardia lamblia*. This has caused scientific advisory panels in the United States to be somewhat cautious in defining the role of ultraviolet radiation in water treatment disinfection. However, research has indicated that it can be effective for control of viruses and bacteria and its use may be appropriate in cases where exposure to *Giardia lamblia* and other protozoan pathogens is not an issue. While this situation may not occur in many surface water supplies, many groundwater supplies may be protected from the intrusion of protozoan pathogens, which are larger than bacteria and viruses. For these supplies the focus may be on disinfection of bacteria and viruses. Under such conditions, ultraviolet disinfection could be an attractive primary disinfecting alternative that greatly reduces concern for disinfection byproducts formed by chlorine and other chemical disinfecting agents. It also has the advantage of not requiring extensive contact time.

Ultraviolet radiation has been employed more in smaller treatment facilities due to the complexities that can occur in large systems where several thousand lamps may be required. However, the design of ultraviolet systems has continued to improve, thereby extending the possible range of application to increasingly larger systems. Important considerations in its application are features that both enhance the maintenance of electrical components and reduce the number of lamps that must be maintained. Newer, high-intensity lamps are becoming available that greatly decrease the number of lamps required for some systems.

Ultraviolet disinfection is unique in its mode of action in that it does not necessarily kill the target organism. Instead, the predominant mechanism is thought to be the alteration of cell DNA such that the organism cannot reproduce itself. In effect, therefore, the end result of ultraviolet disinfection is to inactivate the target organism with respect to its capability to proliferate and cause disease. This differs from the mechanisms of chemical disinfecting agents, which predominantly act by disrupting cell function, thereby killing the organism.

One phenomenon unique to the ultraviolet mechanism is the capability of certain organisms to *photoreactivate* when subsequently exposed to certain wavelengths of light. As a consequence of this mechanism, some organisms can repair DNA damage and, under appropriate conditions, can revert back to an active state in which reproduction again becomes possible. In general, the extent of this reactivation effect varies between organisms. While it is important for coliform indicator organisms and some bacterial pathogens such as *Shigella,* many other bacteria are not subject to this phenomenon. Also, viruses do not generally have the capability for DNA repair, except when they have infected a host cell that is itself photoreactive (23, 25).

Photoreactivation typically occurs as a consequence of the catalyzing effects of sunlight at wavelengths outside of the effective disinfecting range. Photoreactivation has been observed to occur mostly at wavelengths in the range of 310 to 490 nm, but in some cases, wavelengths between 230 and 240 nm may cause this effect as well. In general, there is a critical period during which photoreactivation can occur since the DNA damage tends to become irreversible over time. Care should therefore be taken to either shield the process stream or limit exposure to sunlight for the period immediately following ultraviolet disinfection, a time when DNA alterations are most susceptible to repair (23).

As discussed, ultraviolet radiation is not thought to be an adequate disinfectant for control of *Giardia lamblia* and other protozoan pathogens at most commercially available ultraviolet dosages. Higher dosages can be effective for this pathogen class, but the major focus for ultraviolet disinfection is on its disinfection capabilities for viral and bacterial pathogens. EPA criteria for viral inactivation are specified to be 21 and 31 mWs/cm^2 to accomplish 2 and 3 log removals, respectively, of hepatitis A virus. These CT criteria include a factor of safety of three (24).

Ultraviolet disinfection is strongly influenced by the actual radiation pattern produced and the associated geometries. For example, at increasing distances from a source of light, the quantity of light must be spread over an expanding arc. Even if the total quantity of light available remains unchanged by the absorption of the surrounding water, the amount available per square centimeter of area would diminish as a consequence of expanding the area of the arc. Radiation is further diminished as a consequence of losses that result from the inherent absorbance in the solution to be disinfected. Absorbance is increased by the presence of color and turbidity. As a result, the light intensity available in solution varies as a result of a composite of all of the conditions of exposure as follows:

1. Intensity of individual lamps
2. Geometry of lamp arrangement (i.e., number of lamps and overlapping patterns produced)
3. Relative absorbance of solution (color and turbidity)

Poor geometry that creates excessive spacing between lamps can leave dead areas where inadequate disinfection will occur. As a consequence, a key consideration to improve disinfection is the geometry to minimize the amount of such dead area in which limited exposure can occur. Another important feature is the creation of sufficient turbulence to allow cross-mixing of flow as it proceeds through the ultraviolet contactor. In this way, flow can be more uniformly distributed through the varying regions of intensity, allowing exposure to the full range of available ultraviolet radiation. The intent is to achieve a relatively uniform level of disinfection throughout the entire flow, avoiding conditions in which certain portions of the flow might only be marginally disinfected.

Because systems for ultraviolet radiation typically provide a very brief contact, amounting to only a few seconds, it is extremely important that the system configurations limit the extent of short circuiting. In this regard, the features of a system that might relate to short circuiting should be fully considered in the design and selection of equipment. These particular features are discussed in detail in the U.S. EPA publication *Municipal Wastewater Disinfection* (23).

Ultraviolet disinfection provides no residual disinfecting capability and is only applicable for achieving primary disinfecting objectives. Therefore, secondary disinfecting agents will be necessary in situations where a protective disinfecting residual is needed in the distribution system. Ultraviolet radiation is destructive to both chlorine and chloramines, so these secondary disinfecting agents should be applied at a downstream location.

Nondisinfection Uses of Ultraviolet Radiation

The role of ultraviolet radiation for nondisinfection uses is limited since the process is inherently physical in nature and does not provide the opportunity for the beneficial chemical reaction that is afforded by chemical disinfecting agents. However, some photochemical interactions can take place. For instance, ultraviolet radiation has been used beneficially with ozone to produce highly reactive hydroxyl radicals, which can be extremely effective for oxidizing certain organic compounds. This ultraviolet/ozone combination is discussed further in Chapter 7.

Some ultraviolet lamps are capable of emitting radiation at the lower wavelength of 184.9 nm. Light at this wavelength has a capability of producing ozone. However, this phenomenon is somewhat inadvertent in its occurrence and is not always desirable because it wastes output from the ultraviolet system by producing radiation outside of the optimal range for germicidal efficiency. In addition, this phenomenon can represent an interference in some ultraviolet systems where ozone that accumulates in the atmosphere surrounding certain lamps acts as an absorbing agent to diminish the transmittance of ultraviolet radiation. Therefore, lamps that minimize the production of light at this wavelength are often favored (23).

Alternative Ultraviolet Systems

Ultraviolet systems can be categorized according to the contacting configuration. Three types of systems are in use.

Unsubmerged Systems

In these systems, the process flow stream is commonly routed through transparent tubes that are placed adjacent to externally mounted lamps. The geometry of these systems is influenced by the number and location of lamps as well as the size and velocities of the flow tubes. Clear Teflon, which allows for relatively efficient transmittance of ultraviolet radiation, is a commonly selected material for construction of the flow tubes. The entire contacting system is normally housed in an enclosure that protects plant personnel from ultraviolet exposure which can be especially harmful to eyes. These enclosures must have a fan or other means for providing adequate ventilation to avoid excessive heat buildup.

In-channel Submerged Systems

A typical in-channel submerged system is shown in Figure 9–1. Lamps are mounted on racks, which are lowered into position in the flow channel. The selection of type and geometric arrangement of lamps achieves the desired distribution of ultraviolet radiation. Each lamp is inserted in a transparent tube, and wiring is sealed to protect against water. In order to achieve effective distribution of ultraviolet radiation throughout the flow stream, the lamps tend to be relatively closely spaced. Hydraulic characteristics are important for this type of system to avoid short-circuiting effects and maintain effective detention time.

Very careful attention must be paid to hydraulic design of the channel for submerged systems since very precise control of water level over the entire range of flow is particularly important. Typically, water level variations over the entire range of flows from minimum to maximum should be less than 2 inches. If the water level rises above this limitation, the top portion of the lamp battery may be excessively submerged under maximum flow conditions, resulting in short-circuiting the top of the flow that is poorly contacted and not as effectively disinfected. On the other hand, if the level is allowed to drop too low under a minimum flow condition, some of the upper lamps can become exposed to air and a condition can be created that encourages the formation of a scale on the exterior of the upper lamps as a consequence of a "baking-on" effect. This will interfere with ultraviolet transmittance into the process stream.

Enclosed Submerged Lamp Systems

In these systems, the ultraviolet lamps are submerged in the process stream that flows through an enclosed chamber, as shown in Figure 9–2. This approach has been used for both low- and high-intensity ultraviolet lamps. High-intensity lamps used in this type of system have recently been developed using a medium-pressure mercury arc lamp that can pro-

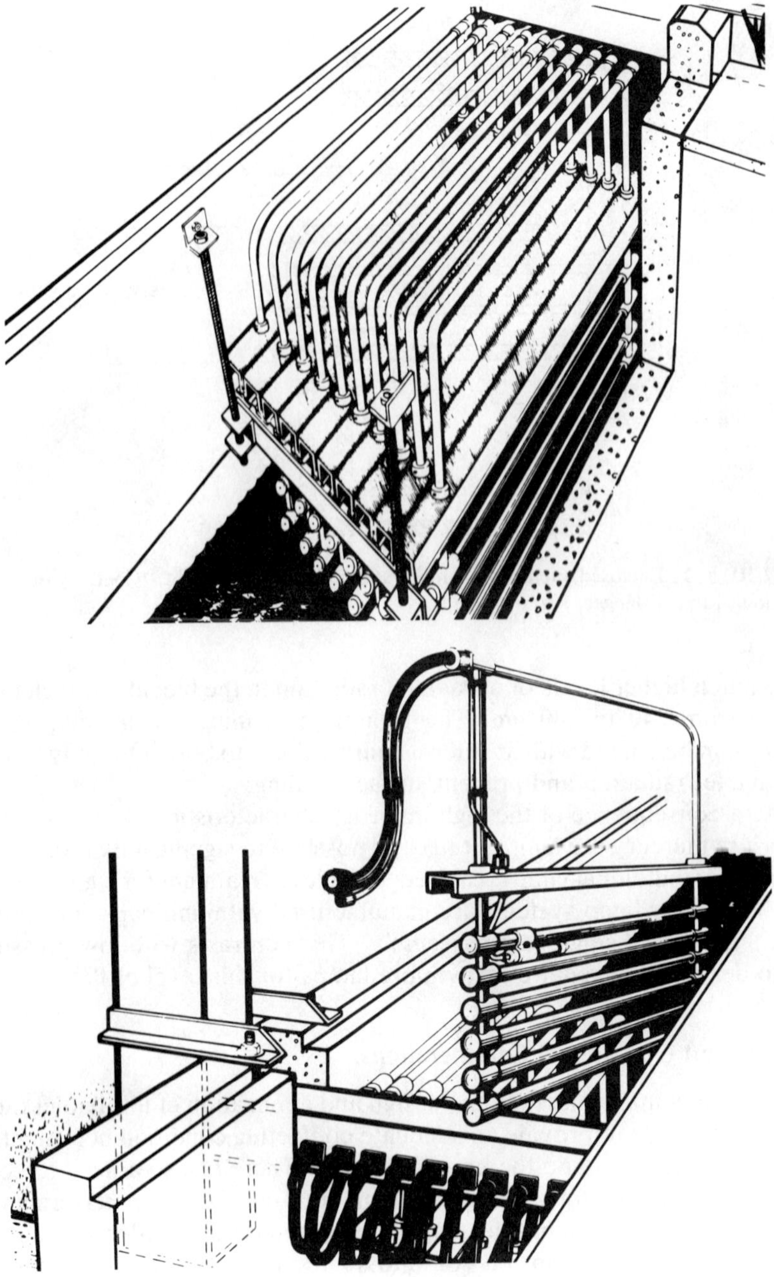

FIGURE 9–1. In-channel submerged system for ultraviolet light. (Courtesy of Trojan Technologies, Inc., London, Ontario N6E 2S8, Canada.)

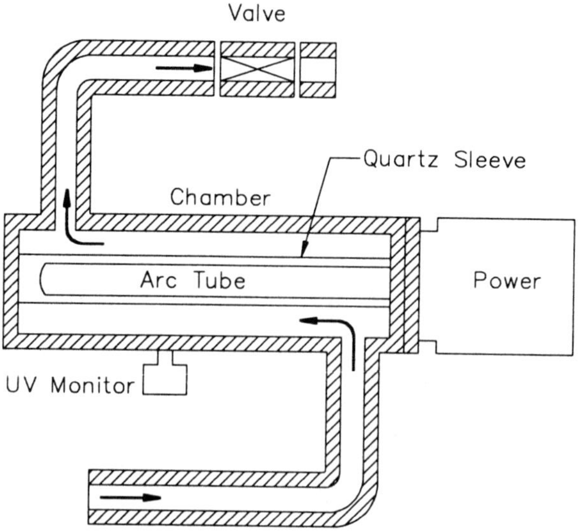

FIGURE 9–2. Enclosed submerged lamp system for ultraviolet light. (Courtesy of Aquionics Inc. Erlanger, KY.)

vide much higher levels of ultraviolet radiation in the biocidal wavelength range from 240 to 280 nm. The treatment chambers containing these lamps can be coated with an internal mirror finish to both internally reflect ultraviolet radiation and prevent surface fouling.

As a consequence of the high-intensity characteristics of the medium-pressure mercury arc lamps, it may be possible to significantly reduce the number of individual lamps required to achieve treatment for a given flow. High-intensity lamp systems are manufactured with unit capacities of up to 1.8 mgd for a single lamp assembly. This contrasts with low-pressure lamp designs that require many more lamps for this level of flow.

Design and Operational Considerations

The fundamental concern in the design and application of ultraviolet radiation systems is to provide an adequate contacting condition between the source of radiation and the process stream. There is also a need to consider requirements for ancillary equipment to monitor lamp performance and provide for inevitable cleaning of lamps and tubes in order to maintain effective ultraviolet transmission into solution. In addition, an adequate plant electrical feed must always be available to power the system.

The procedure for testing and cleaning lamps should be thoroughly evaluated in design. Pilot studies can be performed to give an indication of the scaling potential and cleaning frequency in a specific water. Waters with high levels of hardness, alkalinity, iron, manganese, and other constituents that may form precipitates are especially susceptible to scaling, which may affect practicability in some cases. Therefore, pilot testing should be conducted where these conditions exist. Hand cleaning of lamps and tubes may be appropriate for small ultraviolet systems. Racks might be provided for holding lamp and tube assemblies to facilitate such cleaning. However, to minimize labor where large numbers of lamps are required, consideration may be given to in-vessel or outside cleaning tanks that allow a number of tubes to be cleaned at one time.

Maintaining reliability in design of ultraviolet radiation is a much greater concern for meeting primary disinfection goals for water treatment than in the case of wastewater systems. Water should be treated to effectively remove particulate matter that might shield pathogenic organisms before ultraviolet radiation is applied in a water treatment system. In addition, design should consider the possibility for light attenuation due to the presence of color and other materials that can absorb ultraviolet radiation. This should be much less of a problem in a drinking water system than in a wastewater system, where color removal is not normally practiced. In any case, ultraviolet radiation should be applied at a downstream point in the process stream where there is an opportunity for minimizing the presence of radiation absorbing substances. Also, note that ultraviolet radiation does not provide color reduction as many other methods of disinfection do. Therefore, supplemental addition of oxidizing chemicals may be required in cases where color cannot be adequately reduced with coagulation processes alone or where coagulation is not provided.

One of the predominant means of increasing reliability in water treatment is by providing redundancy. In this regard, it would be appropriate to operate with ultraviolet contacting units in an arrangement that includes at least one redundant or spare unit. It would also be appropriate to monitor lamp outputs to ensure that the system is operating properly.

From a safety standpoint, ultraviolet radiation can be harmful to eyesight, therefore, design should take into account the need for minimizing this type of exposure. To a certain extent, some protection is afforded when lamps are immersed since water has an inherent capability for absorbing radiation, even when color is absent. However, additional measures are prudent, and special care should be taken to avoid exposure to nonsubmerged lamps.

MEMBRANE PROCESSES

Membrane processes, which have been used in Florida for some time (6), are rapidly developing water treatment technologies that were initially developed to achieve desalting objectives. However, in recent years, these processes have demonstrated capabilities for achieving high levels of removal of disinfection byproduct precursors. Under appropriate conditions, these separation processes can represent a significant component of an overall disinfection/disinfection byproduct strategy. The applicability of membrane processes varies according to source water quality. For example, membranes have been more readily applied in treatment of certain groundwater sources where the fouling by particulates is less likely than in surface waters. Variations in such effects will occur according to membrane types, and as membrane processes continue to improve, source water characteristics that are appropriate for this type of treatment will expand.

In many cases, the attractiveness of a membrane process may depend on the capability for achieving multiple process objectives that includes rejection of undesired inorganic constituents as well as removal of organic precursors. The discussion of membrane processes presented here, therefore, includes an overview of both types of uses.

Alternative Membranes

Membrane processes use synthetic films that act as a type of barrier to certain substances found in water. These processes are typically subdivided into the categories of reverse osmosis, filtration, and electrodialysis. Membrane filtration processes are further characterized into three groups according to the size of particles removed: nanofiltration, ultrafiltration, and microfiltration. Of the three, nanofiltration is capable of removing the smallest particle and rejecting precursors and some inorganic ions. Ultrafiltration removes slightly larger particles, including most viruses and bacteria, and is capable of some degree of precursor removal, although not with the same effectiveness as nanofiltration. Microfiltration, which removes still larger particles and bacteria, is predominantly associated with particulate removal.

Both reverse osmosis and the filtration-type systems involve the transport of water through a membrane, which acts as a barrier to the passage of constituents to be removed from solution. Electrodialysis relies on a somewhat different principle in which water is channeled between two membranes that segregate the main flow from cells in which positively and negatively charged ions are accumulated. Electrical charges are superimposed in these cells to attract oppositely charged ions. On one side is a cation-permeable membrane that allows the passage of positively charged ions, which are attracted to a negative cathode, while on the other side an anion-permeable membrane allows the passage of negatively charged ions, which are attracted to a positively charged anode. Therefore, electrodialysis relies on these electrical charges to draw positive and negatively charged salt species out of solution, leaving a desalted product water to remain in the center compartment. This contrasts with other membrane processes, which pass the main process flow stream through the membrane, leaving removed substances behind.

While membrane systems were originally developed for removal of inorganic salts, a capability for removing organic material has also been observed. Typically, organic compounds above a specified molecular weight are removed by a given membrane composition. Removal appears to occur as a result of a straining-type mechanism that would be mostly applicable for reverse osmosis and nanofiltration membranes. In the case of ultrafiltration and microfiltration, the molecular weight cutoff appears to be relatively high, and these membranes have yet to demonstrate efficient removal of organic precursor material associated with trihalomethane-formation potential (2, 22). Because the main process flow is not routed through a membrane in electrodialysis processes, straining-type removal for organics is not available, thereby reducing the effectiveness of electrodialysis as a control strategy for removal of precursors. However, it should be noted that some degree of organic removal has been observed for this process as well.

Because of the limitations of electrodialysis, ultrafiltration, and microfiltration for removing organics, reverse osmosis and nanofiltration processes will tend to be the focus of the remainder of this section. Some research is being performed to assess the potential for eliminating disinfection agents by using ultrafiltration processes to achieve a particulate-based removal of pathogens (11). However, although this type of approach may be plausible, reliability must be established as compared with multiple barrier systems that use filtration in conjunction with disinfection. Moreover, membrane filtration processes would still require the subsequent addition of a disinfecting chemical to meet goals for secondary disinfection.

Basically, membrane processes require the application of water at a pressure that is required for achieving the desired flow rate across the membrane. The pressure requirement involves two groups of forces. The first group of forces can be associated with mechanical requirements for pressure drop across the membrane at a given flow rate. This involves the water flow through the membrane openings. The second group of forces involves the natural pressure gradient that develops between two solutions of different salt content. Differences in salt content are inherent to reverse osmosis, and concentrations can build up to relatively high levels on the inlet side of the membrane, whereas a relatively desalted product water exists on the outlet side. Natural osmotic forces are capable of creating significant pressure gradients under these conditions since the concentration differences of the two solutions create an essentially unbalanced condition in which a pressure must be maintained to prevent water contained in the relatively dilute outlet solution from reversing its path to try to equilibrate the salt concentration on both sides of the membrane. This pressure is referred to as the osmotic pressure and must be added to the pressure associated with mechanical forces in order to arrive at the total pressure requirement.

The natural osmotic pressure is determined by the salt content of a given solution. For a common brackish water, with a total salt content of 1,500 mg/l the natural osmotic pressure is on the order of 15 psi, whereas a typical seawater total with a dissolved solids level of 35,000 mg/l has a natural osmotic pressure of approximately 350 psi (1). Even if the mechanical forces across the membrane could be reduced to negligible levels, these natural osmotic pressures would still need to be overcome, and it is not possible to operate a reverse osmosis system at zero pressure.

In fact, the mechanical pressure component is not negligible and can be quite significant. In this regard, one of the areas of advance has been the reduction of this pressure component to allow operating pressures to be progressively reduced, with an ultimate objective of approaching an operating pressure as close to the natural osmotic pressure as possible.

Another significant area in the development of membrane technology is the efficiency of a membrane for removing or rejecting salts. In general, salt-removal efficiency improves as the membrane structure is made tighter. However, this tends to increase the mechanical pressure requirements. Therefore, the goals for minimizing pressure while increasing salt rejection tend to come into conflict. In a sense, many of the developments in membrane technology over the years have been related to attempts to resolve this conflict.

Although reverse osmosis has been recognized as a natural process for more than 200 years, the development of commercially available membranes is relatively recent (1). A cellulose acetate membrane material, which successfully rejected sodium chloride, was first developed in 1959 at the University of Florida. However, the rate at which water could permeate the membrane was not sufficient to make this development economically feasible (18). Subsequent work was performed by others to modify the molecular structure of the cellulose acetate in order to allow a rate of permeation more attractive for commercial operation (13).

Membranes originally evolved into a tubular configuration in which the feed stream entered the center and was transported across a membrane that was either inserted into or coated onto a porous tube. Product water was then collected on the outside of the tube, leaving a concentrated brine solution remaining on the inside. This approach limited the surface area to that available on the inside of tube structures. Subsequently, a layered, flat film type of arrangement was developed in which the membrane layers overlie an inner channel that collects product water. This material can be wound in a spiral (known as *spiral-wound configuration*) and inserted into a cylindrical housing, thereby providing a high surface area availability within a given volume of housing.

An alternative development that also increased available surface area was the production of small hollow-fiber membrane structures that could be bundled together and packaged in a pressure vessel. Both the spiral-wound and the hollow-fiber configurations are now in wide use, while the earlier tubular types of membrane are less common. Another configuration that is sometimes still considered is a flat-film, plate-and-frame type of housing.

While cellulose acetate is still a widely used membrane material, several new membrane compositions have been developed (16). These include thin-film composite membranes that consist of a thin, very tight membrane structure that is coated over a more porous backing material that provides structural support. The tight structure of the membrane provides good salt rejection, while the mechanical pressure drop is minimized by keeping the membrane thin. A common membrane material is a polyamide formulation. Polysulfone formulations are commonly used for the porous support layer, which is typically attached to a backing that provides additional structural integrity. These newer compositions provide some advantages over the original cellulose acetate compositions, which are subject to chemical degradation if the feed solution is not properly controlled in a moderately acid pH range of 4 to 6. Cellulose acetate also is subject to a biological attack that requires the addition of a disinfecting agent to the feed stream for control.

The newer membranes can be operated over a wider range of pH from 4 to 8. They also are not as susceptible to biological attack. However, these new materials have the disadvantage of being intolerant to exposure to chlorine and other oxidizing chemicals, a problem that does not occur with acetate membranes. As a result, this limits the alternatives for control of biological fouling, which still can be a problem even though direct biological attack of a membrane might be precluded. Intolerance for chlorine usually requires that a dechlorination step be provided in cases where such a prior chlorination step occurs in the process sequence. In some cases shock treatment with sodium bisulfite can be used with chlorine-sensitive membranes as an alternative method for control of biofilms.

No one membrane system is without disadvantages. As a consequence, either cellulose acetate or alternative membrane compositions can be used, depending on site-specific conditions. Selection will vary depending on water quality goals and operational considerations inherent to maintaining the different membrane compositions.

Low pressure membranes are another development that provides benefits for specific applications. These membranes do not have the tight structure (and associated higher mechanical pressure requirements) needed for extremely high levels of salt rejection such as might be required in a seawater desalination application. They can be used to advantage for lower-salt-content waters that do not require the same level of salt rejection, allowing for a much reduced mechanical pressure component. Similar low-pressure applications have developed around softening type, nanofiltration membranes, which can be used to treat high-hardness, low-total-dissolved-solid waters. In these applications, the main goal is to remove the larger +2 charge ions such as calcium and magnesium. These membranes are, therefore, configured with a structure that will not have a high rejection characteristic for singly charged ions such as sodium and chloride, but will still reject a significant quantity of the calcium and magnesium hardness. These membranes actually fall somewhere between reverse osmosis and filtration in character since the smaller, singly charged ions are not efficiently rejected. Membrane softening is being widely considered for application to high-hardness Florida groundwaters. Many of these groundwaters are highly colored and contain large quantities of organic precursor compounds that can be removed by the membrane-softening process as well.

Concepts for Inorganic Removal

Concepts for inorganic removal by membranes are associated with osmotic forces that occur when two solutions of different salt concentrations are separated by a semipermeable membrane that inhibits the transfer of salt but not water. The osmotic pressures of these two solutions are different and therefore out of balance. As a consequence, an osmotic flow of water will tend to develop from the solution of lower concentration to dilute the solution of higher concentration, thereby bringing the solutions into balance. Unless an external pressure can be applied that will offset the differential in osmotic pressure between the two solutions, this transport of water will continue until the two solutions are equal in concentration. When an external pressure is applied the osmotic pressure difference can be offset, thereby bringing the system into balance without requiring flow between the two solutions. The balance point for this type of condition can be described by the following expression:

$$dh = \pi_1 - \pi_2 = d\pi \qquad (9\text{–}1)$$

where
dh = differential head or pressure applied to the solutions
π = osmotic pressure for a given solution concentration
$d\pi$ = differential osmotic pressure

If a pressure greater than $d\pi$ is applied, the direction of flow will be reversed so that water is transferred against the osmotic gradient and will be moved from the concentrated side to the dilute side. This is the condition that occurs in a reverse osmosis system. Because these systems involve a continuous flow of water instead of a system in balance, flow-related friction or mechanical forces also come into play in order to maintain a continuous transport of flow through the membrane. Therefore, the pressure required to overcome friction forces must be added to the osmotic pressure requirements in order to sustain the desired level of flow.

While several specific theories have been developed to explain salt removal by the reverse osmosis process, it is generally thought that some form of physical-chemical interaction is operative in inhibiting salt passage. Therefore, salt exclusion is affected by chemical properties. Organic material, on the other hand, appears to be more strongly influenced by physical screening or sieving, with efficiency significantly affected by molecular size (9, 14, 18, 20). While a series of complex mathematical models can be developed to predict the performance of a specific membrane, some simple equations are available for general characterization of the process (5).

Rate of water passage through a membrane:

$$Q_w = K_w(dp - d\pi)A/T \qquad (9\text{–}2)$$

where
Q_w = water flow rate through membrane
K_w = membrane permeability coefficient
dp = hydraulic pressure differential across membrane
$d\pi$ = osmotic pressure differential across membrane
A = active membrane surface area
T = membrane thickness

Rate of salt passage through a membrane:

$$Q_s = K_s(dC)A/T \qquad (9\text{–}3)$$

where

Q_s = quantity of salt bleed through a membrane per unit time
K_s = membrane permeability coefficient for a given salt
dC = differential salt concentration across membrane

Note that Equation 9–2 indicates that flow rate across a membrane is related to the applied pressure, while Equation 9–3 indicates that the rate of salt bleed is proportional to the concentration gradient and is not directly related to pressure. As a consequence, there is a diluting effect in which the salt concentration in the product water is reduced as flow is increased with increased pressure. This diluting effect is partially offset by a degree of increase in salt bleed due to an increasing salt concentration gradient that occurs when flow is increased. However, the end result is a general trend of improved product water quality with increased flow. Therefore, proper selection of operating pressure and hydraulic loading rate are critical to achieving treatment objectives for salt concentration in the product water. This will vary depending on treatment goals and characteristics of the membrane.

Important considerations for the reverse osmosis process are chemical phenomena that occur in concentrated salt streams at the inlet side of the membrane. If the concentrations are allowed to increase beyond a certain level, some of the salts will start to precipitate and scale the membrane, thereby interfering with the process. In design and operation, the level of concentration for the most insoluble salt should be calculated to determine the allowable level of concentration before this type of effect occurs. Chemicals can be added to reduce some precipitation.

From a practical standpoint, the level of salt buildup on the inlet side of a membrane is limited by wasting a portion of the flow. Wasting is also required to control the osmotic pressure gradient across the membrane. As a consequence, two separate flow streams exit the process. These consist of a desalted product or permeate stream, which is transported across the reverse osmosis membrane, and a waste or concentrate discharge that is necessary for avoiding excess salt accumulation. The ratio of treated product water to the total inlet feed water to a membrane module is one method of describing the productivity of a reverse osmosis system in terms of a percent recovery, *Y*:

$$Y = \frac{Q_p}{Q_f} 100 \qquad (9\text{–}4)$$

where
Q_p = permeate or treated product water flow
Q_f = feed flow to the system

Salt rejection in the treated product water is not complete, and a similar expression can be used to characterize the percent salt passage through a system (SP):

$$SP = \frac{C_p}{C_f} 100 \tag{9–5}$$

where
C_p = salt concentration in permeate stream
C_f = salt concentration in feed stream

It is not uncommon for reverse osmosis units to operate in series, allowing brine that is rejected from an upstream unit to become the feed stream for downstream units, thereby increasing the overall percent recovery. Where series of operation is practiced, a progressive concentrating effect occurs in which salt concentration increases from membrane element to membrane element in a system. Under these conditions, salt passage is calculated using a bulk or average value of C_f, termed C_{fb}. Permeate quality is then described by the following relationship:

$$C_p = \frac{SP \times C_{fb}}{100} \tag{9–6}$$

To calculate C_{fb}, a concentrating factor (CF) for feed concentration in succeeding stages can be developed from a percent recovery relationship and applied as follows:

$$CF = \frac{1}{1/(1 - Y/100)} \tag{9–7}$$

Stage 1: C_{f_i} = initial feed concentration
Stage 2: $C_{f_2} = C_{f_i} \times CF$
Stage 3: $C_{f_3} = C_{f_i} \times (CF)^2$
Stage n: $C_{f_n} = C_{f_i} \times (CF)^n$

C_{fb} can then be roughly estimated as an average:

$$C_{fb} = C_{f_i} \frac{(1 + CF + CF^2 + \ldots CF^n)}{n} \tag{9–8}$$

These equations are based on a crude mass balance that assumes nearly complete rejection of salts. While this approach is instructive, more rigorous calculation requires the development of concentration factors to reflect the actual salt passage for each ion in solution. This type of information is usually available from the membrane manufacturer. In addition, for more precise calculation, especially where a number of reverse osmosis modules are operated in series, a log mean concentration is more appropriate for computing C_{fb}.

When membranes are manufactured, the manufacturer tests each membrane or a sampling of a production run under standard test conditions. Since these conditions may vary from manufacturer to manufacturer and the conditions existing in a system also will be very different, a technique called *normalization* is used to compare membrane performance with standard conditions of Q_p and SP as follows:

$$Q_p = (\text{PCF})(\text{TCF})(\text{MFRC})Q_i \qquad (9\text{–}9)$$

$$SP = SP_i(\text{SPCF}) \qquad (9\text{–}10)$$

where

PCF = pressure correction factor
SPCF = salt passage correction factor
TCF = temperature correction factor
MFRC = membrane flux retention coefficient
Q_i = initial permeate flow under standard conditions
SP_i = initial salt passage under standard conditions

PCF and SPCF can be adjusted to system conditions, but TCF and MFRC must be obtained from the membrane manufacturer. The MFRC is based on clean membrane operation, and only testing at system conditions can provide a coefficient modified to reflect the effect of membrane fouling.

Process Concepts for Organic Precursor Removal

Although reverse osmosis was originally developed for the removal of inorganic salts, it has long been recognized for its capability to remove certain organic compounds. Early work was performed to characterize the separation of various organic compounds from relatively dilute solutions using cellulose acetate membranes (19). Rejection varied considerably from compound to compound and was generally related to the molecular weight. For example, in one particular test, a higher molecular weight dextrose was rejected at greater than 99 percent, while lower molecular weight acetic acid was rejected at only 20 percent. Rejection of sodium chloride was at higher levels than experienced for all of the organics tested (12, 19). Because the molecular weights of sodium chloride and acetic acid are similar, it was concluded that a different mechanism of rejection prevailed for organic removal.

Other studies indicate that properties in addition to molecular weight could have an effect. For example, organics such as phenol, with vapor pressures significantly higher than water, can pass through membranes to a significant extent (8). Simple straight-chain organics, with four carbons or less, pass through membranes if they have a hydrogen-bonding capability. However, within each of these classes of compounds, removal can increase as molecular weight increases as observed in some of the initial work (10). In other cases, organics can actually be absorbed into the membrane structure itself to reduce permeability, which is an undesired effect.

Membrane technology research has begun to demonstrate and evaluate capabilities for removing naturally occurring organic DBP precursor compounds. Testing of highly colored groundwaters in Florida has demonstrated reverse osmosis membranes and nanofiltration membranes, as are often used for groundwater softening applications (4), can perform very well for removing these precursor compounds. Many of these tests have indicated a potential for removal of the formation potential of trihalomethane and other byproducts (haloacetic acids, chloral hydrate, chlorinated ketones, and haloacetonitrites) at levels in excess of 90 percent when using membranes with molecular weight cutoffs of 500 or less. Total organic halide formation potential was also reduced by greater than 90 percent in these tests (15).

Some testing of membrane processes for surface water sources has also been performed. However, while this testing has shown that trihalomethane formation potential can be rejected from surface waters by both reverse osmosis and nanofiltration types of systems, the water flux or flow-through capability can be severely reduced over time, raising questions of practicality for this type of application (2, 22).

Nanofiltration membranes are presently being considered as a potential softening process alternative for many Florida groundwaters (3, 7, 17, 26). In some other cases, low-pressure reverse osmosis membranes are being considered for treating the moderate levels of total dissolved solids found in brackish water aquifers. In both instances these membranes may also remove precursors.

Salt rejection based on a standard test with sodium chloride is frequently used as a basis for predicting finished water quality in terms of removal of inorganic compounds. However, because of increasing interest in the use of these membranes for removing organic precursors, many manufacturers have also established a screening classification based on molecular weight cutoff (MWC). While MWC does not give a definitive indication for removal of specific organic constituents, it is still a useful tool for establishing the potential effectiveness of the membrane. Low-pressure, reverse osmosis membranes have an MWC of about 100, while the MWCs of softening-type nanofiltration membranes commonly range from 300 to 500. Ultrafiltration, which primarily addresses the removal of very fine particles by physical means, offers little or no salt rejection. These membranes, which have high MWCs ranging from 1,000 to 100,000, have not been able to lower the THM formation potential below 100 μg/l in limited tests performed to date (3, 21).

The major focus for applying membrane technologies to control disinfection byproducts has been directed at the removal of the precursor compounds and not the disinfection byproducts themselves. Limited work in some seawater applications in the Middle East, where chlorination/dechlorination of feedwater is practiced for control of biological activity, has indicated that high concentrations of trihalomethanes (>800 μg/l) have been identified in the product water. These membranes have very tight pore structures, and such a finding suggests that the low-pressure reverse osmosis membranes and the softening membranes, both with larger pore structures, would also be ineffective for trihalomethanes.

Design and Operational Considerations

Membrane Alternatives

Design begins with the selection of an appropriate range of membranes to meet treatment goals. Ideally, membrane configurations can be selected with the correct rejection or removal characteristics for the targeted chemical species, while not having a needlessly tight membrane structure that restricts the flow of water to a greater degree than is necessary. In the case of desalination of seawater, where high salt concentrations require very high levels of rejection, much tighter membranes would be necessary than for brackish water applications in which moderate levels of salt are encountered. Low-pressure reverse osmosis membranes with a looser structure are more appropriate for brackish water systems and allow much lower operating pressures for salt removal. These structures are also capable of efficient precursor removals.

Decisions must also be made with respect to the compatibility of alternative membranes with chemical conditions found in the feed stream. As has been discussed, some membranes are extremely sensitive to pH and biological attack, while other membranes are intolerant of the presence of oxidizing species such as chlorine. These factors will affect both the selection of membranes and the types of pretreatment processes required. Where chlorination is practiced ahead of oxidant-sensitive membranes, an effective dechlorination step must be applied ahead of the membrane.

Membrane selection and operating conditions are normally dictated by water quality. A relatively complete assessment of the ionic content of a water should be performed to determine which alternative membrane should be considered and to develop a preliminary basis of design. Often this is done based on consultation with the membrane suppliers. Typical water quality parameters that should be evaluated include calcium, magnesium, sodium, potassium, strontium, barium, iron, bicarbonate, sulfate, chloride, fluoride, carbonate, phosphate, nitrate, silica, carbon dioxide, pH, and total dissolved solids. A balance between positively and negatively charged ions should be achieved in evaluating these analyses since a major imbalance indicates an incomplete or incorrect analysis. These analyses provide the input necessary for preliminary evaluations of pretreatment needs and rejection characteristics.

Evaluation of chemical analyses is normally only a first step that leads to selection of conditions to be tested in a subsequent field or pilot investigation phase. This test phase is used to confirm the rejection properties of the membrane and also can be useful to assess pretreatment requirements and the extent to which the brine stream must be wasted to maintain proper performance for rejection and avoidance of scaling problems. In many cases, several alternative membranes might be evaluated to determine the most suitable for a given application.

Fouling Features

An important and frequently limiting consideration in the design of a membrane system is the need to avoid the formation of chemical precipitates that can occur due to the concentrating effect on the inlet side of the membrane. A relatively complete characterization of the feed stream should be performed to assess the scaling potential. Silica (SiO_2) scaling, particularly troublesome in some systems, may require pretreatment to either remove or to bind silica compounds in a soluble form. A number of other precipitates have also proved to create similar problems. This group includes calcium carbonate, calcium sulfate, barium sulfate, strontium sulfate, calcium fluoride, and iron precipitates. Strategies for controlling these problems include the addition of scale inhibitors to prevent precipitation by binding troublesome constituents into solution, adjustment of feed stream pH to a range where solubility is increased, and pretreatment steps to remove constituents from solution.

Colloidal particles can also cause fouling of membrane devices. The potential for this concern is sometimes indicated by a silt density index, which is a standard determination based on the rate of pressure loss across a membrane filter. In general, colloidal particles should be removed by pretreatment processes. As a consequence, a coagulation process is sometimes required to remove a significant portion of this material through agglomeration along with the frequent need of filtration to remove the larger particles. In small plants, particle removal often can be accomplished with cartridge filters with ratings from 5 to 25 μm (1). These filters are intended to remove residual coagulated particles, as well as other larger particles in the feed stream. In many cases, filtration alone may be adequate and filters in a size range of 1 to 20 μm are used, 5 μm being a common size (27).

Principal System Elements

A representative membrane softening system is shown in Figure 9–3. In this case, raw water is obtained from a hard groundwater source, and a pretreatment system applies scale inhibitor and sulfuric acid to maximize the solubility of troublesome constituents that might otherwise precipitate at the membrane surface. A cartridge filter is also used to remove particulate matter. High-pressure feed pumps are then used to provide the pressure necessary to transport flow across the membrane softening step. Capability is provided for the addition of a cleaning solution and sodium bilsulfite to the membrane surface. The cleaning solution allows for peri-

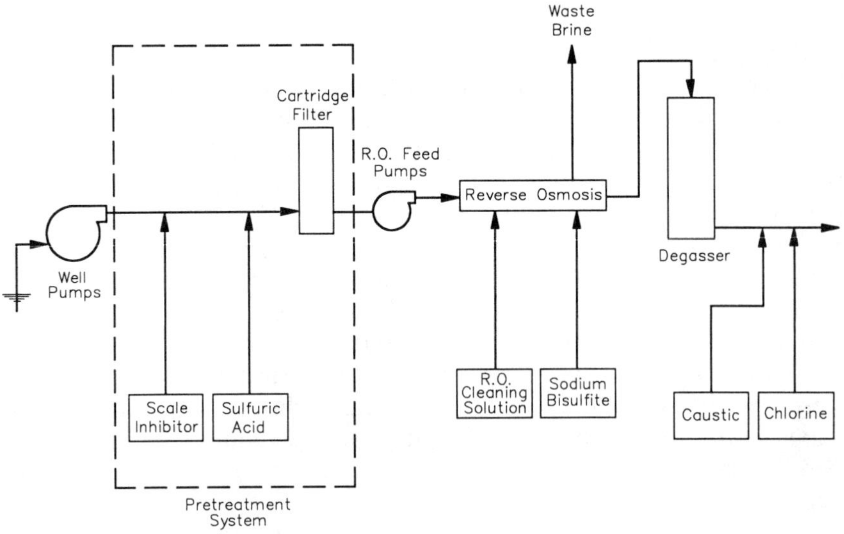

FIGURE 9–3. Typical membrane softening process.

odic cleaning of the membrane, while the sodium bisulfite (a reducing agent) is used as a disinfectant for removing attached biological growth. This treatment is appropriate for membrane configurations that are not directly attacked biologically and are not compatible with the feed of strong oxidizing-type disinfectants.

In cases where cellulose acetate membranes are used, the addition of a strong disinfecting agent to the feed stream may be required to prevent biological attack inherent to this type of membrane composition. These particular membranes are tolerant of exposure to oxidants and do not exhibit the deterioration that might occur with other membrane compositions.

Because of the removal of a number of dissolved salts, a relatively aggressive water is usually produced by membrane systems. In addition, the pretreatment step may include the feed of acids to adjust pH to a moderately acid region to reduce the solubility of problem constituents that might precipitate. This further increases the aggressive nature of the product water. To address these problems, a degassing step is often applied for removing carbon dioxide that could be formed, and the pH is increased with the addition of a caustic solution.

As with all membrane desalting systems, a waste brine stream must be removed from the inlet side of the membrane (see Figure 9–3). Without such removal, excessive salt buildup would occur. The extent of buildup affects both the osmotic pressure that must be overcome and the potential for scale-forming precipitates. In many cases, a minimum level of wasting is desired so that production can be maximized. There is a trade-off between this goal and the adverse effects of salt buildup that occurs when the waste brine stream is reduced in quantity. In many instances, it is often desirable to minimize disposal of the waste brine stream in order to reduce costs and associated disposal problems. In fact, the disposal of waste brines is a major consideration in the selection and cost evaluation of membrane systems and should be thoroughly evaluated as a part of any study or design process. In some cases, the inability to dispose of waste brines or the excess cost for such disposal may mitigate against the use of membrane systems.

Principal Operating Considerations

Major operating costs for membrane processes involve electrical power associated with pumping pressure as well as costs for chemicals that include acids and caustic to adjust pH and costs for scale inhibitors. Membrane replacement is another principal cost consideration since most existing membranes have a life of 3 to 5 years. The need for replacement is a result of deterioration in membrane capability for rejecting salts and reduced flow capacity. With the appropriate cleaning protocols, membrane life can be extended, but cleaning does not fully restore the membrane to its initial capabilities, so that membrane replacement will be necessary at some point. However, the degree of recovery of capacity achieved following each cleaning makes the cost of this maintenance procedure worthwhile.

System Configurations

Membrane systems are often configured in modules of convenient flow increments since it is difficult to maintain proper performance over a wide range of flows for any given membrane. For example, if the flow rate is increased, the salt buildup on the inlet side will be increased, thereby affecting the scaling potential and the osmotic pressure that must be overcome. On the other hand, if the flow rate is decreased too much, the quantity of product water available for diluting the salts that break through the membrane is also decreased, and the concentration of undesired constituents in the product stream will increase. The extent to which flows can vary and still produce acceptable results depends on specific site conditions and membrane characteristics.

One approach to consider with membrane systems is to gradually increase capacity over time by progressive installation of modules with capacities that roughly match production needs. Otherwise, membranes that are held off-line for extended periods may need to be stored under appropriate conditions to minimize degradation. Many membranes are hydrophobic in nature and, unless stored in a wet condition, require proper wetting protocols before they can be put back in service. For wet storage in excess of 3 days, consideration should be given to storage in a sodium bisulfite solution together with scheduled refreshment of this biocidal solution to prevent biological growth.

The complexity of storage makes it advisable to give careful consideration to the manner in which membrane modules can be operated. In some cases, a large volume of finished water storage may be required to compensate for limitations in the extent to which flow can be varied in the membrane modules to meet different demand conditions. Costs for this type of storage should be included in evaluating and designing membrane systems.

Flexibility for Source Quality Changes

Membrane processes are particularly applicable where a relatively constant water quality is encountered, such as in groundwater treatment. This, however, may not always be the case even with groundwater sources because, with continued withdrawal, the quality of some groundwaters can change over time. This type of change can affect the suitability of a given membrane or pretreatment approach. As a consequence, the extent of possible water quality changes needs to be considered as a part of the evaluation/design effort. In some cases, this may require a water quality modeling effort in groundwaters that are susceptible to change in quality.

In many cases, gradual changes in water quality can be compensated by simply allowing flexibility for variation in the feed pressure. Brine disposal rates can also be varied to adjust the quality on the inlet side to the membrane, thereby controlling the osmotic gradient that must be overcome. Flexibility in these adaptations can be considered when gradually changing quality is anticipated. Where changes in water quality can occur, it may be necessary to provide a planning/design approach that allows flexibility to use a different type of membrane at some future time.

Ultimately, the potential for significant changes in source water quality may affect the viability of a membrane approach. This is particularly true for many surface water supplies that are especially susceptible to short-term variability. These sources tend to exhibit water quality variations due to runoff conditions, as well as seasonal variations. Surface water sources also can have a much higher level of colloidal particles and may require more stringent pretreatment to avoid membrane plugging problems. As a consequence, it has been much more difficult to apply membrane systems to surface waters. For these reasons, the focus for the application of membrane technologies has largely been in treating groundwater and seawater, where source water quality is more consistent. This limitation may change as advances are made in membrane technology.

AIR STRIPPING

Air-stripping processes are specifically applicable for removing many organic constituents that have low solubility in water and are also susceptible to dispersal into surrounding air. These compounds are said to be volatile and are readily transferred from solution to air under appropriate contacting conditions. The air stripping process may be implemented in many different forms, including diffused aeration, mechanical aeration, packed column air stripping, tray stripping columns, and venturi air stripping columns. For disinfection byproduct applications, this process is essentially limited to the removal of volatile byproducts such as the trihalomethane, chloroform. Brominated trihalomethanes also can be removed, but the extent of removal declines as volatility decreases with increased bromine content in the molecule.

For potable water systems, certain site-specific considerations have favored the use of packed column air stripping processes for the removal of target volatile organic compounds (VOCs). A typical packed column air stripper is illustrated in Figure 9–4. A relatively new modification to this process is a cascade air stripping approach that involves the addition of fresh air along the full depth of a column. The concentration gradient from the liquid to the gas can be increased by introduction of air at these intermediate locations, increasing the rate of stripping and allowing for the removal of less volatile compounds. General concepts presented in this section will emphasize the more conventional packed tower approach. Additional information on cascade air stripping may be found in *Cascade Air Stripping System for Removal of Semi-Volatile Organic Contaminants: Feasibility Study* published by the AWWA Research Foundation (28).

Under proper conditions, volatile compounds in water will evaporate (be transported) from exposed surfaces into the adjacent air. If the surface area exposed to air is increased, the transport will also increase. If the air accepting the volatilized compounds is moved away or replaced with uncontaminated air, the rate of evaporation from the surface will also increase. Air stripping of volatile compounds from water is based upon

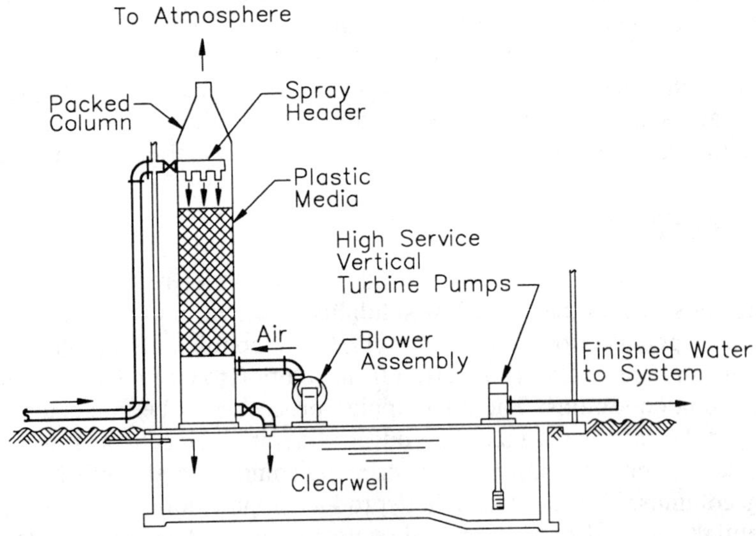

FIGURE 9–4. Typical packed column air stripper. (Reprinted from Ref. 25, with permission of U.S. EPA.)

these two basic premises. In air stripping, the water flows through a bed of packing installed in a vertical column. The packings used in the column or towers may be made of glass, plastic, or metal material. They may be shaped as open cylinders, saddles, or rings with a complex inner structure of struts and vanes. Size of the individual packing units may range from several inches in overall dimension to a fraction of an inch. In all cases the packing is designed to break up the downflow of water through the tower and provide a large surface area over which the water can flow. Air passes up through the tower flowing counter to the liquid. The design intent is to provide ideal surface conditions for volatilization and removal of the volatile organics.

Process Theory

Henry's law relationship defines the extent of volatility of a compound, thereby indicating its susceptibility to air stripping. In this relationship, the ratio of the concentration of a contaminant in the gas phase to the contaminant concentration in the liquid phase at equilibrium is defined as Henry's law coefficient:

$$H = \frac{C \text{ air}}{C \text{ water}} \tag{9–11}$$

The Henry's law coefficient of a specific compound, also known as the Henry's constant, can be determined in a laboratory.

For most drinking water applications, the contaminant concentration occurs in a low concentration range in which the Henry's law coefficient is approximately constant and does not vary significantly with concentration. However, the Henry's law coefficient may be affected by temperature, exhibiting a tendency for decrease as temperature is decreased.

In the case of increases in temperature, the Henry's law coefficient may be dramatically influenced, with higher temperatures enhancing the out-gassing of the organic compounds. This strong temperature coefficient has been empirically described by the following equation:

$$\log H_c = A - B - T \tag{9–12}$$

where T is the absolute temperature and A and B are constants.

The Henry's law coefficient is a direct indicator of the tendency for removal of a target compound by air stripping. For example, the larger the Henry's law coefficient, the lower the water solubility and the more amenable the compound is to removal by the air stripping process.

In addition to the Henry's law coefficient, another important concept is the mass transfer coefficient, which defines the rate at which an equilibrium condition can be approached. This coefficient is normally related to the diffusion coefficient of the target compound through water and through air. When combined with equilibrium relationships, mathematical models of air stripping columns can be developed in terms of tower heights and air and liquid loading rates.

There are several different ways to estimate the mass transfer coefficient using empirical equations from handbooks. However, it is sometimes necessary for the estimated values to be verified by field testing. If an air stripping facility at the nearby location has been evaluated, the data may, under limited situations, be applied to the subject site. Otherwise, pilot testing might be appropriate, especially where removal of uncommon volatile compounds is involved.

Design and Operational Considerations

Modeling approaches allow evaluation of combinations of water and air loadings that are capable of achieving target levels of removal. The selection of conditions can be viewed as an optimization. In general, the height of packing has the most profound influence in increasing tower performance. However, costs substantially increase with tower height, and an optimum height occurs where the incremental benefits from further increase are outweighed by incremental additions to cost.

A major design decision involves selection of a packing material, which affects the removal efficiency per unit height, the back pressure on the air blower, and the maximum allowable liquid loading per unit area. Other considerations include the local cost of power and site-specific constraints regarding the structural integrity of existing facilities.

For many applications, a mixture of organic compounds is encountered, each with its own Henry's law coefficient. The individual compounds typically do not interact and are removed independent of each other. An individual tower design can be developed for each compound to be removed, but the design that controls is that required for the worst-case compound. This will result in a tower design capable of achieving the desired removals for all compounds. Therefore, it is important to identify the limiting compound as a key step in design and evaluation.

For multiple compound designs, a useful first approach is to compare the Henry's law constant for all compounds and identify the compound with the lowest Henry's law coefficient. This is the compound that is most reluctantly air stripped and, if the percent removal requirements are approximately the same for all compounds, this compound will be the limiting component.

Where different removal percentages are required for different compounds, an initial evaluation to determine the limiting component can be accomplished by multiplying the Henry's law coefficient by the required fractional removal. The number with the lowest value generally indicates the limiting compound. If no other compound is within an order of magnitude of this number, this is probably the process-limiting compound. If, however, the numbers are very similar, much more detailed calculations and perhaps a pilot investigation may be required to determine the actual limiting compound.

Air stripping has several site-specific features to be considered. For example, water temperature can play an important role in determining the efficiency of air stripping, with lower winter temperatures presenting a severe limitation to both the process efficiency and possible freezing of the unit. Therefore, minimum or lowest temperature is an important design consideration.

Air pollution concerns represent another site consideration. Costs can be significantly affected if spent air must be treated prior to discharge to the surrounding atmosphere. When this becomes a concern, it is sometimes possible to increase the air flow rate or alter the tower height or exhaust gas velocity so that greater dilution is achieved. Under more stringent conditions, treatment of the exit air may be required. Such treatment can include the following processes: thermal destruction, catalytic incineration, ozone destruction, and carbon adsorption. The addition of these processes can significantly increase the cost of air stripping systems and in some cases can double the cost (25).

Another feature that can affect the location and operability of air stripping columns at various points in a process train is the presence of constituents that can precipitate within a column and require periodic tower cleaning. Iron and manganese are the more common constituents that cause such problems. This type of problem may require that air stripping systems be located at downstream locations in a treatment train so that as much of these constituents as possible can be removed before introduction to the tower.

Depending on the particular volatile contaminants present, it is often sufficient to submit analyses of the water source to the designers and manufacturers of air stripping equipment for quotations and proposals for installation. Where more complex or difficult-to-remove volatiles may be present, pilot testing may be necessary to develop the required design coefficients. Cascade air stripping methods also may be a consideration for treating these more difficult compounds.

References

1. Applegate, L. E. 1984. Membrane separation processes. *Chem. Eng.* 91(12): 64–89.
2. Conlon, W. J. 1985. Pilot field test data for prototype ultra low pressure R.O. membrane. Proceedings of the Second World Congress on Desalination and Water Reuse, Vol. 3, International Desalinization Association.
3. Conlon, W. J., et al. 1988. Membrane softening facilities in south Florida—A cost update. 62nd Annual Tech. Conference, FS/AWWA/FPCA and FW and PCOA, November 1988.
4. Culler, P. A., and S. A. McLellan. 1976. A new approach to partial demineralization. 50th Annual Tech. Conference, FS/AWWA/FPCA and FW and PCOA, October 1976.
5. Dupont Co. 1982. *Permasep engineering manual.* Wilmington, DE: E. I. Dupont de Nemours and Company.
6. Dykes, G. M. 1983. Desalting water in Florida. *JAWWA* 75(3): 104–7.
7. Edwards, E. D., I. C. Watson, and D. C. McKenna. 1988. Softening membranes, testing shows a strong municipal application for THM control. Biennial Conference National Water Supply Improvement Association, August 1988.
8. Hindin, E., G. H. Dunstan, and P. J. Bennett. 1968. Water reclamation by reverse osmosis, Bulletin 310. Tech. Extension Service, Washington State University.
9. Hodgson, T. D. 1970. Selective properties of cellulose acetate membranes toward ions in aqueous solution. *Desalination* 8: 99.
10. Kaup, E. 1973. Design factors in reverse osmosis. *Chem. Eng.* 4: 46–55.
11. Jacangelo, J. G., et al., 1991. Evaluation of low-pressure membrane filtration as a water treatment alternative for the removal of *Giardia* and microbial indicators. Presented at 1991 AWWA Conference, Philadelphia, PA, June 1991.
12. Krem, S. S. 1975. Reverse osmosis makes high quality water now. *Environ. Sci. & Tech.* 9(14): 315.
13. Loeb, S., and S. Sourirajan. 1960. UCLA Dept. of Engr. Report No. 60-60. University of California, Los Angeles.
14. Lonsdale, H. K., and H. E. Podall. 1972. *Reverse osmosis membrane research.* New York: Plenum Press.
15. Mulford, L. A., P. S. Jones, and J. S. Taylor. 1990. Disinfection by-product control by nanofiltration. Presented at 1990 AWWA Convention, Cincinnati, OH, June 1990.
16. Peterson, R. 1986. *The expanding roster of reverse osmosis membranes.*

Proceedings of the National Water Supply Improvement Association, Washington, DC.
17. Post, Buckley, Shuh and Jernigan, Inc. 1988. City of Boynton Beach Membrane Process Test Study Report, Boynton Beach, FL, May 1988.
18. Reid, C. E., and E. T. Breton. Water and ion flow across cellulosic membranes. *J. Appl. Polymer Sci.* 3(2): 133–43.
19. Sourirajan, S. 1963. The mechanism of demineralization of aqueous sodium chloride solutions by flow, under pressure, through porous membranes. *I&EC Fundam.* 2(1): 51–5.
20. Sourirajan, S. 1970. *Reverse osmosis*. New York: Academic Press.
21. Taylor, J. S., et al. 1986. Cost and performance of in-plant trihalomethane control techniques. U.S. EPA Report EPA/600/52–85/138, January 1986.
22. Taylor, J. S., et al. 1988. *Long-term performance, cost and modeling of membrane processes used for THM control on an organic groundwater source*. Proceedings of the National Water Supply Improvement Association, San Diego, CA.
23. U.S. EPA. 1986. *Design manual: Municipal wastewater disinfection*. EPA/625/1-861/621. Cincinnati, OH: U.S. Environmental Protection Agency, Office of Research and Development.
24. U.S. EPA. 1989. *Guidance manual for compliance with filtration and disinfection requirements for public drinking water systems using surface water sources*. EPA/68-01/6989. Washington, DC: U.S. Environmental Protection Agency, Office of Drinking Water.
25. U.S. EPA. 1980. *Technologies for upgrading existing or designing new drinking water treatment facilities*. EPA/625/4-89/023. Cincinnati, OH: U.S. Environmental Protection Agency, Office of Drinking Water.
26. Watson, I. C. 1988. *Membrane system applications and economics*. Proceedings of the Annual Meeting, American Water Works Association, Orlando, FL.
27. Taylor, J. S., S. J. Duranceau, W. M. Barrett, and J. F. Goigel. 1989. *Assessment of potable water membrane applications and research needs*. Report for AWWA Research Foundation, Denver, CO, December 1989.
28. Jang, W., N. Nirmalakhandan, and R. E. Speece. 1989. *Cascade air stripping system for removal of semi-volatile organic contaminants: feasibility study*. Report for AWWA Research Foundation, Denver CO, December 1989.

10

Activated Carbon

with contributions by

James P. Black and Dennis O. Rester
American Norit Co., Inc.
on *Manufacture/Properties/Regeneration*

Francis A. DiGiano, Prof.
University of North Carolina
on *Modeling/DBP Removals*

A. David Nickols
Hazen and Sawyer
on *Design Concepts*

Activated carbon provides an effective method for adsorbing a wide range of organic compounds and can be considered for use in the removal of organic disinfection byproducts and organic precursors. Adsorption involves the removal of an adsorbing compound (adsorbate) from solution by attachment to an adsorbing surface (adsorbent). Attachment results from attraction that may be physical, chemical, or electrical, or a combination of all three. In dilute solutions such as those typically found in drinking water sources, physical adsorption is the most prevalent form.

Adsorption phenomena are enhanced by the porous nature of activated carbon, which exposes a large internal surface over which the adsorption can take place. One pound of activated carbon can have a total surface area of about 150 acres. Activated carbon particles also have an irregular shape, which provides an external surface to which microbes can readily attach, resulting in the biological removal mechanisms for many compounds that occur in conjunction with adsorption. These effects will be described in this chapter and in Chapter 11 as well.

The capability of activated carbon to adsorb materials was recognized as early as the 1770s by Carl Wilhelm Scheel. However, modern practice dates from 1900 when a German patent was issued for the manufacture of steam-activated carbon from various carbonaceous raw materials. Actually, the first significant application of activated carbon was in 1909 in sugar refining, which continues to be a major market. Production of activated carbon became significant in Holland in 1911 and in Germany in 1913. In the United States, production began with the manufacture of activated carbon from peach pits and nutshells. These were principally used for adsorption of vapors and were used in gas masks during World War I (1914–1918).

After World War I, production in the United States grew rapidly, and activated carbon began to be used in liquid adsorption applications as well. New grades of activated carbons were manufactured from black ash, a paper pulp waste residue, and from lignite coal. These were used predominantly in sugar refining. In 1929, the use of activated carbon for control of tastes and odors in potable water was initiated in the United States.

Today, activated carbon is used worldwide. In addition to the United States, producers are located in England, France, Holland, Germany, Mexico, Belgium, Italy, Russia, India, and Japan. Activated carbon is now produced from coal, sawdust, wood chips, petroleum coke, peat, fly ash, and coconut shells. Between 6 and 8 million pounds of activated carbon are placed in water treatment plants each year. This is, for the most part, virgin carbon, since very little regenerated carbon is used in water treatment at this time.

Activated carbon (AC) is used in two basic forms, powdered and granular. In water treatment, granular activated carbon (GAC) can either be contained in separate contactors or included as part of filter media, where it replaces sand and/or coal filter media. Use of GAC can be relatively expensive, especially where separate contactors add capital cost of about the same order of magnitude as regular filters or where high operating costs are incurred for periodic replacement or regeneration. However, the method of application is varied, and no single process arrangement can represent GAC costs or its effectiveness for all water treatment scenarios.

Powdered activated carbon (PAC) is often added to the process flow as a first treatment, preferably ahead of disinfectants and coagulants. However, it can also be added with coagulants or just before filtration. Whether PAC is more economical than GAC depends upon frequency of use and the feed rates needed. PAC has been particularly effective in treating periodic increases in source water organics or tastes and odors. Although past effectiveness for removal of disinfection byproduct precursors has been mixed, recent studies show that PAC performance might be improved if the proper size and type of PAC is chosen and adequate contact time and agitation is available. However, there is still no clear indication of the success of these modifications for high levels of precursor removal.

TREATMENT MECHANISMS OF ACTIVATED CARBON

Adsorption

Adsorption occurs when the attraction at the adsorption surface is stronger than the solution forces available to keep the contaminants dissolved in solution. The solubility of compounds is a relative measure of the solution forces, so that the more soluble compounds tend to be less readily adsorbed. The principal attributes that promote adsorption are low water solubility, high molecular weight, and neutral charge. A condition that affects solubility is characterized by the concept of polarity. Under this concept, molecules with a net neutral charge can still have centers of positive and negative charge at different locations along the molecule. Some compounds can have fairly distinct positive and negative charge centers at different locations in the molecule. These compounds are said to have a polar character, with water providing a good example of a common polar molecule. Water is efficient in solubilizing other polar or ionic materials, since the water molecule's positive and negative charge centers will exert attractive forces on oppositely charged centers in the molecules of the other materials. Therefore, polar compounds are more soluble in water than nonpolar compounds due to this added *solution force* and are generally less readily adsorbed.

Although adsorption of a dissolved impurity from water may be enhanced by low solubility, several forces of attraction are involved at the adsorbing surface. Three particular phenomena cause adsorption: electrical attraction (exchange adsorption), van der Waals attraction (physical or ideal adsorption), and chemical reaction (chemisorption or chemical adsorption) (22). In most cases, adsorption results from some combination of all three of these conditions, with physical adsorption, possibly enhanced by low solubility, playing the dominant role for many organic compounds.

As an adsorption process proceeds, compounds are removed from solution until an equilibrium is reached between the concentration in solution and the quantity adsorbed by or adhered to the physical surface. An adsorption isotherm expresses the equilibrium relationship between the amount adsorbed per unit weight of carbon (adsorbent) and the concentration remaining in solution. This equilibrium can be altered if other compounds present can compete for adsorption sites, thereby reducing the capacity available for a given compound.

In adsorption, an undesirable process called *sloughing* is caused by competing contaminants that may displace an already adsorbed target contaminant. When the target contaminant is displaced, it moves farther down in the bed until it finds an unused spot at which to reattach. Finally, as the bed becomes depleted of available adsorption sites, the desorbed contaminant has nowhere to go and passes out or breaks through the bottom of the media. Under this desorption condition, the concentration of the contaminant in the effluent sometimes can occur at levels considerably higher than in the influent.

An adsorption isotherm provides a graphic plot showing the distribution of a contaminant between the adsorbed phase and the solution phase at equilibrium. Although the practical detention time used in most treatment applications does not provide sufficient time to achieve true equilibrium, isotherms are still important first steps in evaluating the applicability of activated carbon alternatives. The ultimate condition that will be continually approached with increased contact time is described by isotherms, making them essential for any characterization of adsorption behavior.

Adsorption is, in reality, a dynamic process that involves three consecutive steps for the transport of a compound from the bulk solution to an adsorption site of a porous adsorbent such as activated carbon: (1) transport through a surface film to the exterior of the adsorbent; (2) diffusion within the pores and/or along the pore wall surfaces (intraparticle diffusion); and (3) attachment to an available interior site (22). Each of these steps proceeds at a given speed, and it is possible for one step in particular to be slower than the others. This slower step controls the overall rate of adsorption. In most cases, the overall rate of adsorption of organics onto activated carbon tends to be controlled by one of the first two transport steps. The attachment or adsorption step is typically very rapid and normally is not a controlling condition.

When the overall rate is controlled by a transport through a surface film, the reaction rate should be directly proportional to the difference between the concentration of the adsorbing compound in solution and the ultimate equilibrium concentration. On the other hand, if diffusion within the pores and capillaries of the carbon limits the adsorption rate, the rate would not be expected to be linear with concentration gradient. The effect of concentration gradient still exists but is more complex under this circumstance.

Chemical Reaction

Although the physical adsorption phenomena tend to be the dominant interaction for many organic compounds on activated carbon, chemical reactions significant to disinfection can occur on a carbon surface as well. For example, chlorine is removed from water by reaction with carbon to form chloride ions (8). Activated carbon can also remove chloramines, and the following reactions have been proposed for monochloramine (NH_2Cl) (4):

$$NH_2Cl + H_2O + \overline{C} \longrightarrow NH_3 + Cl^- + \overline{CO} + H^+ \tag{10–1}$$

$$2NH_2Cl + \overline{CO} \longrightarrow N_{2(g)} + H_2O + 2H^+ + 2Cl^- + \overline{C} \tag{10–2}$$

where $\overline{C}$ represents the GAC surface, which initially reacts to form a surface oxide site ($\overline{CO}$). $\overline{CO}$ reacts with monochloramine to form molecular nitrogen (N_2) while $\overline{C}$ reacts to form ammonia (NH_3), resulting in a mix of end products. These reactions are slower than those with free chlorine and require longer contact times.

Reactions also occur with chlorites, a byproduct of chlorine dioxide. However, these may not always be beneficial since the end product for these reactions can be chlorate, which is also an undesired byproduct (7). Chemical reaction is also important in removing some common tastes and odors from drinking water.

Biological Action

Biological degradation processes generally become established on activated carbon surfaces and can provide benefits in addition to those available through adsorption mechanisms. For example, these processes are capable of controlling many taste and odor compounds (2). This has probably been an influence in the past use of GAC to control tastes and odors. Removal of biodegradable organic matter, a concern in relation to bacterial regrowth, is another possible role for biological mechanisms. Phenomena associated with biodegradable organic matter and associated removal processes are discussed in Chapters 2 and 11.

Whether intended or not, most applications of GAC in drinking water treatment have resulted in some inevitable organic removal by biological processes that occur due to biofilms that accumulate at the carbon surface. Where biological mechanisms are a major focus, the process is sometimes termed *biological activated carbon* (BAC). However, even in cases where physical adsorption is an objective, biological removal often occurs and continues after the physical adsorption capacity is reached. This is sometimes termed *steady-state removal* since it levels off at this fairly steady removal rate for a long period of time.

In drinking water, steady-state removals have been observed for TOC and trihalomethane-formation potential. The degree of removal is variable and is inevitably affected by factors such as character of organics, water quality characteristics, and loading conditions for GAC (e.g., bed depth, loading rates, and detention time). Also, prior treatment of water with ozone can make the organic matter more readily biodegradable, thereby enhancing this type of process. Ozonation converts larger molecular-sized organics to those of smaller size, which may be more adsorbable or more biodegradable. In some cases, steady-state removals can exceed 50 percent, but they are typically much less and may not be enough when high levels of control over disinfection byproduct formation are required.

Use of activated carbon for biodegradation can be achieved in two basic configurations: postfiltration contactors and filter contactors. Filter contactor approaches involve the replacement of conventional filter media with GAC, which then performs a dual function: biological activated carbon for adsorption and for biodegradation, and a filtering media for removal of particles. Although this filter adsorbing approach offers potential for significant reduction of capital cost compared to separate filters and contactors, several features of this process need to be considered (10):

- Possible increased rate of head loss buildup in the filters due to biological growths in the media. This will require good filter wash capability. Consideration should be given to air scour for improved wash capability as compared with hydraulic methods. Care should be exercised to avoid excessive air scour that will damage GAC particles.
- Possible increase in mud-ball formation promoted by the growths, again requiring consideraton of appropriate filter wash and air scour methods.
- Corrosive action of GAC on metal parts in the filters, requiring coating with corrosion resistant materials or the use of stainless steel.
- When GAC is used to partially replace conventional media by serving as an upper media layer over a smaller sized sand, a dual media configuration can be achieved. The potential may exist for premature wear and breakdown of the GAC media by the sharp, siliceous sand media particles during backwashing. Selection of an appropriate sand size to provide for the separation of media during backwash can reduce the opportunity for wear.

MANUFACTURE

Activated carbon is manufactured by selective oxidation of a carbonaceous material to produce a highly porous structure; almost any carbonaceous material can be used. In the United States, granular activated carbon is generally derived from some form of coal: bituminous, subbituminous, or lignite. At least one supplier is now providing a wood-based activated carbon that has a porous structure intended to increase surface area available for biofilms in BAC applications.

Carbonaceous materials are activated by either high-temperature steam or chemical dehydration. High-temperature steam activation is more common, and water-grade granular activated carbon is typically manufactured by this process. It involves heating the raw material to high temperatures (800 to 1,000°C) under very carefully controlled conditions in the presence of steam, which acts as an oxidizing gas.

Chemical activation consists of heating the raw material to a lower temperature (400 to 500°C) in the presence of a strong dehydrating agent. The most common agent is phosphoric acid, although zinc chloride and others are used in Europe and Asia.

The choice of raw materials, the activation method, and the manufacturing conditions control the pore size distribution and other properties of the final activated carbon. In a particular application, the effectiveness of an activated carbon is most often influenced by the pore size distribution.

ACTIVATED CARBON SELECTION CRITERIA

In the past, activated carbon selection has been based on a comparison of published properties or single-component isotherm tests. Testing of spiked water samples at higher-than-normal concentration levels has also been used for activated carbon selection purposes. However, the best way to choose an activated carbon is by conducting tests on the actual water to be treated at the contaminant concentration levels most likely to be encountered in plant operation. This is the only way to ensure that the best match of carbon is selected for the specific water being treated.

For activated granular carbon, the testing should consist of multiple pilot columns where the effluent from each column is analyzed to accurately determine the effective life of the carbon bed. Adsorption isotherms can be used as supplemental information for screening purposes, but should not be relied upon for system design.

Pore Size Distribution

Pores within activated carbons may vary significantly in size. Measures of the amount of pore volume available and the size distribution are, therefore, important for characterizing different activated carbons. This distribution affects carbon selection for a given application, since maximum adsorption normally occurs in pores that are approximately the same size as the molecules being adsorbed. A small-pore carbon, which characteristically tends to have a high surface area, is generally more suitable for gas phase removals since the molecules being adsorbed are relatively small. In liquid phase applications, however, removals may be hindered if pores are too small and may become blocked by the larger molecules. A lower-surface-area, large-pore carbon is often more suitable for many liquid phase applications.

Activated Carbon Properties

Physical properties of granular activated carbons typically available in the United States are listed in Table 10–1; adsorptive properties of these same activated carbons are listed in Table 10–2. More detailed characteristics for a specific product are available from the manufacturer. The most significant difference in both physical and adsorptive properties of coal-based carbons is found to occur as a consequence of the type of coal used for preparation. Lignite-based carbons have a mean pore radius of over 30 Å, whereas the bituminous based carbons have a mean pore size less than 20 Å. In terms of adsorptive characteristics for liquid applications, the bituminous-based coal carbons have a higher capacity for small molecules, whereas the lignite carbons have a higher capacity for larger molecules such as those that can act as disinfection byproduct precursors. The bituminous-based coal carbons adsorb more iodine, phenol, and atrazine; the lignite-based carbons adsorb more humic acid, tannic acid, and molasses color.

Many activated carbons are characterized by the capability to adsorb low molecular weight organics, which is based on the capability to adsorb iodine from a standard solution (known as the iodine number). This parameter tends to favor the smaller-pore activated carbons, which have a large total surface area. However, the molasses number, which characterizes the availability of large pore diameters, may be more appropriate for characterizing an activated carbon for removing the higher molecular weight precursor compounds. For many of the lower molecular weight SOCs and most disinfection byproducts (DBPs), smaller-pore activated carbon may be more appropriate.

In addition to pore size, the overall particle diameter of the granular activated carbon has an effect. The smaller the particle size, the faster the rate of removal, whether by adsorption or chemical reaction. This is because, in smaller-sized particles, the contaminant has less distance to travel through the pores to reach the adsorption sites in the interior of the carbon particle.

The effect of particle size on performance is illustrated by a test in which a 5 mg/l chlorine solution was run through GAC beds with an empty

TABLE 10–1. Physical Property Data for Potable Water Granular Carbons

Carbon Type	Moisture (wt %)	Ash (wt %)	Vibrating Feed Density (lb/ft^3)	Backwashed and Drained Density (lb/ft^3)	Mesh Size	Uniformity Coef.	Effective Size (mm)	Mean Particle Diameter (mm)	Approximate Mean Pore Radius
Lignite 1	8 max.	16	25	24	10 × 30	1.7	0.8	1.1	30
Lignite 2	8 max.	16	25	24	8 × 30	1.9	0.9	1.5	33
Bituminous 1	2 max.	8	33	30	8 × 30	<2	0.8–0.9	1.6	17
Bituminous 2	2 max.	8	33	30	12 × 40	<1.8	0.55–0.65	1.0	17
Bituminous 3	2 max.	5	28	26	8 × 30	<2	0.8–0.9	1.6	16
Bituminous 4	2 max.	5	28	26	12 × 40	<2	0.55–0.65	1.0	15
Bituminous 5	2 max.	8	36	30	12 × 40	<1.8	0.55–0.75	1.0	17
Bituminous 6	2 max.	8	36	30	8 × 30	<1.8	0.85–1.05	1.6	17
Bituminous 7	2 max.	8	28	25	12 × 40	<1.8	0.55–0.75	1.0	15

All carbons measured approximately 75 by the AWWA abrasion test method.

Source: American Norit Company, Inc.

TABLE 10–2. Adsorptive Data for Potable Water Granular Carbons

	Relative Efficiency[a]					
Carbon Type	Iodine	Molasses	Tannic Acid	Humic Acid	Atrazine	Phenol
Lignite 1	68	285	213	1,000	53	50
Lignite 2	62	285	213	1,000	53	50
Bituminous 1	90	29	23	100	42	40
Bituminous 2	90	29	32	100	42	40
Bituminous 3	100[b]	100	100	100	100	100
Bituminous 4	113	129	160	210	105	100
Bituminous 5	87	30	34	200	—	—
Bituminous 6	92	123	87	200	—	—
Bituminous 7	108	149	126	300	63	79

[a] Coal carbon number 3 (a widely used grade) assigned as 100.
[b] Corresponds to 975 Iodine Number.

Source: American Norit Company, Inc.

bed contact time of 10 seconds. A 20 × 50 mesh carbon maintained an effluent of 1 mg/l concentration for 60 hours, but a large 8 × 30 mesh broke through after 5 hours (12).

In general, particle size should be as small as possible, while avoiding excessively small carbon particles that will be susceptible to high loss of head and plugging. Loss of carbon in backwashing carbon contactors is also a consideration in selecting particle size, since there is more of a tendency for smaller-sized particles to be carried away in backwash flow.

Powdered Activated Carbon

Reported results regarding the removal of disinfection byproduct precursors by powdered activated carbon (PAC) have often been discouraging. This may be the result of using PAC with small pore diameters that do not readily accommodate the larger precursor molecules. Some improvement in performance might occur with use of larger pore size materials. Inadequate contacting conditions may represent another problem in these evaluations.

Although PAC generally involves the same theoretical adsorption process as GAC, it is contacted as a suspension as opposed to the fixed position condition that occurs in GAC columns. Water quality conditions, intensity of mixing, and contact time all have significant effects on PAC adsorption efficiency. The conditions in many flocculation units, where PAC is usually added, can conflict with the adsorption process. Surfaces of the carbon can be plugged by coagulants or floc, and, in addition, flocculation employs gentle agitation, whereas a vigorous mixing is better for adsorption. Separate contact basins, ahead of coagulation and possibly with PAC recirculation provisions, have been suggested for improving PAC performance. However, experience with this type of operation is limited.

Particle size is another important factor in PAC adsorption. Commercial PAC has a nominal diameter of 44 μm. It was observed in one study that when a carbon with a 7-μm radius was used, the adsorption rate was greatly increased. This would mean that much smaller doses of PAC would be required. However, it is not clear whether it is feasible for manufacturers to supply such smaller sizes (13).

BREAKTHROUGH CURVE RELATIONSHIPS FOR GAC

The progression of adsorption in a GAC column is shown in Figure 10–1. As the loading of the GAC column increases over time, the concentration

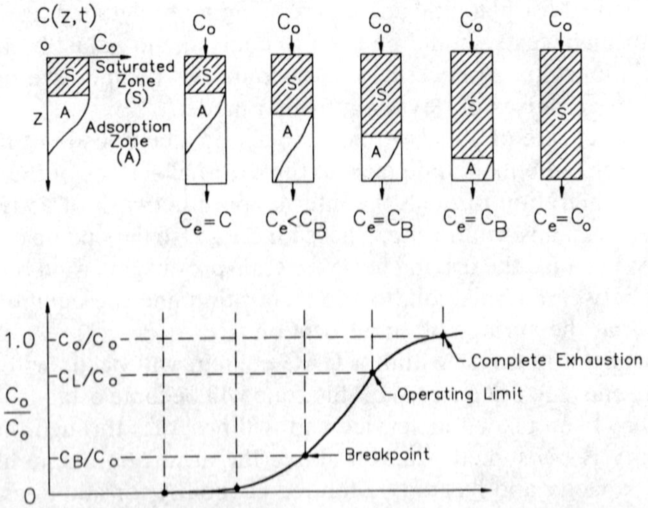

FIGURE 10–1. Breakthrough characteristics of a fixed bed adsorber. (Reprinted from W. J. Weber, *Physicochemical Processes for Water Quality Control*, Copyright © 1972 Wiley Interscience, by permission of John Wiley and Sons, Inc.)

at the effluent of the bed begins to increase, illustrated by the breakthrough curve. This phenomenon is frequently shown as a plot of the ratio of effluent concentration to feed concentration (C_e/C_O) versus the loading to the column expressed either as volume of water processed or the time of operation. The objective of process analysis is to estimate the service time before GAC regeneration or replacement is necessary. A target concentration or C_e/C_O along the breakthrough curve, most likely established by regulatory requirements, will determine this service time.

The shape of the breakthrough curve, and thus the nature of the rise to the target concentration, is dictated both by the equilibrium capacity of the carbon and the rate at which this capacity is approached. These phenomena, which are described by adsorption kinetics, will describe the shape of the curve beginning with a low initial concentration and extending to the point of complete column exhaustion. Typically, the target concentration occurs at some intermediate point along the curve.

Mathematical relationships exist for describing adsorption kinetics, although their use is often quite difficult because of the competition between other adsorbing compounds that often occur in natural waters, which greatly complicates the evaluation. Therefore, mathematical modeling evaluations should be performed in conjunction with testing. Despite this complication, mathematical modeling provides important insights critical for planning and establishing more detailed testing protocols. Pilot plant tests should be used to confirm and adjust breakthrough curve relationships as necessary to account for competitive adsorption and any other causes of deviation from a model.

The overall rate of an adsorption process is a composite of the rate of transfer from the bulk liquid phase to the external surface of the GAC and the rate of migration through the internal pore network of activated carbon to reach an adsorption site. These kinetics also depend on equilibrium principles because the driving force for transport is governed by a driving gradient between a bulk solution concentration and the equilibrium concentration at the surface of an adsorption site.

Much of the removal within a GAC column will occur within an adsorption zone (see Figure 10–1). This zone will become established once a column has been placed in service and will progress through the column as capacity is consumed. Carbon above the adsorption zone has nearly reached capacity and has only a limited capability for additional adsorption. The exhausted portion of the column that precedes the adsorption zone provides little opportunity for removal. Therefore, flow enters the adsorption zone at a concentration nearly equal to that of the column influent. As this flow enters the adsorbing zone, it encounters carbon with progressively increasing adsorption capacity remaining. Significant adsorption begins to occur and continues until most of the adsorbing constituents are removed as the flow reaches the lower part of the adsorption zone. Carbon located beyond this zone remains relatively fresh. The adsorption zone will progress through the column as an adsorption front with the adsorptive capacity being consumed as the front passes. In mass transfer calculations, the adsorption zone is often referred to as the *mass transfer zone* (MTZ).

The total breakthrough curve within a carbon column can be approximated by focusing on changes that occur in the MTZ since only limited changes in concentration occur at other locations in the bed. As a consequence, some simplified adsorption models concentrate on defining the changes that occur in the MTZ. This can significantly simplify the mathematical analysis. Because external (outside the particle) and internal (within the pores) diffusion occurs in series, the slowest of these mechanisms will control the overall rate of adsorption and the shape of the MTZ. Two extremes of shape are shown in Figure 10–2. When external diffusion is the slower step, the breakthrough curve tends to be S-shaped. If internal diffusion is slower, the breakthrough curve rises without a clear inflection point and tends to tail off very slowly as the effluent approaches the influent concentration. In either case, the faster the adsorption process, the steeper the breakthrough curve.

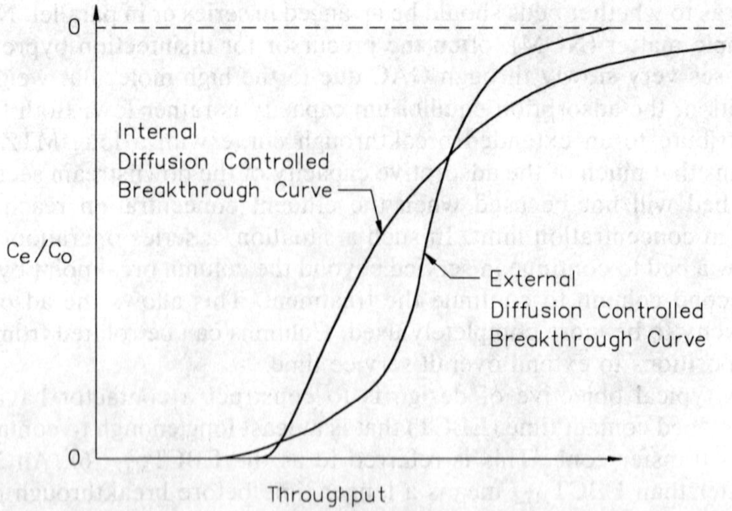

FIGURE 10–2. Extremes of typical breakthrough curves. (Courtesy of F. A. DiGiano.)

Mass transfer rates and, thus, the steepness of the breakthrough curve depend on several conditions, including the concentration and relative diffusive rate of the target compound within the bed, the hydraulic loading through the bed, the GAC particle size and shape, the pore size distribution of the GAC, and the adsorption equilibrium properties of the target compound. Two important design decisions to be made are particle size and hydraulic loading. Pore size distribution and adsorption equilibrium properties will depend on the types of GAC selected. Particle size affects the available external surface area; external area increases as particle size is decreased. Smaller particles also provide for less distance or resistance to internal pore travel to adsorption sites for internal mass transfer processes. Therefore, there is a potential for increasing rates by using smaller particles.

Hydraulic loading affects the level of turbulence at the particle interface, thereby increasing the external mass transfer rate from the bulk solution. For a given column volume, increased hydraulic loading, with a decrease in the required cross-sectional area, must be compensated for by increasing column height. Beyond a point, the mass transfer advantages of increased hydraulic loading begin to be offset by increased head losses and the increased cost for construction of taller columns.

The steepness of the breakthrough curve, dictated by the mass transfer rate and the hydraulic loading, is an important consideration in the decision as to whether beds should be arranged in series or in parallel. Natural organic matter (NOM), often the precursor for disinfection byproducts, diffuses very slowly through GAC due to the high molecular weight. In addition, the adsorption equilibrium capacity is rather low. Both factors contribute to an extended breakthrough curve with a long MTZ. This means that much of the adsorptive capacity of the downstream section of the bed will not be used when the effluent concentration reaches the design concentration limit. In such a situation, a series operation would allow a bed to continue in service beyond the column breakpoint by using a second column to continue the treatment. This allows the adsorptive capacity to be more completely used. Columns can be rotated from lead/lag positions to extend overall service time.

A typical objective of design is to construct a contactor having an empty bed contact time (EBCT) that is at least long enough to contain the mass transfer zone. This is referred to as the $EBCT_{MTZ}$ (6). An EBCT greater than $EBCT_{MTZ}$ means a longer time before breakthrough begins and, thus, a longer service time and more complete utilization of activated carbon capacity. Therefore, it is desirable in practice to design an EBCT that is longer than the minimum so as to have a reasonable exhaustion frequency. Also, activated carbon in the MTZ is only partially exhausted, and the extent to which activated carbon capacity can be fully utilized is determined by the ratio of the volume of the MTZ to the volume of carbon that resides in the exhausted portion of a GAC column upstream of the MTZ. The lower this ratio, the higher the cost for activated carbon replacement and regeneration. This ratio is increased by increasing the size of the contactor. However, incremental economic benefits in terms of reduced replacement/regeneration costs are offset by added costs for larger contactors, and a point is reached at which the added incremental cost for increasing the contactor volume exceeds the incremental savings in carbon replacement/regeneration (reactivation) costs. Because improved economy is achieved up to this point, this becomes the optimal design condition. Therefore, proper sizing of a contactor can be viewed as an optimization process that balances the costs of extra contact volume versus the reduced replacement/regeneration costs.

Table 10–3 lists $EBCT_{MTZ}$ values calculated from an analysis of mass transfer using the homogeneous surface diffusion model approach (HSDM) (6). The $EBCT_{MTZ}$ is specific for a given contaminant and bed design because it depends on external and internal diffusion, equilibrium adsorption characteristics, GAC particle radius, and hydraulic loading condition. In actual practice, competing substances will be present, and these effects will also have to be taken into account in developing a revised $EBCT_{MTZ}$.

TABLE 10–3. Calculated Empty Bed Contact Time vs. Bed Volumes Fed Before Breakthrough

Adsorbate	Feed Conc. (μg/l)	$EBCT_{MTZ}$ (min)	BVF_{max}
PFA	6,000	686	1,080
CCE	300	1.74	13,100
Benzene	300	0.88	21,600
m-Xylene	5.2	2.64	4,640,000
TCE	77.3	9.22	119,000

PFA = peat fulvic acid; CCE = carbon tetrachloride; TCE = trichloroethene; MTZ = mass transfer zone.

Source: Ref. 6. Reprinted from *Journal American Water Works*, Vol. 79, No. 1 (January 1987), by permission. Copyright © 1987, American Water Works Association.

All except one of the $EBCT_{MTZ}$ values listed are less than 10 minutes. The exception is 686 minutes calculated for peat fulvic acid (PFA), a commonly used chemical model for naturally occurring precursors. Slow internal diffusion of PFA and poor adsorbability account for the unusually long $EBCT_{MTZ}$. Also, the feed concentration (6 mg/l) is higher than would be encountered in most waters and some variation would be expected as a consequence. The typical range of EBCT for most applications is from 10 to 20 minutes, long enough to contain the MTZ of many synthetic organic compounds (SOCs) of interest and to give service times on the order of years. However, these service times are not normally available when GAC is applied for removal of NOM. As will be discussed later, service times based on removal of NOM are typically on the order of months rather than years.

Estimating Service Time

Equilibrium Modeling

Although kinetics are important in determining the shape of the MTZ, rough approximations of service time can be made from estimates that neglect kinetic effects and rely upon equilibrium calculations. With this approach, the assumption is made that mass transfer occurs fast enough so that the $EBCT_{MTZ}$ can be ignored and the carbon bed is completely saturated at breakthrough. This condition will yield the maximum number of bed volumes that can be fed (BVF_{max}) prior to the breakthrough at a time of breakthrough (t_B):

$$BVF_{max} = \rho_B q / C_O \quad (10\text{–}3)$$

$$t_B = BVF_{max} \times EBCT \quad (10\text{–}4)$$

where q is the equilibrium solid phase loading on GAC in terms of mg adsorbed/g of GAC, ρ_B is the bulk density of the bed, g of GAC/l of bed volume, C_O is the feed concentration of material to be adsorbed, mg/l, and t_B is the time to reach complete breakthrough. The equilibrium solid phase loading, q, is often related to the feed concentration, C_O, by the Freundlich equilibrium adsorption equation:

$$q = kC_O^{1/n} \qquad (10\text{–}5)$$

where k and $1/n$ are compound and activated carbon-specific constants that are empirically derived based on experimental results.

Inspection of Equation 10–4 shows that the computed t_B for this simplified condition is directly proportional to the EBCT once the BVF_{max} value has been determined for a particular contaminant. Values of BVF_{max} at representative concentrations are given in Table 10–3. Note that PFA, a material similar to many naturally occurring THM precursors, has the smallest value because it exhibits weak adsorbability and is introduced to the GAC bed at a relatively high concentration as compared with available capacity. As in determinations of $EBCT_{MTZ}$, equilibrium modeling may need to be modified to account for competitive adsorption. In addition, the assumption of a negligible MTZ can be overly simplistic for less strongly adsorbed materials. Therefore, equilibrium models often represent a beginning point in the attempt to assess adsorption phenomena, but additional methods will be required to improve the level of understanding.

Dynamic Modeling

Dynamic models are far more complex mathematically than equilibrium models because they must account for mass transfer mechanisms at each location in the bed. Thus,

$$C = fn(z, t, r)$$

where z is length along the bed, t is time, and r is radial position in a GAC particle. Predictions of SOC breakthrough are possible with a homogeneous surface diffusion model (HSDM) or a pore-surface diffusion model (PSDM). The effects of competition between SOCs can be included with equilibrium relationships contained within these models.

There is ample evidence that reasonably good agreement between model and data can be obtained with a minimum of calibration when dealing with well-characterized SOCs. However, the presence of NOM complicates mass transfer and equilibrium considerations greatly. It has, in fact, been suggested that surface diffusion coefficients must be greatly reduced to reach agreement between model and data. Moreover, the predominant mechanism of internal diffusion for many SOCs may be pore diffusion rather than surface diffusion due to probable fouling of the surface by NOM. As will be discussed later, this will have implications for use of GAC for the removal of specific disinfection byproducts in the presence of NOM.

The simplified HSDM (6, 26) is often used to calculate the breakthrough curve and provides a good approximation when the EBCT is long enough to establish a constant wave pattern, i.e., unchanging shape of the concentration profile within the MTZ. This is referred to as the minimum EBCT, or $EBCT_{min}$, which is somewhat larger than the $EBCT_{MTZ}$ shown in Table 10–3. In fact, the $EBCT_{MTZ}$ is calculated directly from the $EBCT_{min}$ by accounting for only that portion of the adsorption zone that is bounded by concentrations between $C/C_O = 0.05$ and $C/C_O = 0.95$ (26).

Once a constant pattern is achieved, the shape of the breakthrough curve will remain relatively unchanged for most compounds and it is then possible to calculate the time to reach selected concentration in the effluent for an actual EBCT ($EBCT_{act}$):

$$t = t_{min} + (EBCT_{act} - EBCT_{min})(D_g + 1) \qquad (10\text{–}6)$$

where t is the actual time to breakthrough of the target C/C_O, and t_{min} is the time to breakthrough at the selected EBCT for the target C/C_O, starting from a time beginning at the edge of the MTZ. The values of $EBCT_{min}$ can be obtained from nomographs of HSDM model solutions for mass transfer conditions in the bed and by using Freundlich constants to characterize adsorption equilibria. D_g is the solute distribution parameter (a ratio of the mass of the adsorbing compound on the solid to that in water at equilibrium). It is defined by the following equation:

$$D_g = \rho_B q / E C_O \qquad (10\text{–}7)$$

where E is the pore volume in the bed.

The breakthrough time, t_B, can be very long even if $EBCT_{act}$ is only slightly larger than $EBCT_{min}$, because D_g is usually a large number (typically ranging from about 15,000 to more than 10,000,000). While an accurate solution is obtainable only when $EBCT_{act} > EBCT_{min}$, this approach also can give reasonable approximations when $EBCT_{act}$ is smaller.

Accounting for Fouling Effects

Recent work has measured the so-called fouling effect of NOM on the adsorption of SOCs (20). The empirical observation is that GAC particles withdrawn from a given position in the bed during contact with NOM have less equilibrium capacity as characterized by the Freundlich *k* value (the *n* value remains about the same) than fresh GAC. Moreover, the capacity decreases with time of bed operation until some minimum level is reached.

Capacity decrease occurs first in the influent end but eventually spreads throughout the bed. The reason is that, because of its poor adsorbability, the adsorption front for NOM moves much more quickly through the bed than does that of most SOCs. While NOM may not interact directly with the SOC, it may preadsorb onto GAC and thereby inhibit penetration of the slower advancing SOCs to otherwise available sorption sites.

Empirical findings are not easily incorporated into dynamic process modeling, but they may nevertheless be useful in estimating the reduced equilibrium capacity of a specific SOC (or disinfection byproduct) in theoretical models for estimating service time. One approach for estimating this effect is to preload a small laboratory GAC bed with NOM and then remove GAC particles for use in measuring the adsorption isotherm for the organic compounds of interest. The preloading time needed to get the maximum reduction in sorptive capacity is estimated to be about 1 day in a properly designed small column test (20). If this maximally reduced Freundlich *K* value is used in Equation 10–5, it should give a conservative estimate of service time.

The extent of reduction in SOC adsorption by NOM fouling depends very much on the adsorbability of the SOC. Those SOCs that are strongly adsorbed have adsorption fronts that advance very slowly, thus allowing for much more preloading of NOM before interactions with SOCs occur, especially in long columns (long EBCT). This will produce a greater reduction in the capacity of the SOC than if the SOC is weakly adsorbed, in which case less preloading of NOM occurs before the SOC front arrives at some position in the column.

The Rapid Small-Scale Column Test (RSSCT)

Crittenden and co-workers have advanced the idea of using very small columns (containing only a few grams of GAC) to obtain breakthrough curves that can be used directly to calculate service time in pilot and full-scale operations (27, 28). The essence of their concept rests in dimensional analysis of the HSDM, which leads to dimensionless groups that determine proper scaling of column experiments to maintain similitude. The RSSCT relies on scale-up relationships to extrapolate from a smaller

TABLE 10–4. Comparison of RSSCT and Full-Scale Column Design and Operation Parameters

	RSSCT	Large Column
GAC particle diameter	0.01 mm	0.5 mm
Column diameter	1.1–2.5 cm	2.5 m
Column length	0.06–0.4 m	0.4 m
EBCT	10–60 s	300 s
Application Rate	4–25 m/h	5 m/h
Flow rate	0.1–0.5 l/s	6.5 l/s
Required volume to simulate 50,000 bed volumes of feed	300–2,000 l	8×10^6 l
Required time to simulate 50,000 bed volumes of feed	5–30 days	150–170 days

Source: Ref. 27, with permission of the American Society of Civil Engineers.

particle size, higher application rate, and less EBCT than pilot or full-scale operation. This is illustrated in Table 10–4. Alternative designs are derived from assumptions about the dependence of internal surface diffusion on particle diameter (independent or linearly proportional) and changes in turbulence with particle size, indicated by the Reynolds number. It is then possible with 1 or 2 days of operation of small columns to obtain the breakthrough curve and project these results to larger-scale operation. While the principle is reasonable, difficulties can arise with uncertainties about the dependency of internal diffusion on particle size and with competitive adsorption, especially between SOCs and NOM. Nevertheless, the breakthrough curve obtained with the RSSCT has been shown to agree fairly well with that from pilot scale tests, both with SOCs in a mixture (Figure 10–3) and for NOM (Figure 10–4).

GAC FOR CONTROL OF DISINFECTION BYPRODUCTS

GAC can be used either to remove disinfection byproducts or to remove the NOM that acts as a precursor. In spite of low absorbability as compared with many SOCs, NOM is more adsorbable than many of the disinfection byproducts. As a consequence, the service time will generally be longer for removal of NOM, and this is frequently the preferred strategy. However, even this approach may have some limitations due to the large

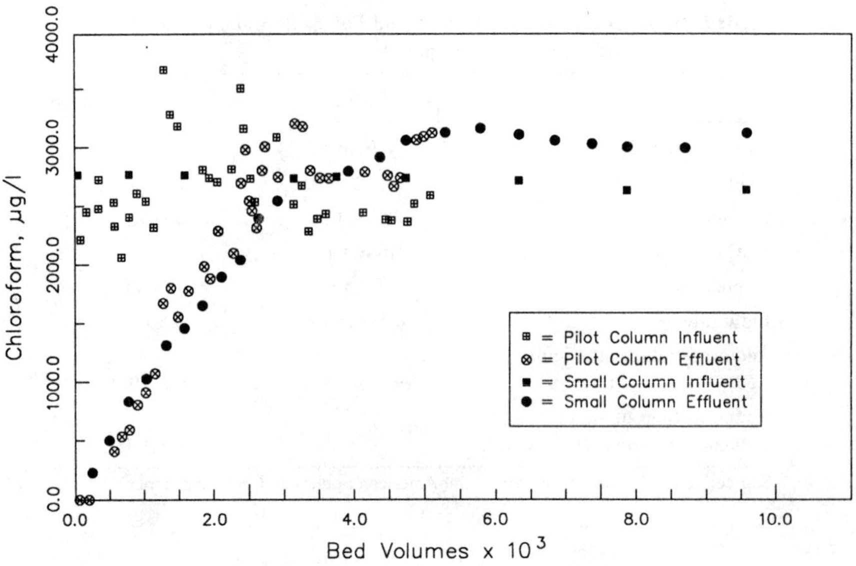

FIGURE 10–3. Comparison of chloroform effluent profiles predicted from rapid small-scale column test with long term pilot scale columns. (From Ref. 28. Reprinted from Crittenden, J. C., Berrigan, J. K., et al. Figure 2 from "Design of Rapid Small-Scale Adsorption Tests for a Constant Diffusivity." *Journal of Water Pollution Control Federation* 58: 312–9 (1986), by permission.)

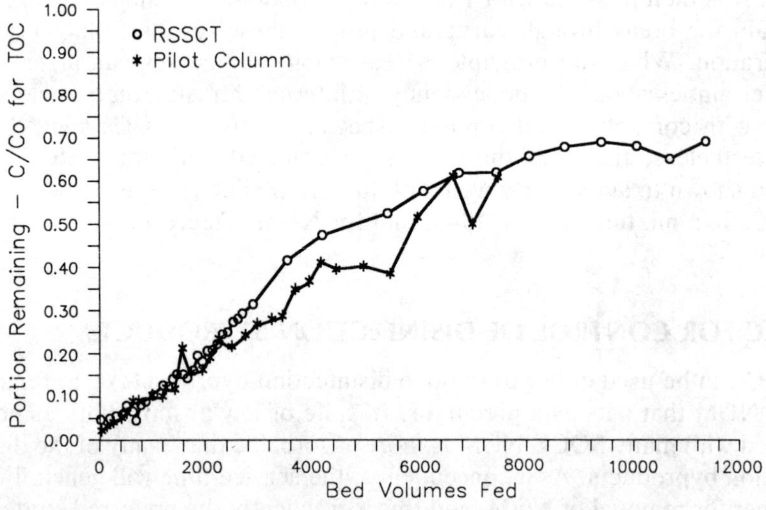

FIGURE 10–4. Comparison of the TOC breakthrough profile predicted by RSSCT with pilot GAC contactor data. (From Ref. 11. Reprinted from *Proceedings of AWWA Annual Conference*, by permission. Copyright © 1988, American Water Works Association.)

size of many NOM molecules in relation to the pore size available in many activated carbons.

Adsorption of Naturally Occurring Organic Matter Precursors

The adsorption characteristics of NOM are not easily generalized, owing to the complex macromolecular nature and seasonal variability of these constituents. Evidence shows that NOM is poorly adsorbed compared with many SOCs (not disinfection byproducts) of interest. A very rough estimate of sorptive capacity for NOM in calculating BVF_{max} in Equation 10–3 is 10 mg/g. Note that this work was based on smaller-pore-diameter carbons that may be inappropriate for the larger molecules of the NOM. More recent developments indicate that large-pore activated carbon may have a significantly larger capacity for such molecules (5).

The breakthrough of some measure of the total trihalomethane formation potential (TTHMFP) is often of direct interest in design rather than the breakthrough of total organic carbon (TOC). Some differences in performance in regard to these two parameters have been observed. The effects of feed concentration of THM precursors and EBCT on service time as determined at several pilot plant locations are given in Table 10–5

TABLE 10–5. Length of GAC Operation for Various Combinations of EBCT and Feed Concentrations of THMFP

Location	Term (days)	Day[a]	Conc.[b]
Cincinnati, OH (15.2 min EBCT)	3	208	70
Jefferson Parish, LA (18.8 min EBCT)	5	63	170
Manchester, NH (23 min EBCT)	3	98	65
Evansville, IL (9.6 min EBCT)	3	56	53
Miami, FL (24.8 min EBCT)	6	17	580

[a] Day to GAC exhaustion for THM goal.
[b] GAC influent concentration.

Source: Ref. 29. Reprinted from *Journal American Water Works*, Vol. 80 (May 1988), by permission. Copyright © 1988, American Water Works Association.

(29). In this table the criterion for service time is a target of 50 μg/l for TTHMFP. From simple equilibrium modeling (Equations 10–3 and 10–4), service time will decrease as EBCT decreases and feed concentration increases. The extremely high TTHMFP of 580 μg/l in the feed at Miami, Florida, produced a service time of just 17 days despite the very long EBCT (24.8 minutes). This contrasts, for example, with results from Cincinnati where the service time was 208 days, owing, in part, to a much lower TTHMFP in the feed (70 μg/l); in fact, service time was longer than at Miami even though the EBCT was much shorter (15.2 vs. 24.8 minutes) (29). The EBCTs at Cincinnati and Jefferson Parish are roughly the same and so allow more direct comparison of the effects of TTHMFP feed concentration. Because the TTHMFP is much higher at Jefferson Parish (170 vs. 70 μg/l), the service time was reduced considerably (63 days vs. 208 days). These results underscore the importance of characterizing the nature of THM precursors at a given location before selecting the EBCT that will give economically acceptable service times (29).

In a study by the Los Angeles Metropolitan Water District, the concept of simulated distribution system THM (SDSTHM) was used to assess the service time before exceeding a target level for total THMs (TTHM) in the distribution system (11). This is a modified approach in evaluating formation potential where conditions for holding the sample are based on actual disinfection conditions anticipated in the distribution system. The relationship of EBCT and GAC service time is shown schematically in Figure 10–5. Service time prior to regeneration was based upon an effluent blending concept. In effluent blending, beds are operated in parallel with some kept in operation even though the effluent concentration exceeds the target, while the effluent concentrations of other beds are below the target. The net effect is an average formation potential that meets the goal. However, even with such enhancement, the study concluded that GAC was not economical if the target for TTHM was less than 50 μg/l, since very large contactors would be required for reasonable regeneration cycles.

Another potential means of extending the service time is to encourage microbial degradation of NOM by addition of ozone ahead of GAC. The question of whether ozone byproducts are a problem or whether they can be removed by GAC is a consideration for this approach. Some concern has been expressed that bacteria that are attached to GAC fines appear to be difficult to inactivate. However, there are several facilities where bacterial inactivation is routinely practiced without difficulty, so no firm conclusion can be drawn as to the significance of these concerns. In some cases, a sand layer can be installed at the bottom of the GAC media in order to provide a degree of filtration of GAC fines that might otherwise

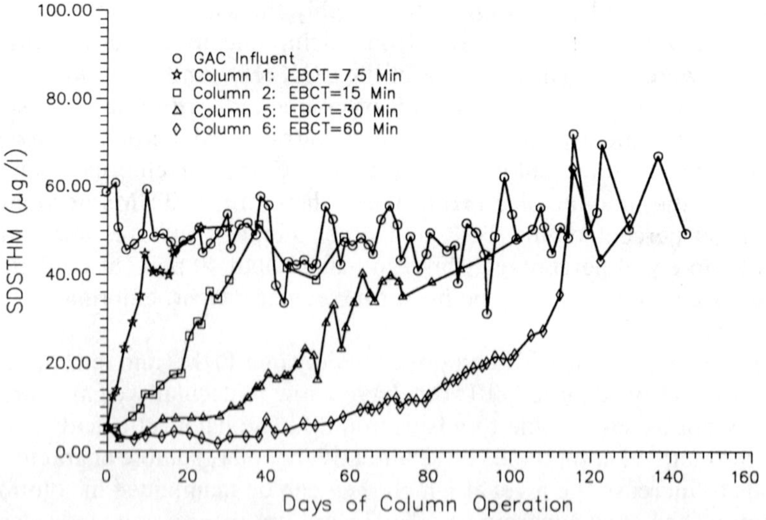

FIGURE 10–5. Simulated distribution system THM concentrations vs. days of operation of GAC column operation for various EBCTs. (From Ref. 11. Reprinted from *Proceedings of AWWA Annual Conference,* by permission. Copyright © 1988, American Water Works Association.)

exit a GAC bed with bacteria attached. The possible mixing of the sand with GAC may make regeneration difficult.

Adsorption of Chlorination Disinfection Byproducts

The applicability of GAC for removal of disinfection byproducts depends upon concentration and adsorptive capacity. At the moment, only TTHMs are regulated, but additional byproducts are of health concern (3).

A survey of water utilities showed that TTHMs represent approximately 30 percent of the total organic halides (TOX) produced (both parameters expressed on an equivalent chlorine basis) (15). TTHMs constitute the major portion of volatile components, and the remaining TOX appears to be predominantly nonvolatile. Thus, nonvolatile byproducts make up about 70 percent of the TOX, or about 2.5 times that contributed by THMs. At this ratio, if TTHMs are 100 μg/l, the TOX is about 350 μg/l.

The possible health concerns about nonvolatile TOX are of interest in determining the feasibility of adsorption. In recent research the major nonvolatile compounds were found to be dichloro- and trichloroacetic acid, which together accounted for roughly the same amount of TOX as TTHMs, whereas contributions from trichloroacetone and dichloroacetonitrile were less than 1 percent of the TOX (16). Another study showed that on a weight basis, the amount of compounds with relatively simple identifiable structures such as haloacetonitriles, haloketones, haloacetic acids, chloropicrin, chloral hydrate, and cyanogen chloride is nearly equal to the amount of TTHMs (30). Therefore, if THMs account for about 30 percent of the TOX and other simple structures account for nearly an equal percentage, this can leave about 40 percent unidentified TOX, some of which may be higher molecular weight, chlorinated fulvic material.

The 60 percent of TOX comprised mainly of TTHMs and the haloacetic acids is poorly adsorbed. TTHMs have a low molecular weight character that is not as susceptible to adsorption (9). The haloacetic acids and the other identified compounds have a relatively polar, soluble character that tends to increase the level at which they can be maintained in solution in the presence of an adsorbing media. Therefore, these compounds also are not likely to be readily removed by GAC.

To illustrate the poor adsorbing capabilities of the THMs, the equilibrium adsorption of any of these compounds is at least two orders less than that for simple ring structures such as phenol, nitrobenzene, and xylene and even below that for trichloroethylene, a simple, two-carbon chlorinated compound (31). In particular, the adsorption capacity for the THM chloroform used by the U.S. EPA to estimate breakthrough time with an equilibrium model (see Equations 10–3 and 10–4) is 0.35 mg/g (at a solution concentration of 75 μg/l) (21). This would give an initial breakthrough time of just 15 days at a typical EBCT of 10 minutes.

THMs other than chloroform (i.e., the chlorobromoform species) have higher adsorptive capacities (approaching 2 mg/g), but they are usually present in lower concentrations except in waters with significant bromide levels. Although their breakthrough times may be somewhat longer, the total maximum contaminant level (MCL) for THMs can still be exceeded due to earlier breakthrough of chloroform. In fact, the poor adsorbability of chloroform suggests that a breakthrough can occur even earlier than calculated by the simple, single solute model because of competitive adsorption in practical operation.

Field evaluations under EPA-sponsored pilot plant studies at representative EBCTs have shown that service times based on selected target concentrations of THMs are in the order of 1 to 2 months. Actual operation might be extended somewhat beyond breakthrough in an individual contactor if the effluent blending concept already described is used. However this strategy probably will not achieve sufficient improvement to make this a reasonable application for GAC.

Data regarding GAC removal characteristics for other specific byproducts is limited. Some information is available for removal of TOX, which serves as a general surrogate for other chlorinated byproducts. A breakthrough curve for TOX obtained at Jefferson Parish, Louisiana, illustrates a general trend for removals (Figure 10–6) (29). THMs often appear early in bed operation and comprise most of the initial TOX (14).

The capacity of GAC for nonvolatile TOX (NVTOX) was investigated at Jefferson Parish by removing GAC from various positions in the pilot plant adsorber (EBCT = 19 minutes) and measuring adsorbed NVTOX (14). The maximum value found was about 1 mg/g. While this capacity is lower than seen typically for TOC (5 to 100 mg/g), equilibrium had not been reached in the GAC bed. Moreover, the feed concentration of NVTOX is considerably less than TOC (<0.5 mg/l compared to 3 mg/l). Both factors suggest a longer service time if the design is to be based on removal of NVTOX rather than TOC.

Comparison of GAC Methods for Disinfection Byproduct Control

Not only are most DBPs formed by chlorination poorly adsorbed, but there is also the question of whether it is prudent to use chlorination ahead of GAC. Some research has shown that chlorine may react with sorbed organics to produce undesirable byproducts. Moreover, chlorine residuals are dissipated by GAC, thereby requiring further addition of chlorine (or chloramines) for achieving secondary disinfection goals. The

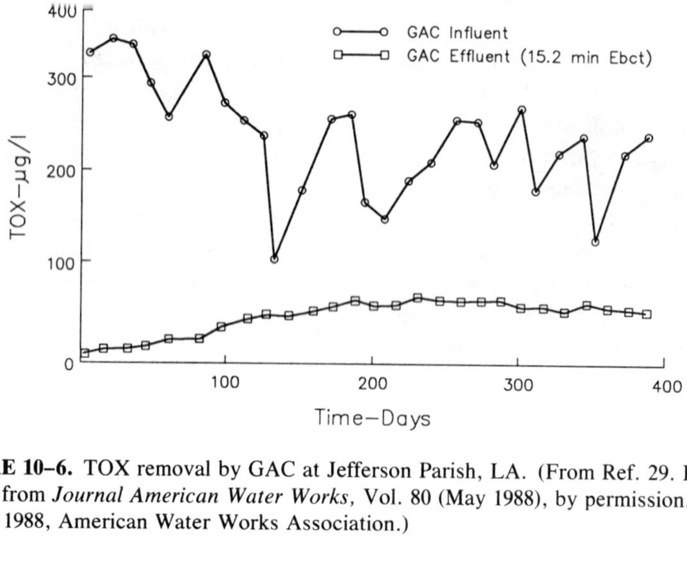

FIGURE 10–6. TOX removal by GAC at Jefferson Parish, LA. (From Ref. 29. Reprinted from *Journal American Water Works*, Vol. 80 (May 1988), by permission. Copyright © 1988, American Water Works Association.)

trend appears to be use of alternative oxidants when necessary ahead of GAC, which means that chlorine DBPs will not appear at this point in the treatment train. Furthermore, reserving chlorine addition until downstream points can result in significant reduction in chlorine demand with an associated reduction in DBP formation.

DESIGN CONSIDERATIONS

GAC Contactors: Filter Adsorbers vs. Postcontactors

In filter adsorbers, GAC replaces a conventional filter media and combines both particle removal and dissolved organics adsorption in one unit process. Postcontactors are located behind or downstream of the filters, allowing prior removal of particulates and optimization of GAC operation specifically for adsorption goals.

The selection of the approach depends primarily on the required EBCT and costs. Filter adsorbers generally have low capital cost, are compact, and can often be converted from existing filters. However, existing filters may provide insufficient EBCT, requiring a deeper filter box than is available in existing filters. Compatibility of metal surfaces is also a consideration due to the highly corrosive nature of GAC. The coagulants may obscure some GAC pores and can affect performance of filter adsorbers.

Postcontactor adsorbers can provide greater EBCT and better use of the adsorptive capacity of the GAC than retrofitted filters, but may have higher capital cost. Postcontactor adsorbers also allow use of a smaller size carbon, which can provide greater use of adsorptive capacity.

A general comparison between filter and postcontactor adsorbers has been made based on the TOC removal (24). Filter adsorbers can be effective and economical at existing plants where the filtration rate is low (around 2 gpm/sf) and an EBCT of about 10 minutes or less is provided. For high-rate filters (4 to 5 gpm/sf), the typical EBCT of 5 to 7 minutes is frequently insufficient, unless the design of the filter box allows the media depth to be increased or it is economical to construct additional filters to increase the EBCT. In some cases, EBCT might be increased somewhat through conversion to a more compact underdrain system that affords more volume in the overlying filter. It is important to note that GAC, when properly designed, is at least as effective as sand or dual media beds for particulate (turbidity) removal.

Effect of Backwashing on Adsorption Front

Various researchers have evaluated the effect of backwashing on the adsorption front in the GAC (17, 24). Research tends to consider two extreme cases for the GAC bed: completely stratified and undisturbed (no backwashing), and fully mixed (with backwashing). The two extreme cases demonstrate that any backwashing (even if only monthly) widens the MTZ as compared with a fixed or undisturbed bed (see Figure 10–7) and leads to an early initial breakthrough. These research conclusions must be used with caution when applied to full scale plants, because (1) backwashing does not usually fully mix the media, and (2) backwashing will almost certainly be necessary prior to GAC replacement or regeneration, even in postcontactor adsorbers. This is due to head loss development, resulting from biological growths and particulate removal. It is also possible that backwashing to a bed expansion (40 percent or more) and then allowing the media to settle slowly may fully restratify the bed so that a portion of the adsorption front is retained.

Adsorber Configuration

The two fundamental types of GAC adsorbers are classified as fixed bed and fluidized or moving bed. In a fixed bed adsorber, the GAC remains stationary, operating in either a downflow or upflow mode. In a fluidized bed adsorber, the GAC is held in suspension by a flow of process water

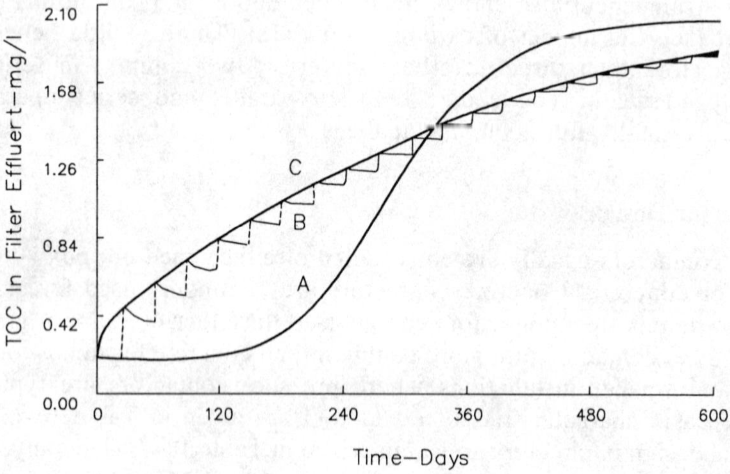

FIGURE 10–7. Simulated breakthrough curves for GAC filter operation with and without periodic backwashing: (A) no backwashing; (B) monthly backwashing; (C) daily backwashing. (From Ref. 24. Reprinted from *Journal American Water Works*, Vol. 79, No. 12 (December 1987), by permission. Copyright © 1987, American Water Works Association.)

that is at a rate adequate to lift the particles. Since the fluidized bed is suspended and the carbon does not remain in fixed positions, it will not have a distinct MTZ and therefore cannot achieve as low an effluent concentration as a fixed bed. As a result in drinking water treatment, fixed bed adsorbers are more commonly used than moving bed adsorbers, although fluidized beds may have other applications (19).

For filter adsorbers, the arrangement will almost always consist of multiple fixed beds in parallel, as this is the normal arrangement for filters. For postcontactor adsorbers, multiple beds can be arranged either in parallel or in series. The choice will depend upon whether the treatment objectives are moderate or stringent. For moderate objectives (e.g., moderate organics removal), it may be advantageous to operate the adsorbers in parallel and to blend the effluent of parallel operating adsorbers that have been in operation for different times.

For stringent treatment objectives, it may be advantageous to use multiple adsorbers operated in series. In this system, the lead adsorber is removed from service when breakthrough is reached. The lag adsorber, which should have some capacity remaining if the breakthrough front has not fully penetrated this column, is then moved to the lead position by valving, and a fresh adsorber is placed on line as the lag unit. This allows greater utilization of the GAC, as the most exhausted carbon in the lead position column is exposed to the highest concentrations of organics. The series arrangement also allows smaller bed depths and can, in this manner, reduce the impact of carbon fouling (18). There is little benefit in having more than three adsorbers in series; two columns in series is usually adequate. The choice between parallel and series operation should be made after economic analysis.

Contactor Design

GAC contactors usually are constructed of either lined or epoxy-coated steel or concrete. Concrete contactors are commonly used for gravity flow, whereas steel contactors can be used for either pressure or gravity flow. Steel contactors are more common than concrete for upflow operation and smaller installations where pressure contactors are typically used. Basic characteristics of contactors are given in Table 10–6, and typical design parameters are summarized in Table 10–7. Generally, economies of scale favor concrete contactors for plants of over 15 mgd capacity and steel pressure contactors for lower capacity plants.

Contactor flow rates are usually between 3 and 10 gpm/sf, with media depths ranging between 2.5 and 15 feet. Conversion of existing filters to first-stage adsorbers generally provides only 2 to 4 feet media depth.

TABLE 10–6. Basic Characteristics of Adsorbers

Adsorber Type	Material	Volume Range (ft^3)	Diameter	Remarks
Steel, gravity flow	Lined carbon steel	6,000–20,000	20–30 ft	Field fabricated by welding or bolting preformed steel plate. Mounted on concrete slab foundation.
Steel, pressure flow	Lined carbon steel; stainless steel	2,000–50,000	Up to 12 ft	Shop fabricated; over-the-road transportation constraints limit size.
Concrete, gravity flow	Standard reinforced concrete	1,000–200,000	Usually rectangular	Field constructed. Designs vary. A 2 : 1 length-to-width ratio is common.

Source: Reprinted from Ref. 18, by permission. Copyright © 1988, American Water Works Association.

TABLE 10–7. Units and Typical Values for GAC Adsorber Parameters

Parameter	Symbol	Units		Typical Values in Practice (metric)
		English	Metric	
Volumetric flow rate	V	gal/min	m^3/h	50–400
Bed volume	V_F	ft^3	m^3	10–50
Cross-sectional area	A_F	ft^2	m^2	5–30
Length	l	ft	m	4–18
Void fraction		ft^3/ft^3	m^3/m^3	0.38–0.42
Filter density	Q_F	lb/ft^3	kg/m^3	350–550
Filter velocity	V_F	$gal/min/ft^2$	m/h	5–15
Effective contact time		min	min	2–10
Empty bed contact time	EBCT or t_A	min	min	5–30
Operation time	t_F	days	days	100–600
Throughput volume	V_L	gal	m^3	10^4–10^5
Specific throughput	V_{sp}	gal/lb	m^3/kg	50–200
Bed volumes	BV	gal/gal	m^3/m^3	2,000–20,000

Source: Reprinted from Ref. 18, by permission. Copyright © 1988, American Water Works Association.

Therefore, this approach may not be adequate in cases where greater depth is required for treatment. New filters can be designed for greater depths.

Several contactor arrangements are shown in Figures 10–8 through 10–10 (19, 23). A typical steel pressure contactor is shown in Figure 10–8, and a concrete gravity contactor is shown in Figures 10–9 and 10–10. Design for either postcontactors or existing filter conversion must consider the following:

- EBCT requirements
- Constraints for surface loading and associated effects on bed depth
- Adsorber configuration
- Backwashing
- Materials of construction
- Underdrain system
- GAC installation, removal and transport
- Storage of fresh, spent, and reactivated carbon

EBCT requirements and adsorber configuration have been previously discussed. A backwashing system is required for all contactors, even if it is used only at the time of GAC installation to remove fines. As far as backwash appurtenances (e.g., valves and piping) are concerned, GAC contactors do not differ very much from conventional filters. Air scour should be used in addition to water backwash, but not simultaneously,

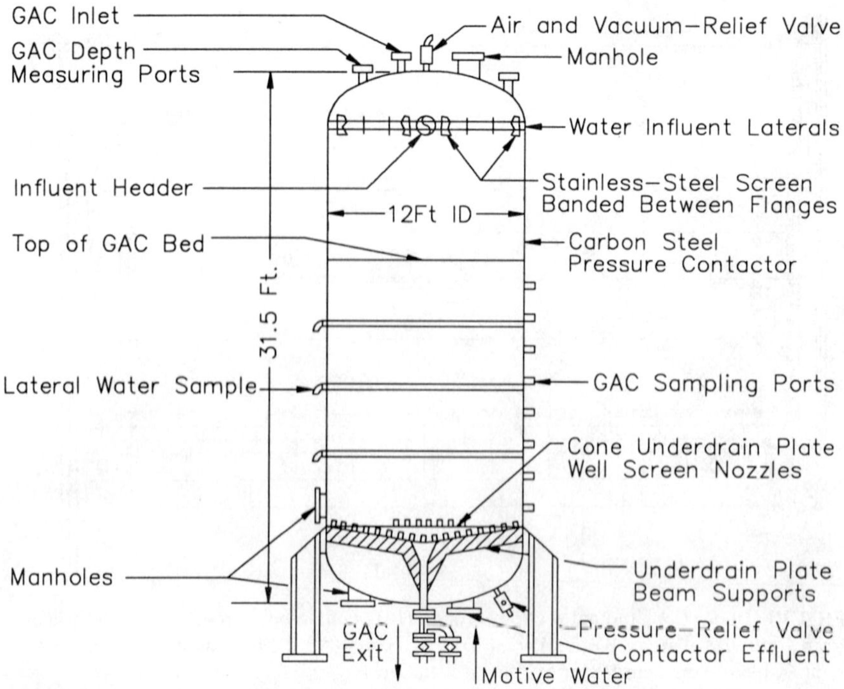

FIGURE 10–8. Typical GAC pressure filter. (From Ref. 25. Reprinted from *Journal American Water Works,* Vol. 82, No. 1 (January 1990), by permission. Copyright © 1990, American Water Works Association.)

otherwise GAC carryover will occur. Backwash systems must have provision for the gradual variation of flow rate between and during washes. In order to fully stratify the bed, the backwash flow rate and contactor should be sufficient to allow 40 percent bed expansion.

GAC (in water) is both corrosive and abrasive, which needs to be taken into account in selecting materials of construction. Concrete, stainless steel, and plastics are satisfactory, but carbon steel may require special coatings such as organic polymers.

Although many plants use GAC media placed directly on underdrain nozzles with a slot size of 0.2 mm, some engineers consider a sand or gravel support layer essential to protect the underdrain from penetration by GAC. However, elimination of this layer avoids problems of separating the GAC and gravel before regeneration. If no sand or gravel is used, a low rate backwash should be provided during installation of GAC in a contactor, a proprietary nozzle system should be used, and, in the event

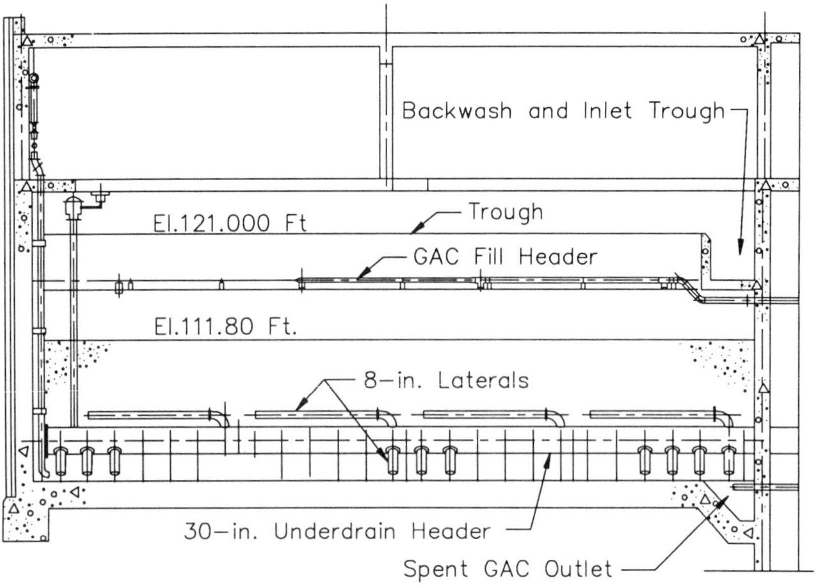

FIGURE 10–9. Longitudinal section through GAC contactor. (From Ref. 23. Reprinted from *Journal American Water Works*, Vol. 78, No. 4 (April 1986), by permission. Copyright © 1986, American Water Works Association.)

that plugging occurs, the backwash and air scour piping should be provided with pressure-relief systems.

There are many suitable underdrains for use with a sand or gravel layer, including nozzles in suspended floors, nozzles and headers, or plastic "tile" systems. Some form of pressure-relief system would still be advisable, and suspended floor systems should be pressure tested prior to media installation.

Although many manual and semiautomatic GAC handling systems are in use, GAC removal from fixed bed contactors and storage tanks is relatively complicated. Pneumatic transport is feasible, but hydraulic transport as a slurry is more common. Care should be taken in design of transport systems to minimize GAC losses due to excessive abrasion. This tends to mitigate against extensive use of pneumatic systems and requires careful design of hydraulic transport systems.

The most successful transport systems use 6- or 8-inch pipes through the wall of the contactor, located either immediately above a suspended floor or 4 to 6 inches above any gravel layer. GAC is removed through these pipes using either an eductor or recessed impeller pump, aided by intermittent low rate backwash. Alternatively, a flexible suction pipe can be used, lowered into the filter from above and moved about manually.

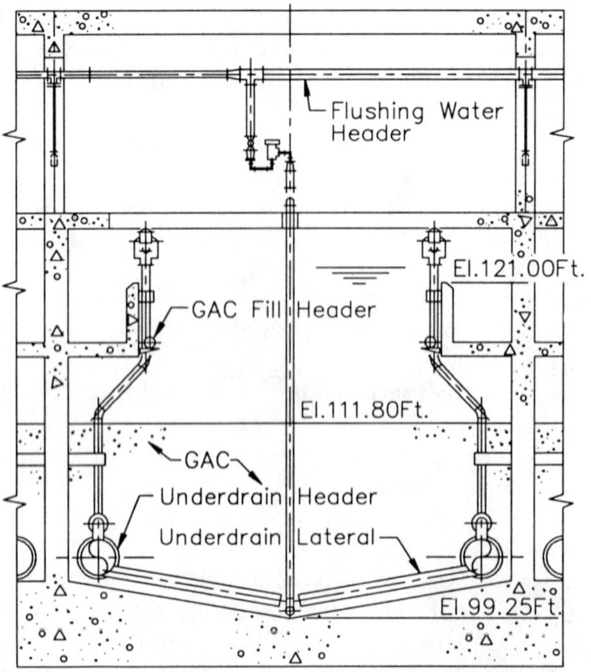

FIGURE 10–10. Cross section through GAC contactor. (From Ref. 23. Reprinted from *Journal American Water Works,* Vol. 78, No. 4 (April 1986), by permission. Copyright © 1986, American Water Works Association.)

Flat-bottomed filters make GAC removal more difficult. In removal, slurry concentrations should be around 1 to 2 lb GAC/gal, with a transport velocity between 4 and 6 ft/sec. If the velocity is too low, the GAC will settle out of the slurry; velocities that are too high will cause excessive carbon abrasion and pipe erosion. Piping is generally stainless steel, with sweep bends, with provision for flushing after use.

REGENERATION/REACTIVATION

Selection of the reactivation method for GAC is significant in planning and design of a system. Because of economy-of-scale considerations, on-site regeneration is frequently not practiced at small facilities. These facilities can either purchase new carbon or enter into contracts for off-site regeneration, depending on relative costs and availability of services.

There are a number of reactivation methods available for large-scale facilities. Although chemical reactivation of activated carbon is possible, the most widespread method is thermal regeneration. Multihearth furnaces have commonly been used to reactivate carbon in the past, but fluidized bed and electric infrared tunnel furnace methods are also being utilized (25). Other methods include rotary kiln, indirect heated vertical moving bed, and steaming processes.

Although regeneration recovers some of the original adsorptive capacity, some loss occurs with each reactivation cycle. One significant effect of multiple reactivations of activated carbon may be the loss of capacity in small pores due to the following phenomena:

- Adsorbed organics deep in pores are difficult to reach with oxidizing gases so that small pores tend to become plugged, with a resulting loss in total surface area.
- Some small pores are "burned out" by the oxidizing gases during regeneration.
- Inorganic residue can be deposited in the pore structure during the drying and regeneration process.
- Some organics are irreversibly chemically adsorbed.

As a result, service GAC will have a somewhat reduced capacity for adsorption of small molecules. This reduction can be as much as 50 percent in some cases. However, this capacity loss can be offset for some applications by an increase in the availability of large pores with an associated capacity increase for larger molecules. This increase, which can be as great as 40 to 50 percent, can be advantageous for adsorbing large molecular weight precursor material.

Because of the transfer and handling of the GAC during the regeneration cycle, there will be some particle breakdown. This will typically cause a 20 to 30 percent reduction in particle size and a degree of loss that will require addition of fresh carbon. If pressure drop is a potential problem, the particle size decrease can be offset by using a coarser grade of carbon for makeup. However, some carbon manufacturers resieve the regenerated carbon to achieve the original grading specification.

In addition to the basic reactivation process, regeneration requires facilities to store, transport, and dewater carbon. Also, air pollution control devices such as scrubbers may be required for furnace emissions. All of these facilities can represent a substantial added investment and will require added space as well.

GAC FACILITIES PLANNING

Contactor costs and equipment for GAC replacement/regeneration and storage are the two principal costs in determining the feasibility of adopting GAC process. The frequency of GAC replacement varies greatly with contact time and the surface loading rate. To determine the most economical combination of the size of contacting facilities and the replacement/regeneration costs requires modeling and pilot testing evaluations based upon actual water quality conditions. The modeling approaches outlined earlier in the chapter provide useful information and are instructive for evaluating applicability of GAC in many installations. A degree of conservatism should be applied to the models, and accuracy of the prediction improves with more detailed pilot testing. The expense of pilot testing, however, may not be warranted for many installations. Even in cases where pilot testing is to be performed, minicolumn operation in conjunction with mathematical modeling can provide useful information for planning the pilot plant effort.

Pilot plant data should be adequate to plot curves showing percentages of target compounds remaining for various contactor loading rates and empty bed contact times (see Figure 10–11 for an example of the relationships that should be generated). These curves will be the basis for determining frequency of regeneration under a given loading condition (1).

Often the data from pilot studies will need to be adjusted for anticipated operating protocols. For example, if it is assumed that the regenera-

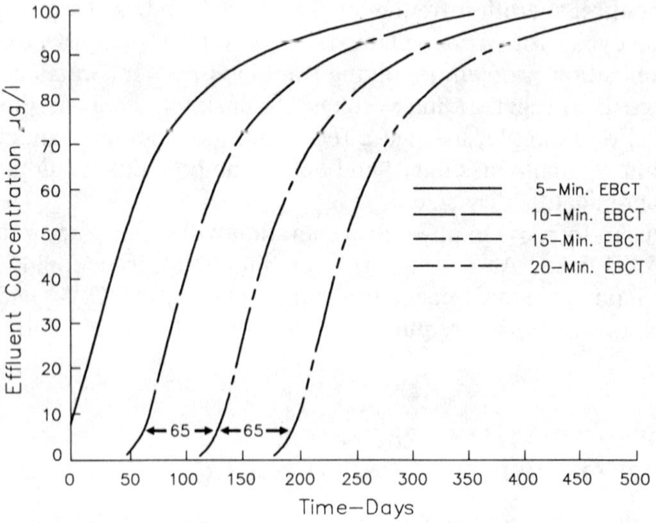

FIGURE 10–11. Effluent concentrations vs. days for various EBCTs. (From Ref. 1. Reprinted from *Journal American Water Works,* Vol. 81 (April 1989), by permission. Copyright © 1989, American Water Works Association.)

TABLE 10–8. GAC Cost vs. Regeneration Rates

Plant Size (mgd)	Regeneration Cycle (months)	Cost[a] (cents per 1,000 gal)
1	24	41
1	11	55
10	24	27
10	1	75
100	24	14
100	1	48

[a] Costs are 1988 dollars (ENR construction costs index = 421).

tion of contactors can be spaced at equal intervals, it may be possible to extend the regeneration cycle by effluent blending.

System cost estimates should include all housing, tanks, piping, siting, and so forth. An allowance for reactivation furnace downtime should be made in sizing and developing costs for these units. This will be dictated by anticipated operating protocols for furnace operation and projected downtimes that include an allowance for maintenance. Total downtimes can range between 25 and 40 percent.

Several factors may be involved in arriving at the most economical sizes. Larger beds (higher EBCT) cost more to construct but decrease the replacement/regeneration frequency Table 10–8 shows the effects of regeneration cycles for various plant sizes. Therefore, sizing is essentially a cost optimization problem involving trade-offs between costs of contactors and costs of regeneration systems. A sensitivity analysis should also be made. For example, assume a regeneration cycle approximately half the amount originally assumed, and determine how this would affect the most economical facility size.

A decision to provide on-site regeneration will depend upon the quantity of GAC used. As a rough rule of thumb, the breakpoint in costs between having on-site regeneration or replacing the GAC with virgin GAC occurs when GAC requirements are about 140 to 160 lb/day (6 to 7 ft^3/day).

ROLE OF ACTIVATED CARBON FOR CONTROL OF DISINFECTION BYPRODUCTS

The specific role of activated carbon as an adsorbing media for control of disinfection byproducts is not clear. Although it is generally more effective for removing precursors and might be more logically applied in this role than for removal of specific byproducts, even this approach has some limitation due to the poor adsorbability of some of the high molecular weight compounds in the confined pore openings of many activated carbons. Enhancements that might be achieved with larger-pore-size activated carbons remain to be established. Therefore, in spite of provisions of the 1986 Amendments of the Safe Drinking Water Act that encourage the use of granular activated carbon as the yardstick process for removal of organic contaminants, other processes may be more effective and at less cost.

In spite of a somewhat unclear role as an adsorbing media, a role may be emerging for GAC as a biological support media for use in BAC applications. This approach can remove biodegradable organic carbon (BDOC), biologically reduce precursor content, and lower chlorine demands to allow lower chlorine dosages that will form fewer disinfection byproducts. Additional discussions of the use of GAC in a BAC mode are included in Chapters 2 and 11, and discussion of BAC use with ozone processes may be found in Chapter 7.

References

1. Adams, J. Q., R. M. Clark, and R. J. Miltner. 1989. Controlling organics with GAC; A cost and performance analysis. *JAWWA* 81(4): 132–40.
2. Bouwer, E. J., and P. B. Crowe. 1988. Biological processes in drinking water treatment. *JAWWA* 80(9): 82–93.
3. Bull, R. J. 1980. Health effects of alternate disinfectants and their reaction products. *JAWWA* 72(5): 299–303.
4. Byung, R. K., and V. L. Snoeyink. 1980. Monochloramine-GAC reaction in adsorption systems. *JAWWA* 72(12): 488–9.
5. Chudyk, W. A., V. L. Snoeyink, D. Beckman, and T. J. Temperly. 1979. Activated carbon versus resin absorption of 2-methylisoborneol and chloroform. *JAWWA* 71: 529–38.
6. Crittenden, J. C., D. W. Hand, H. Arora, and B. W. Lykins, Jr. 1987. Design considerations for GAC treatment of organic materials. *JAWWA* 79(1): 74–82.
7. Dixon, K. L., and R. G. Lee. 1990. Chlorite and chlorate removal in water treatment processes. Presented at 1990 AWWA Conference, Cincinnati, OH, June 1990.
8. Feige, W. A., and J. DeMarco. 1980. Water treatment process modifications for trihalomethane control and organic substances in the Ohio River. EPA-600/2-80-028. Cincinnati, OH: U.S. Environmental Protection Agency.
9. Giusti, D. M., R. A. Conway, and C. T. Lawson. 1974. Activated carbon adsorption of petrochemicals. *JWPCF* 46(5): 947–65.
10. Graese, S. L., V. L. Snoeyink, and R. G. Lee. 1987. *GAC filter adsorbers.* Denver, CO: AWWA Research Foundation.

11. McGuire, J. J., et al. 1988. Optimization and economic evaluation of granular activated carbon for organic removal. *Proceedings of AWWA Annual Conference,* Orlando, FL (1988): 263–88.
12. Mazzoni, A. F., and R. T. Deithorn. 1988. Activated carbon: What is it, how does it work? *Water Technol.* 9(11): 26–9.
13. Najm, I. N., V. L. Snoeyink, M. T. Suidan, C. H. Lee, and Y. Richard. 1990. Effect of particle size and background natural organics on the adsorption efficiency of PAC. *JAWWA* 82(1): 65–72.
14. Quinn, J. E., and V. L. Snoeyink. 1980. Removal of total organic halogen by granular activated carbon absorbers. *JAWWA* 72(8): 483–8.
15. Singer, P. C., and S. D. Chang. 1989. Correlations between trihalomethanes and total organic halides formed during water treatment. *JAWWA* 81(8): 61–5.
16. Reckhow, D. A., and P. C. Singer. 1990. Chlorination by-products in drinking water: From formation potentials to finished water concentration. *JAWWA* 82(4): 177–80.
17. Sontheimer, H., J. C. Crittenden, and R. S. Summers. 1988. In *Activated carbon for water treatment,* 2nd ed., pp. 507–10. Denver, CO: OVGW-Forschungstelle/AWWA Research Foundation.
18. Sontheimer, H., J. C. Crittenden, and R. S. Summers. 1988. In *Activated carbon for water treatment,* 2nd ed. Denver, CO: OVGW-Forschungstelle/AWWA Research Foundation.
19. Sontheimer, H., J. C. Crittenden, and R. S. Summers. 1988. In *Activated carbon for water treatment,* 2nd ed., pp. 597–604. Denver, CO: OVGW-Forschungstelle/AWWA Research Foundation.
20. Summers, R. S., et al. 1989. The influence of background organic matter on GAC adsorption. *JAWWA* 81(5): 66–74.
21. Symons, J. M., et al. 1981. Treatment techniques for controlling trihalomethanes in drinking water. EPA-600/2-81-156. Cincinnati, OH: U.S. Environmental Protection Agency.
22. Weber, W. J., Jr. 1972. *Physicochemical processes for water quality control,* Chapter 5. New York: Wiley, Interscience.
23. Westerhoff, G. P., and R. Miller. 1986. Design of the GAC treatment facility at Cincinnati. *JAWWA* 78(4): 146.
24. Weisner, M. R., J. J. Rook, and F. Fiessinger. 1987. Optimizing the placement of GAC filtration units. *JAWWA* 79(12): 39.
25. Koffskey, W. E. 1990. GAC adsorption and infrared reactivation—a case study. *JAWWA* 82(1): 49.
26. Hand, D. W., J. C. Crittenden, and W. E. Thacker. 1984. Simplified models for design of fixed-bed adsorption systems. *J. Environ. Eng. Div. ASCE* 110: 444–57.
27. Crittenden, J. C., J. K. Berrigan, D. W. Hand, and B. Lykins. 1987. Design of rapid fixed bed adsorption test for non-constant diffusivity. *J. Environ. Eng. Div. ASCE* 113: 243–53.
28. Crittenden, J. C., J. K. Berrigan, and D. W. Hand. 1986. Design of rapid small-scale adsorption tests for a constant diffusivity. *JWPCF* 58: 312–9.

29. Lykins, B. W., R. M. Clark, and J. Q. Adams. 1988. Granular activated carbon for controlling THM's. *JAWWA* 80(5): 85–92.
30. Krasner, S. W., et al. 1989. The occurrence of disinfection byproducts in U.S. drinking water. *JAWWA* 81(8): 41–53.
31. James M. Montgomery Consulting Engineers. *Water treatment principles and design,* pp. 185–6. New York: John Wiley.
32. Fulton, George P. 1988. Contending with filter media problems. *Public Works* (June).

11

Relationship between Disinfection and Baseline Water Treatment Processes

INTRODUCTION

A baseline process is that drinking water treatment required to remove and/or reduce both particulate and dissolved solids to the levels required to achieve the established water quality goals. By providing oxidation capabilities that are of some value for certain of these treatment functions, many disinfecting agents become an integral part of these baseline processes. This interactive consideration may be distinguished from the separate purpose of disinfecting agents to achieve microorganism inactivation or kill. In any case, disinfection processes cannot entirely be separated from baseline processes even in this inactivation role. It is, therefore, important to understand the relationships between disinfection and baseline water treatment processes. Many of the important relationships that exist between disinfection and baseline water treatment processes are site specific. The variations in quality between different source waters and, indeed, the variations that may occur in a single source can influence the baseline treatment and disinfection routines that may be adopted. In fact, a review of the controlling issues that follow will indicate that treatment routines acceptable for many types of waters may not apply in other situations.

The predominant baseline processes for achieving drinking water quality goals typically have included particulate removal processes to produce a clear water that is esthetically acceptable to the consumer. Chemicals traditionally added to these process trains for disinfection purposes have been strong oxidants that also achieve important nondisinfection goals such as control of color, tastes, odors, iron, and manganese. In addition, disinfecting chemicals can influence the behavior of the baseline process train in achieving clarification goals. For example, depending upon the nature of the source water organics, in some applications oxidation by disinfecting chemicals can result in decreased coagulant requirements and achieve more effective filtration.

Baseline processes can also provide an important supplemental disinfection role in the removal of waterborne pathogens. This role is especially important in the removal of some critical pathogens that have proved to be resistant to disinfecting agents. As an example, substantial disinfection credits can be achieved by filtration systems for removal of *Giardia* and viruses, thereby decreasing reliance on disinfecting agents as the sole barrier against waterborne disease. These capabilities are also likely to be important for other disinfectant resistant pathogens such as *Cryptosporidium*.

Some membrane filtration processes (e.g., ultrafiltration) are also being evaluated for nearly complete removal of pathogenic organisms by filtration mechanisms so as to eliminate the need for primary disinfecting agents. The need for secondary disinfecting agents to establish residuals, however, would not be eliminated by these approaches. This means that the opportunity for disinfection byproduct formation may still exist since the membrane compositions used for this type of filtration may not efficiently remove precursors.

The removal of disinfection byproduct precursors can affect selection of baseline processes. For example, conventional coagulation and lime softening processes can remove a portion of the precursors, thereby reducing the formation of undesirable disinfection byproducts upon the subsequent addition of disinfectants. As discussed in Chapter 9, certain membrane processes (i.e., reverse osmosis and nanofiltration) can achieve high levels of precursor removal and may be advantageous at some sites.

With increasing concern for biodegradable organic carbon (BDOC), as discussed in Chapter 2, it is likely that baseline processes may also be evaluated for capability to remove this component as well. Slow sand filters are particularly well suited to this type of application because of the biological activity that is inherent in these systems. Rapid rate filters also may be modified to remove some BDOC, but compatibility with other essential goals needs to be considered in this regard. Other filtration systems may offer less potential for BDOC removal.

An important function achieved with some baseline processes is the removal of color. This can reduce the need to rely on the oxidation capability of disinfectants to achieve such removal, thereby reducing the formation of disinfection byproducts. Among the filtration processes, coagulation-based rapid rate filter systems offer the greatest capability for color removal. Other filter systems are generally less effective and may require greater oxidation.

In some cases, where a choice between alternative baseline processes exists, such choices may be influenced by the range and acceptability of disinfection techniques that can be accommodated. Selection of alternative approaches to disinfection may require comparisons of several baseline systems that are specifically suited to optimize disinfection.

Baseline processes can generally be placed into one of the following categories:

- Clarification to remove turbidity (particulates) and color
- Softening to remove hardness
- Oxidation processes to precipitate or remove undesired substances such as iron, manganese, and sulfides
- Ion exchange and membrane processes to remove dissolved components
- GAC and air stripping processes for removal of organic contaminants and radon

The baseline and disinfection process objectives that can be achieved by typical processes are listed in Table 11–1. In many situations, a combination of the baseline processes may be required to meet multiple treatment objectives. Because of their widespread use, particulate removal systems are discussed in greater detail in the remainder of this chapter.

TABLE 11–1. Alternative Water Treatment Process Systems—Comparison of Relative Capabilities

Clarification/Filtration Systems

1. Rapid rate filtration using coagulant chemicals
   - Capable of removal of turbidity, color, and some disinfection byproduct precursors. Has potential for conversion to permit biological growth in media to remove BDOC, but care must be exercised to maintain other filter functions.
   - Often important for manganese removal in plants that add chlorine or other oxidants to filter influent, thereby producing an oxidized coating that can adsorb manganese. (This strategy may conflict with the strategy of locating chlorine downstream of filters for BDOC reduction.)
   - Capable of removal of pathogens.
2. Slow sand filtration
   - Capable of removal of turbidity and BDOC.
   - Limited removal of color and disinfection byproduct precursors. In one situation, higher removal of disinfection byproduct precursors has been observed in a modification of the process in which GAC was used in place of sand (42). Preozonation also can increase color and precursor removal by making this material more subject to removal by biodegradation in slow sand filters (53).
   - Capable of removal of pathogens.

TABLE 11–1. *(Continued)*

3. Precoat filtration
   - Capable of turbidity removal.
   - Limited removal of color, disinfection byproduct precursors, and BDOC without pretreatment, conditioning of media, or body feed supplement.
   - Capable of removal of pathogens.
4. Cartridge filters
   - Capable of turbidity removal.
   - Limited removal of color, disinfection byproduct precursors, and BDOC.
   - Capable of removal of pathogens.
5. Membrane processes
   a. Filtration membranes
      - Capable of turbidity removal.
      - Limited removal of NOM associated with color, disinfection byproduct precursors, and BDOC. One study has shown that improved removals of organics associated with disinfection byproducts formation could be achieved by pretreatment with powdered activated carbon (41).
      - Capable of removal of pathogens.
   b. Reverse osmosis and nanofiltration membranes
      - Capable of high degrees of removal of turbidity, color, and disinfection byproducts. Salt rejection more limited with nanofiltration membranes, although hardness ions are rejected.
      - Capable of removal of pathogens.
      - Turbidity should be removed by pretreatment to minimize membrane blinding.
      - Pretreatment may be needed to prevent some salts from precipitating on the membrane.

Softening Systems

1. Lime softening
   - Capable of removal of hardness, turbidity, color, and some disinfection byproduct precursors.
   - Limited removal of BDOC.
   - Capable of removal of pathogens. High pH should make this process more effective in deactivating most viruses but not protozoa. As a result it could require lower CT values in waters where protozoa are not present, such as groundwater not under direct influence of surface water.
2. Ion exchange softening
   - Capable of removal of hardness.
   - Limited removal of turbidity, color, disinfection byproduct precursors, and BDOC. (Some ion exchange may have capability for removal of DBP precursors in nonsoftening resins.)
   - Probably not applicable for removal of some waterborne pathogens.
3. Membrane softening processes
   - Capable of removal of hardness, color, disinfection byproduct precursors, and dissolved organic carbon, some of which could include biodegradable matter.
   - Turbidity should be removed by pretreatment to minimize membrane blinding.
   - Pretreatment may be needed to prevent some salt from precipitating on membranes.
   - Capable of removal of pathogens.

Discussions of membrane desalting, air stripping, and GAC processes are presented in Chapters 9 and 10.

PARTICULATE REMOVAL PROCESSES

Predominant particulate removal processes emphasized in drinking water treatment include slow sand filtration, rapid rate filtration, and precoat filtration systems (see Figure 11–1). Cartridge filters also can be considered for some small plants, and the technology for membrane filtration application is improving. For hard waters, lime softening processes can achieve particulate removal as well as providing for removal of hardness. All these systems are discussed as potential processes into which disinfection must be integrated.

The filtration process has become the most common baseline system for water treatment. In the evolution of drinking water filtration, rapid sand filter systems followed slow sand filtration. Slow sand filters use a finer size of filter media and rely primarily on physical mechanisms in concert with a biological growth that is developed in the bed. On the other hand, rapid sand filtration requires pretreatment by chemical coagulation to condition particles prior to application to the filter. As a consequence of this conditioning, the rapid sand filtration process can be operated at higher flow rates and through a larger-sized filter media than slow sand filters.

Rapid Rate Filters

A number of different rapid rate filtration configurations, with various combinations of media, have been developed in recent times. While older single-media filters are still encountered in water treatment plants, newer dual and multimedia approaches often offer improved performance at higher hydraulic loading rates. Other concepts include coarse monomedia filters that have a greater depth to compensate for the increased media size. In all cases, the concept of the newer approaches is to encourage particulate removal throughout much of the depth of a filter bed, as opposed to surface removal mechanisms that predominated with the original single-media filters. With in-depth penetration and storage, the length of filter runs is increased, and turbidity breakthrough caused by shear is reduced.

Coagulation/Flocculation

The most significant feature of the rapid rate filter is the use of coagulation and flocculation to condition particulates before filtration. This is com-

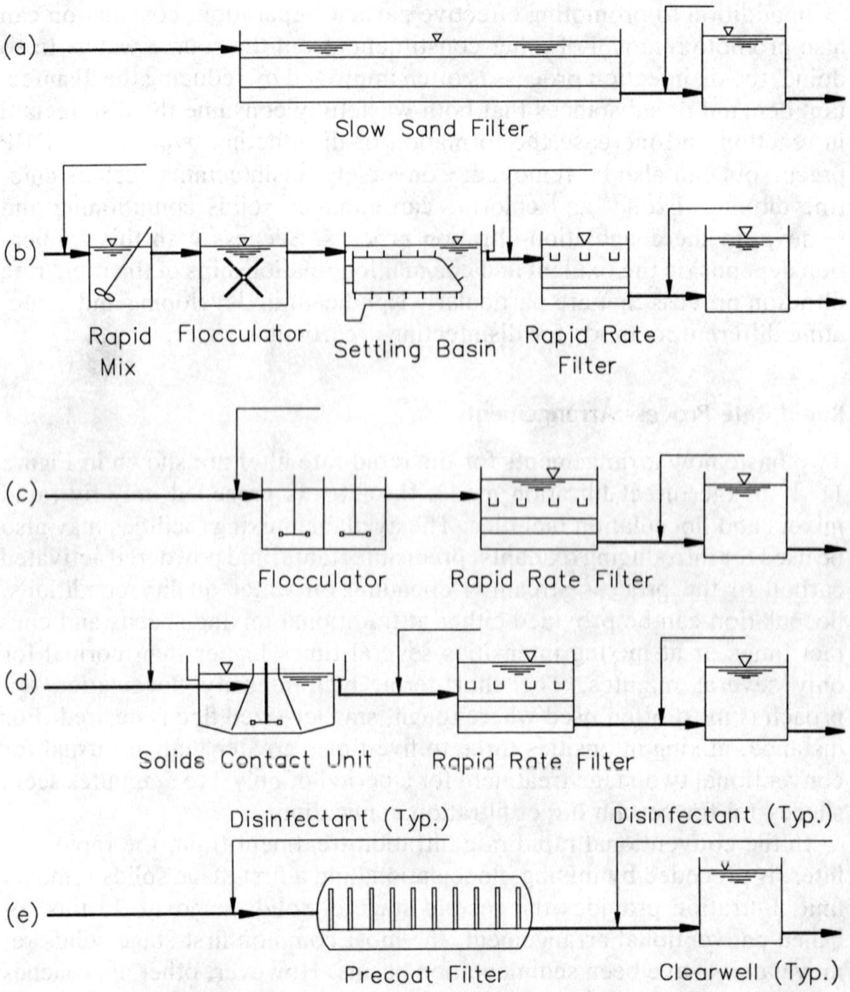

FIGURE 11–1. Typical water treatment process schematics: (a) slow sand filtration; (b) conventional rapid rate filtration; (c) direct filtration; (d) lime softening; (e) precoat filtration.

monly achieved through the addition of metal coagulants such as alum, ferric chloride, and ferric sulfate, or by lime softening of hard waters. A number of new coagulants have been developed so that the range of options has increased. Proper coagulation will promote agglomeration of the particles in flocculation, improving both the attachment and separation (removal) of solids in granular media.

In addition to promoting effective particle separation, coagulation can also promote removal of other constituents from the source water. In so doing, the disinfection process is often improved by reducing the disinfectant demand of substances that both wastefully consume the disinfectant in reaction and increase the formation of disinfecting byproducts. DBP precursors can also be removed. Conversely, disinfectants such as chlorine dioxide, ozone, and chlorine can enhance solids conditioning and removal in the coagulation-filtration process. Success with this application depends on the oxidant and coagulation relationships of the rapid rate filtration process that are particularly significant in developing and evaluating different methods for disinfecting a particular water.

Rapid Rate Process Arrangements

Two basic flow arrangements for the rapid rate filter are shown in Figure 11–1. In the direct filtration mode, the filter is preceded only by rapid mixers and flocculation facilities. The available mixing facilities may also be used for introducing oxidants, predisinfectants, and powdered activated carbon to the process stream. Depending on water quality conditions, flocculation can be provided either at traditional mixing speeds and contact times or at mixing intensities several times higher than normal for only several minutes. The short-term, high-intensity flocculation approach is most often used where tough, smaller-sized floc is desired. For instance, mixing intensities three to five times greater than are usual for conventional two-stage treatment for a period of only 3 to 5 minutes seem successful for certain direct filtration applications.

In the conventional rapid rate filtration treatment train, the rapid rate filter, is preceded by mixing, flocculation, and a first-stage solids removal unit. Filtration provides the second stage of solids removal. In this so-called conventional arrangement, the most common first-stage solids removal units have been sedimentation basins. However, other approaches are now available, including upflow, sludge blanket clarifiers; solids contact clarifiers; plate and tube settlers; air flotation; and high-rate adsorption or contact clarifiers.

Particulate Removal Performance

In general, sedimentation removes between 65 and 90 percent of the total solids loading in a conventional two-stage solids removal system. The primary reason for including sedimentation or an alternative particulate removal process is to reduce the solids loading on the filter, thereby extending the length of run and improving the product water quality.

These approaches are generally required for waters where source water turbidity averages above 5.0 NTU or where the required metallic salt (aluminum and iron) coagulant feed exceeds 20 to 25 mg/l. Direct filtration may be considered for water with lower turbidities and coagulant demands.

The two-stage solids removal arrangement can sometimes provide a significant advantage over the direct filtration mode, especially in regard to disinfection contact time. Flocculation and the first-stage solids removal basins provide significant detention time that is not available in the single-stage, direct filtration process train. In general, however, these issues may not determine which rapid rate filtration mode is selected, as some states do not give credit for this time as part of the CT requirements. Selection is more likely to be influenced by the overall capability for effectively treating a given source water.

Cold Lime Softening

In many respects, the lime softening process is an alternative form of rapid rate filtration. In this process, lime is added to precipitate calcium and magnesium hardness. When present, turbidity particles can be entrained in the precipitate and are removed as well. Under certain conditions, the precipitates formed by this process can also be effective in removing source water organic matter associated with color and disinfection byproduct formation.

Because of the large volume of solids usually produced by lime softening, a first-stage solids removal facility is always installed ahead of filtration. Solids contact clarification units are often favored for softening because the recirculation of solids in these units serves to accelerate the precipitation processes. Depending on source water conditions, the preliminary removal effectiveness of both the carbonate precipitates and organic matter can be affected by the degree of recycle of solids. Preliminary removal can also be enhanced by the addition of supplemental coagulants such as organic polyelectrolytes and inorganic metallic salts.

The lime softening process will generally exhibit turbidity and coliform bacteria–reduction capabilities similar to the conventional coagulation-related processes. However, a major influence on disinfection needs can be imposed by the effect of operating pH. For example, higher CT levels are required under the EPA Surface Water Treatment Rule for free chlorine when operating at the higher pH levels, and no CT credit is given for pH levels greater than 9.0, which are typical of lime softening processes. Some adjustment of this final pH can be achieved by the use of recarbonation, a process in which CO_2 is added, which acts as an acid.

CHEMICAL COAGULATION

Particulates encountered in drinking water treatment generally range from around 0.01 to 100 μm in size. The larger particles are easily removed by settling or filtration. The smaller, colloidal portion (0.01 to 5 μm) presents the most difficulty. Settling rates for these particles are almost imperceptible, and without conditioning many of these particles would also pass through filter media.

Coagulation processes are used to create chemical conditions that facilitate the agglomeration or flocculation of small colloidal particles into larger particles to improve removals in settling and filtration. Colloidal particles of natural origin typically have a net negative surface charge that causes them to repel one another; that is, the particles in raw water are said to be electrostatically stabilized and, therefore, do not aggregate (see Figure 11–2a). A primary role of chemical coagulation processes is to neutralize or reduce the charge-related repulsive forces between particles, thereby allowing the flocculation process to proceed, as shown in Figure 11–2b.

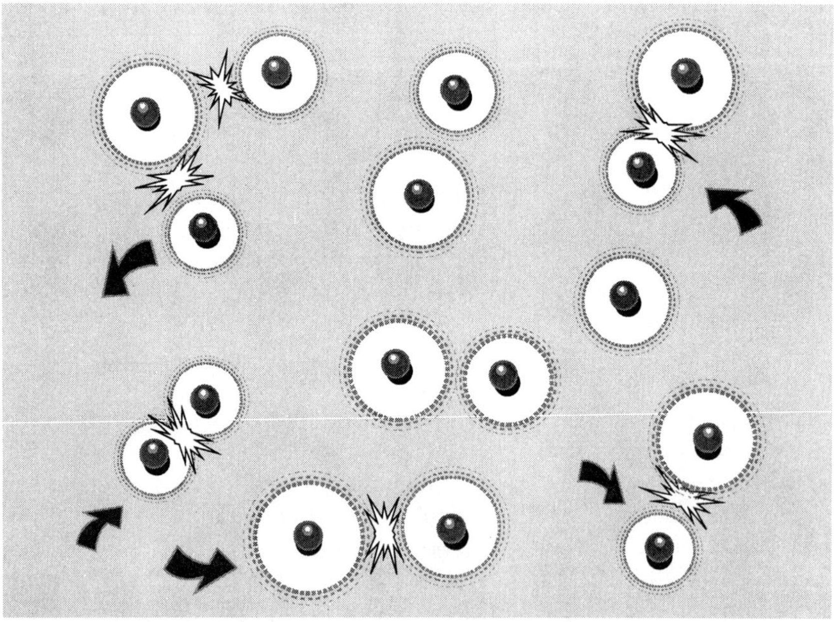

(a)

FIGURE 11–2. Flocculation. (a) Charged particles repel each other. (b) Charge neutralized particles are free to collide and aggregate. (c) Sweep flow-colloids become enmeshed in growing particulate. (Courtesy of Zeta-Meter, Inc., Long Island City, NY.)

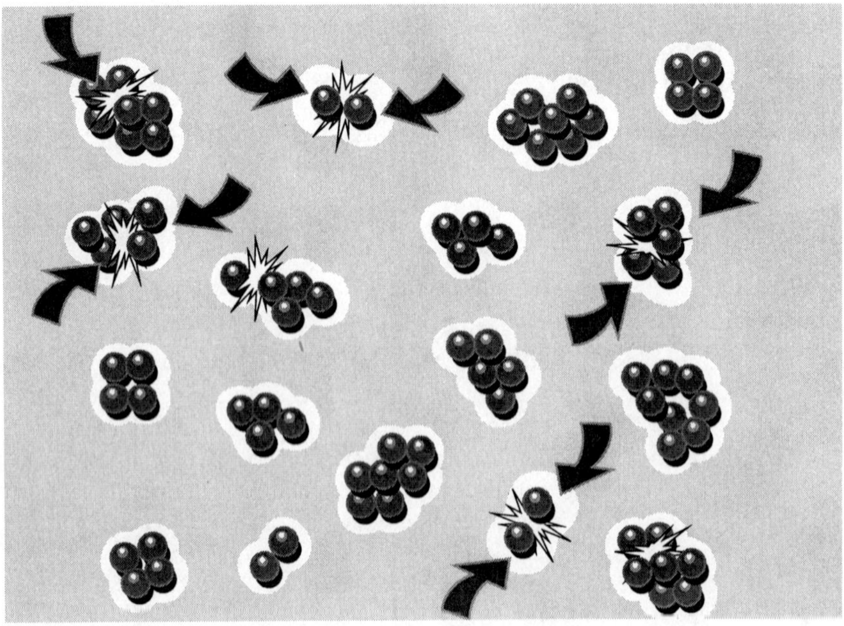

(b)

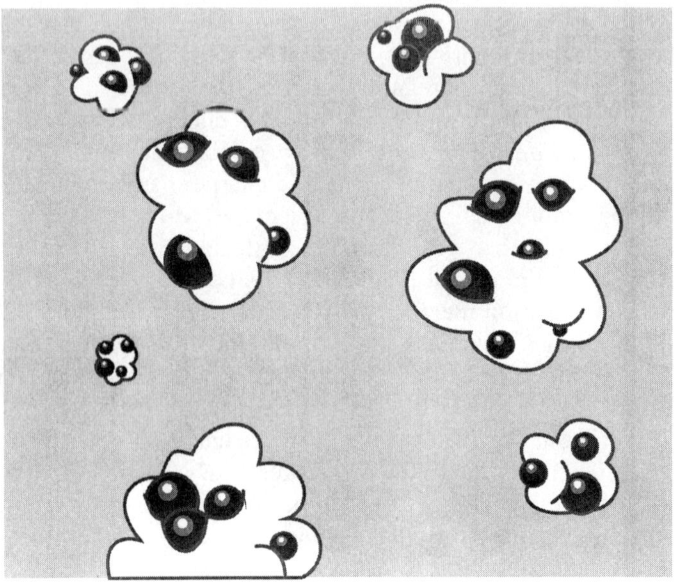

(c)

With charge neutralization, effective coagulation can take place as a consequence of the reduction of the electrostatic repulsion forces. This allows very powerful, but short-range, van der Waals attraction forces to come into play between colloids to enhance coagulation. These van der Waals forces are the result of interactions between individual molecules, which attract approaching colloidal particles. Under appropriate conditions, van der Waals forces permit the aggregation of colloids to eventually form visible floc particles, which may be removed by sedimentation and filtration processes.

Alum ($Al_2(SO_4)_3 \cdot 14.3H_2O$) is the most commonly used coagulant in the United States. Aluminum in alum exists predominantly as Al^{3+} or as chemical complexes formed from Al^{3+} and SO_4^{2-}. Upon addition of alum to water, aluminum hydroxides ($Al(OH)_n^{3-n}$) begin to form. At pH levels less than about 6.5 to 7, n is typically less than 3, resulting in the formation of positively charged dissolved species. Many of these dissolved species are intermediate forms that will subsequently combine to form solid aluminum hydroxide precipitates, which also have a positive surface charge in this pH range.

Dissolved species or ions that have been suggested (2, 6) include $Al_{13}\ (OH)_{34}^{+5}$, $Al_{17}^{+4}\ (OH)_{17}^{+4}$, $Al_8\ (OH)_{20}^{+4}$, $Al_6\ (OH)_{15}^{+3}$, $Al_2\ (OH)_2^{+4}$, $Al_3\ (OH)_4^{+5}$, and $Al_{13}O_4\ (OH)_{24}^{7+}$. These positively charged aluminum ions and the positively charged precipitate surfaces that may subsequently form can adsorb and adhere to negatively charged colloidal particles. This has the effect of directly neutralizing the negative charge on the small particles that are commonly found in most waters. Repulsive forces are thereby decreased, and aggregation of particles by van der Waals and other forces occurs much more rapidly. This charge-neutralization process is often called *destabilization* of the previously stable particles (i.e., particles that contain an adequate negative charge to repulse one another are said to be stabilized in solution since they do not readily settle). Destabilized particles can grow to form settleable flocs that more easily adhere to individual grains of media in filters (see Figure 11–2b).

Under this adsorption mechanism, overdosing of coagulants beyond a zero point of charge can result in a condition of charge reversal. This overdosing condition can cause restabilization of particles to again form a suspension of particles that do not readily coagulate. In other words, there is an optimum dosage beyond which coagulation effectiveness begins to diminish. This is due to the reemergence of repulsive forces, which increase as the level of charge reversal increases. This phenomenon has been observed with alum coagulation under conditions where pH is less than 6.5.

Another mechanism that is important in alum coagulation is the formation of the aluminum hydroxide ($Al(OH)_3$) precipitate that occurs when alum reacts with the source water under an appropriate pH and alum dose range. Aluminum hydroxide coalesces to form a gelatinous precipitate that enhances coagulation by physically entraining particles (as contrasted with charge-related surface adsorption phenomena that occur when dissolved species and small precipitates adsorb at particle surfaces). This predominantly physical enmeshment phenomenon is referred to as a *sweep floc* mechanism (see Figure 11–2c). Unlike the adsorption mechanism, this phenomenon does not exhibit restabilization with increased dose beyond the optimum.

The predominant mechanisms for coagulation with alum can be segregated into regions, as illustrated in Figure 11–3:

1. An adsorption-destabilization region in which aluminum species achieve coagulation (or destabilization) primarily through charge neutralization

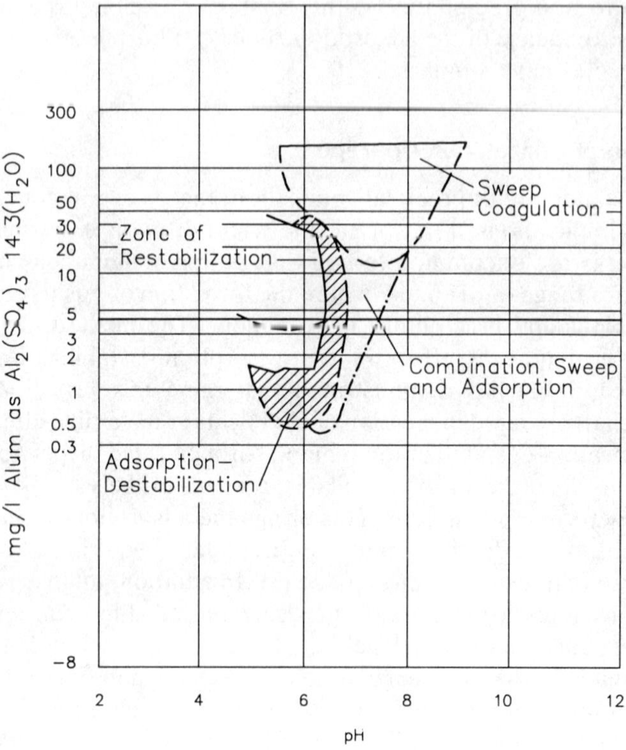

FIGURE 11–3. Stability-coagulation diagram for alum. (From Ref. 2. Reprinted from *Journal American Water Works*, Vol. 74, No. 4 (April 1982), by permission. Copyright © 1982, American Water Works Association.)

2. A restabilization region in which the alum dose is high enough to cause excess adsorption of aluminum species, resulting in charge reversal along with an associated breakdown in the coagulation process
3. A sweep floc region in which enmeshment by aluminum hydroxide precipitates becomes the predominant mechanism
4. A combination sweep and adsorption region in which a mixture of mechanisms occurs

The regions, as shown, represent a generalization, since a number of additional factors can have an influence. For example, high turbidities tend to broaden the destabilization zone, limiting the range of charge reversal–related restabilization. In addition, high sulfate concentrations can catalyze the conversion of the positively charged aluminum ion species to form aluminum hydroxide precipitates, thereby limiting the longevity of many of the adsorbing species that take part in adsorption-destabilization mechanisms. This conversion from soluble aluminum species to form a precipitate has the effect of expanding the sweep floc region at the expense of the adsorption zone (2). Phosphate ions and other anionic species have similar effects.

Application of Coagulation Concepts

From the standpoint of practical application, these general concepts have important implications. First of all, the effect of pH is extremely important, and it is not uncommon to find that optimum alum coagulation occurs within a range of pH 6 to 7 where the formation of positively charged aluminum ions and precipitates is prominent. The method of rapid mix can have a significant effect in the adsorption-destabilization region. Some research (2) has demonstrated that rapid mix processes should achieve relatively rapid dispersion of chemicals to maximize effectiveness in the adsorption-destabilization region. Through rapid dispersion, aluminum cations that are briefly available are more likely to be adsorbed before they form a precipitate. This brings the adsorption-destabilization mechanisms more effectively into play, frequently requiring a lower coagulating dose than usual for sweep floc (3). In addition, intense rapid mixing also promotes a more uniform adsorption of aluminum species for neutralizing charges on all particles.

It is significant that the coagulation regions shown in Figure 11–3 actually lie within the region where aluminum hydroxide precipitate is the ultimate chemical outcome. This leads to some complexities due to the nature of precipitate formation processes. Precipitation reactions do not proceed in a single reaction step, but require progressive linkage between molecules to initially form aluminum polymeric intermediates, some of which are effective coagulating species. The intermediate species will ultimately link to a size that is identifiable as a precipitate. It is often difficult to distinguish charge neutralization by adsorption of soluble cationic species, such as $Al_{13}O_4(OH)_{24}^{7+}$, from the charge neutralization phenomenon that results from the formation of a positively charged colloidal precipitate at a particle surface (15). From a practitioner's point of view, these distinctions are not important since decisions for either concept will lead to the same type of process decisions for control of pH and alum dosage.

Alternative Coagulants

One of the shortcomings associated with the use of alum as a coagulant is the lack of control over the formation of specific coagulating aluminum species; to an extent, pot luck is involved in that the methods of addition within a plant cannot be widely varied to control the types of aluminum species formed. In recognition of this limitation, several alternative coagulants have been developed based on preparation methods that enhance the formation of effective coagulating species prior to addition to the process stream. Important factors in promoting the formation of these species are proper storage time, pH, aluminum concentration, and rate of pH adjustment to the final solution condition (12).

The presence of excess sulfate, a constituent that can interact with aluminum, can have an adverse effect on the preparation and storage of these preformed aluminum-based coagulants. As a consequence, many of the proprietary preparations are made from aluminum chloride to avoid or reduce the sulfate present in the aluminum coagulant, chloride being a much less interactive anion with aluminum. However, this limitation of sulfate is not universal, and sulfate preparations also have been developed and can work well in treating water. In fact it has been found beneficial for some conditions of treatment to include some sulfate in polyaluminum chloride formulation.

Chloride and sulfate preparations are termed polyaluminum chloride and polyaluminum sulfate, respectively, in recognition of their polymeric or linked nature that involves a number of aluminum atoms. The composition of these solutions has been postulated to vary from very large inorganic polymer/particulate species to smaller inorganic polymer species such as $Al_{13}O_4(OH)_{24}^{7+}$ that are thought to dominate in some solutions (21).

In many situations, a lower dosage of these polymerized aluminum species is required than for alum. This may result from the fact that they are preformed under controlled conditions, whereas the operative coagulant species that occur during alum addition are formed under much less controlled conditions that can allow the formation of less effective species as well. As in the case of alum coagulation, coagulation by polymerized species can result from charge neutralization and can also be more effective when rapid dispersal is achieved in rapid mix.

Regardless of the coagulating species, it is a common practice to add organic polymers that will enhance the effectiveness of aluminum coagulants. For example, within the portion of the sweep floc region above a certain pH, the aluminum hydroxide precipitates tend to develop a negative surface charge, causing some charge-related repulsive forces that may reduce the efficiency of particle agglomeration. Addition of an organic polymer can often offset this condition. Organic polymers also may interact with negatively charged colloids, thereby reducing coagulant dose requirements in the adsorption-charge neutralization region. Low to medium molecular weight cationic polymers are often used for achieving this effect. Other high molecular weight organic polymers contain long chains that may actually be able to adsorb onto a particle surface and achieve coagulation by bridging to another particle. This bridging of particles can improve floc strength (13).

While aluminum-based coagulants have been the most widely used, a number of utilities have found iron coagulants to be effective. These include ferric chloride ($FeCl_3$) and ferric sulfate ($Fe_2(SO_4)_3$). In many treatment situations, especially in low-turbidity waters that are more difficult to coagulate, iron coagulants can form a denser, more readily settleable floc than alum. In addition, iron coagulation can often be effective at a pH above 7.0, thereby expanding the range available for coagulation. However, the full-strength iron coagulants are very corrosive and, in addition, can cause staining problems. Therefore, many utilities avoid their use due to associated operating and maintenance considerations, while others find them acceptable despite these problems.

Most of the coagulation phenomena associated with alum coagulation also occur with iron salts. As in the case of alum, pH is important, but not as critical to these phenomena, and both the adsorption and sweep coagulation mechanisms contribute to effective coagulation. However, the effective ranges are wider and can be different than for alum. Iron salts also can be used to preform polymeric iron species similar to those formed from aluminum salts. These can include preparations such as polymerized iron chloride.

Effect of Water Quality on Coagulation

Although the adsorption mechanism can often be used to achieve coagulation, many alum coagulation processes are operated in the sweep floc zone that relies on the precipitation of aluminum hydroxide. A phenomenon associated with this mechanism is the formation of precipitates that can be catalyzed or *nucleated* by the presence of other solids. As a consequence, precipitates often form more readily in high-turbidity waters than in low-turbidity waters. Low-turbidity waters are often found to be difficult to coagulate in the sweep floc region and possibly the adsorption region as well. Clays such as bentonite and kaolinite preparations are sometimes added to supplement the solids content and serve as weighting agents to enhance settling. In some cases, reverting to the adsorption region at a lower alum dose and slightly lower pH can achieve less floc volume for these low turbidity waters and, with sufficient energy input, allow them to be removed as a smaller floc in direct filtration. Supplemental floc conditioning by the addition of cationic polymers with careful attention to avoid a restabilization dose is sometimes required for this approach.

Temperature is another condition that affects coagulation. For example, the formation of intermediate aluminum species appears to be altered by low temperatures resulting in a poor settling floc when alum is used as a coagulant. On the other hand, some of the special polymerized aluminum preparations, which form active coagulating species prior to introduction to the water, have been observed to retain coagulating effectiveness under cold water conditions (14). Deteriorated performance of alum in cold water may prove to be more important than originally recognized. For example, one study has indicated deteriorated filtration performance during winter operation for removal of total bacterial cell counts (39). This study noted that these effects were not indicated by more traditional parameters, such as coliform, heterotrophic plate count (HPC), or turbidity, all of which suggested proper performance. Although the significance of these total bacterial count observations remains to be established, they yield some insight into possible variations in filter performance.

Dissolved organic carbon content also can have a major effect on coagulant dosage. Organic carbon, either when absorbed to the surface of a particle or present in solution, can add a much larger negative charge than that associated with clay or other inert particles alone. This can be especially significant in cases where coagulation occurs principally due to charge neutralization (4). Dissolved organic carbon also can interact with aluminum species to reduce coagulation efficiency. Organic cationic polymers can sometimes be used to offset some of these effects.

Removal of Color and Trihalomethane Precursors by Coagulation

Effective color removal by aluminum and iron coagulants has long been recognized; a number of utilities actually use coagulation processes predominantly for color removal. This is especially true in many coastal areas in the southeastern United States where very highly colored waters can be encountered. Sometimes, when turbidities are quite low and color reduction is the predominant goal, alum dosages in excess of 100 mg/l are required. This particular color has been associated with organic humic material, and the capability to remove at least a portion of these substances has been observed in coagulation processes. Because humic materials are important naturally occurring precursors for the formation of trihalomethanes and other disinfection byproducts, research to evaluate effectiveness of coagulation processes for removing precursors was very logical. Research in 1979 demonstrated that it was possible to remove a significant portion of both humic acids and THM formation potential in laboratory solutions and in some water treatment plants (5, 36).

While removal of the THM-formation potential by coagulation processes has been reported to exceed 50 percent in some cases, experience has indicated that considerable variation can occur. This may be caused by the differences in the character of the organic precursor compounds, which are known to exhibit wide variations in molecular weight. In general, higher molecular weight organic compounds are less soluble and tend to be more easily removed by coagulation processes (10, 30). Therefore, the molecular weight distribution of the organic matter in a source water can give some indication of the likelihood for achieving a high degree of precursor removal by coagulation. A number of other factors are involved, and it is necessary to perform site-specific testing of alternative coagulation approaches to determine actual extents of removal.

Removal Mechanisms

Several mechanisms are thought to be responsible for precursor removal (25):

1. *Removal of particulate organic matter by incorporation into floc.*
2. *Adsorption of dissolved organic matter onto aluminum or iron hydroxide precipitates that are formed in the generation of sweep floc in coagulation.* In many cases, adsorption is difficult to distinguish from coprecipitation processes in which a substance can be concentrated at the surface of another precipitated material and interact to form a precipitate that may not otherwise form in bulk solution. In a practical sense, these distinctions are not important, and the concept of adsorption, as presented here, is intended to encompass these mechanisms as well.
3. *Charge neutralization reactions between aluminum or iron coagulants and soluble precursor organics to form distinct precipitates.*

In general, removal of color and organic precursors by aluminum and iron coagulants is improved at somewhat lower pH levels than those for optimum turbidity reduction. For example, a typical optimum pH range for organic removal is from 5 to 6 with alum as compared with an optimum range of 6 to 7 often encountered for turbidity removal. There is some conflict regarding the reported optimum pH for iron coagulants, as different levels have been reported (25, 32). In either case, reducing pH tends to encourage organic removal up to a point for the following reasons (25):

- Negatively charged organics are progressively neutralized by positively charged hydrogen ions that become more available as pH is lowered. This reduces the negative charge to be neutralized by aluminum or iron. It also can reduce the solubility of many humic materials, causing them to precipitate by independent reactions.
- Aluminum and iron tend to form more positively charged species as pH is decreased. This increases the charge available for neutralizing the negatively charged humic material to form aluminum-humic or iron-humic precipitates. Humic removal by adsorption mechanisms at aluminum or ferric hydroxide surfaces in sweep floc regions also increases at lower pH levels due to an increase in the positive charge on these surfaces.

The soluble portions of the humic materials that are often associated with disinfection byproduct formation are generally segregated into a humic acid fraction that typically contains larger molecules and a more soluble fulvic acid fraction that is comprised of smaller molecules. The distribution among these fractions has an influence on susceptibility for removal since the more soluble fulvic fraction is more difficult to remove. Several laboratory investigations have specifically evaluated the effects of coagulation phenomena on removal of the fulvic acid fraction. For alum, adsorption removal mechanisms appear to predominate for tested fulvic acid fractions within the sweep floc region at a pH greater than 7. The precipitation mechanism tends to predominate below a pH of 5, and both mechanisms can occur in parallel in an intermediate transition region (12). Key water quality characteristics such as sulfate concentration can also have an influence by encouraging the formation of aluminum hydroxide precipitates and extending the sweep floc mechanism to lower pH levels, as discussed previously under mechanisms for particle coagulation (12). Note that most plants operate at a pH in a range of between 5.5 and 7, placing them in the range where mixed mechanisms often occur.

Calcium ions enhance the removal of fulvic acids over a wide range of pH. Other factors can also be involved; one study attributed more effective removals from one source of fulvic acid to the presence of a higher concentration of iron and a lower molecular charge on the fulvic acid fraction under investigation (21).

Coagulant dose requirements increase when higher quantities of fulvic acid are present. However, improved removal percentages also appear to occur at higher fulvic acid concentrations, probably due to the greater opportunity for particle contact during coagulation and flocculation (21) and as a result of the greater quantity of fulvic material that is available to be removed.

Different forms of aluminum coagulants appear to exhibit different regions of optimal performance in laboratory evaluations of the removal of fulvic acid. Selection of coagulant can vary depending on the character of the fulvic acid and pH conditions for coagulation.

In a comparison, polyaluminum chloride tends to be favored over alum for the low-dosage conditions encountered at low fulvic acid levels, as well as for the lower pH condition (5 to 7) where organic precipitation dominates. On the other hand, alum tends to be favored for higher-dosage conditions required by high fulvic acid levels and at higher pH levels (5 to 7). These are conditions that favor organic adsorption/sweep floc mechanisms (12, 21). Obviously, there is no single answer for all treatment conditions.

Water Quality Influences

When the broad variation of organic constituents that occurs in natural waters is considered, molecular weight distribution appears to generally characterize several important features that relate to removal mechanisms for both aluminum and iron coagulants (10, 29). As previously discussed, higher molecular weight molecules tend to be more easily removed by coagulation. In fact, it has been reported that molecular size is a more important characteristic than molecular charge for explaining removals (29).

The chemical nature of the organic material also affects removal. For example, ultraviolet (UV) absorbance at a wavelength of 254 nm is thought to indicate a humic/fulvic type of structure that is more readily removed by coagulation. A high UV/TOC ratio is generally indicative of a high humic/fulvic component of the total organic carbon (TOC). Waters with UV/TOC ratios of 4 to 5 may anticipate reasonably good removal, while lower UV/TOC ratios may indicate a less humic character that might be more difficult to remove. In fact, one outcome of coagulation is the selective removal of the UV component, leaving a lower UV/TOC ratio in coagulated water (17).

In many treatment situations, a higher proportion of the precursor content resides in the more removable, high molecular weight fraction of dissolved organic carbon. This means that precursors often are more effectively removed than the dissolved organic carbon content as a whole. As a consequence of these phenomena, it is prudent to carefully consider the outcome of preoxidation processes. These processes can reduce the molecular weight of organics in a water and may, in some cases, make precursors more difficult to remove through coagulation. This has been demonstrated in some investigations of the effects of preozonation on the removal of precursors by alum coagulation (27). However, these effects are variable, and, as discussed in Chapter 7, preozonation can be beneficial to precursor removal by coagulation under other circumstances. Other oxidants, including chlorine, chlorine dioxide, and potassium permanganate, can also influence coagulation effectiveness.

Polymers

Some research has evaluated the role of organic polymers as primary coagulants for removing precursors (22). In general, cationic polymers can be capable of removing precursor compounds (9). However, comparisons indicate that coagulation with alum may frequently be more effective than with organic polymers alone (22). As in the case of other coagulants, the effectiveness of organic polymers is greater for higher molecular weight organics (9).

Coagulation using organic polymers would tend to be appropriate for TOC levels of less than 5 mg/l and in situations where low turbidities allow direct filtration. Dosage requirements become excessive at higher TOC levels, and it may not be possible to maximize precursor removals with organic polymers alone under such conditions (16).

The effect of organic polymers in combination with alum has also been evaluated (22). Organic polymers with activity based on either long-chain, high molecular weight or on high charge density cationic properties were observed to offer good potential for improved turbidity removal, reduced alum dose, and reduced sludge volume in alum coagulation processes. However, improvements in removal of precursor content and color were not as significant. Therefore, these combinations may be more justified for goals of reducing alum feed rates and sludge quantities and improving turbidity removal.

Activated silica, an inorganic polymeric material that can serve as either a coagulant or a coagulant aid, has been evaluated for precursor removal in a few cases. One study showed significant improvements in precursor removal, indicating a possible role for activated silica in some cases (59).

Coagulation for Disinfection Byproduct Control

It can be concluded that coagulation processes can achieve significant removals of precursor compounds, especially those associated with a high molecular weight humic or fulvic fraction. Lower molecular weight fractions are not typically removed to the same degree. As a consequence of this and other factors that affect the character of precursor compounds, significant variations in the effectiveness of coagulation processes are encountered. Even in cases where testing may indicate effective precursor removal under certain conditions, caution should be exercised in accounting for possible seasonal variation in precursor characteristics that can also include variations in the molecular weight distribution (34). These variations may require other treatment strategies during portions of the year when the effectiveness of coagulation is reduced.

In addition to a role for removing precursors, coagulation processes can sometimes offer an alternative for replacing or reducing the role of chlorine and other oxidants in removing color and can also reduce the overall chlorine demand as well. Many utilities are already using coagulation for these particular goals. This practice can both reduce the level of byproduct formation as well as the cost of oxidizing chemicals.

One application for using coagulants for color goals is the use of ferric chloride to react with the organic color prior to lime addition for a subsequent softening step (31). The precipitated color is then removed in the softening process, which eliminates the need for chlorine as an oxidizing agent for color removal. Because precipitation of color is more favorable at lower pH levels, a period of contact between ferric chloride and the color-containing water was used before pH was raised in the softening process. In this situation, ferric chloride was selected over alum because it is more capable of maintaining a precipitate in the higher pH range encountered in lime softening. While this approach proved satisfactory in this particular application, it has not been shown to have as significant color effect in other situations (19). Use of coagulants should be considered on a site-specific basis based on test results.

Coagulation in Alternative Rapid Rate Filtration Configurations

Alternatives to conventional rapid rate filtration include direct filtration that eliminates sedimentation basins, as well as high-rate sedimentation modifications in which processes such as upflow blanket clarifiers, solids contact units, plate and tube settlers, dissolved air flotation, and adsorption clarifiers replace the conventional sedimentation basin. Most coagulation mechanisms that have been discussed for conventional treatment trains also apply to these alternative technologies.

Each of the technologies has a niche in which its application becomes more favorable. For example, direct filtration and dissolved air flotation approaches are most attractive for treating low-turbidity waters where difficulties can be encountered in generating a settleable floc for removal in conventional sedimentation basins. Direct filtration is already an accepted approach for such conditions, whereas dissolved air flotation is a later innovation. Until recently, the dissolved air flotation (DAF) approach has been more widely used in Europe. DAF was initially adopted in the United States for treatment of a cold, low-turbidity water in New Castle, New York, where its applicability was first demonstrated in pilot testing. DAF is now being considered for wider application. In general, this process is capable of achieving higher levels of turbidity removal than conventional sedimentation systems, while achieving similar removals of organic precursor material. While relative effectiveness can be significantly greater for low turbidity, highly colored water (18), DAF is also effective in removing lighter materials such as algae and organic matter.

Solids contact and upflow blanket clarifiers are applicable under conditions where flow rate and water quality are not susceptible to significant changes. Sudden changes in turbidity or temperature can alter the balance within these units and cause disruption of the solids blankets. In some cases, these problems can be reduced by orifice collectors that withdraw the effluent at a submerged depth rather than by surface withdrawal by overflow weirs. Also, these units can be covered to minimize daily variations in temperature gradients influenced by sunlight.

COAGULATION PHENOMENA IN LIME SOFTENING

Turbidity removal by lime softening is normally quite efficient, but organic removal may be variable depending on water quality and process-related factors. For example, organic removal has been reported to increase with pH and with increased levels of hardness precipitation. The presence of magnesium and phosphate can also improve removals. In particular, the precipitation of magnesium hydroxide, which occurs at the upper end of the lime softening pH region (pH 11), appears to enhance removals (26). This mechanism would not be suitable for many facilities where operation is more typically in a pH range of 9 to 10.

Calcium carbonate precipitates formed in lime softening processes tend to have a negative surface charge, a feature that has an inhibiting influence on the adsorption of negatively charged organic molecules typically found in source waters. Although soluble calcium appears to be capable of directly causing precipitation of organic molecules at elevated pH levels, it has been found that the predominant mechanism for removal of fulvic acid precursors is coprecipitation at the surface of calcium carbonate precipitates (26).

The quantity of organics that can be removed is generally related to the availability of surface area on these precipitates. The surface area of softening precipitates is much lower than that available in the aluminum and iron coagulation processes. As a consequence, the quantity of organic material that can be removed can be more limited. Where low levels of TOC are present, the precipitate surface area may be adequate for achieving a significant removal percentage. However, high TOC levels that greatly exceed the available surface capacity may result in low removal percentages (26).

A common practice in lime softening facilities involves solids recirculation. This allows previously precipitated particles to serve as nuclei to catalyze further precipitation of hardness and also allows for particles to build to a more settleable size. In many cases, this is an important process enhancement that improves the efficiency of lime softening processes. While this solids recycle approach can be important for achieving lime softening goals, research has indicated that excessive recycling can be counterproductive for removal of organic material (23). It is believed that the surface area of precipitates tends to decrease with the aging and particle growth processes that occur with too much recirculation. Agglomeration of particles will reduce overall surface areas. As a consequence, in some treatment situations, it may be advantageous to seek a balance that provides a level of recycle necessary for achieving softening goals, but which is not so excessive that the goals for organic removal are impeded.

Supplemental coagulation using organic polymers, aluminum coagulants, or iron coagulants is often employed to enhance solids removal in the lime softening processes. These combinations can also be considered for improving removal of organic matter (26). The sequence of addition of supplemental coagulants relative to lime can be important. For example, ferric chloride effectiveness for organics removal at one location was enhanced by a period of contact at a more moderate pH level before the pH was elevated by the addition of lime (31).

POWDERED ACTIVATED CARBON AS SUPPLEMENT TO COAGULATION FOR REMOVING ORGANIC CONSTITUENTS

Powdered activated carbon (PAC) has been widely used with coagulation processes for control of certain tastes and odors. When used in this mode, PAC is typically dispersed in the process stream and is then subsequently removed by coagulation, sedimentation, and filtration processes. Because of the capability of PAC for removal of a wide range of organic compounds, its use has been evaluated for removal of organic precursors. Results have been variable and while successful applications have been observed in some studies, others have shown limited precursor removal, especially in the PAC dosage range of 5 to 15 mg/l, which has been typical in water treatment practice for more traditional concerns such as taste and odor control. Higher PAC doses have shown improved success in some applications, but organic removal results still have been variable (57).

Some research indicates that molecular weight distribution of organic matter can affect the applicability of PAC (9). Precursors found in many waters are large, high molecular weight organics which have limited mobility in the porous structure of many activated carbons. Therefore, while PAC can be effective for removal of a wide range of other organic compounds, its effectiveness may be reduced in the removal of higher molecular weight compounds. In contrast, removal by coagulation processes can be quite effective for high molecular weight compounds, while lower molecular weight compounds are not as effectively removed. Therefore, site-specific conditions relative to molecular weight distribution can have an effect on the applicability of both PAC and coagulation for removing precursors. In situations where a significant portion of the precursor content is in the lower molecular weight range, PAC might be advantageously used to supplement removals by coagulation, which are more oriented towards the higher molecular weight component. In other applications, oxidizing agents, such as ozone, might reduce the molecular weight to make the organic material more adsorbable with PAC.

High-pore-volume PACs have been reported to improve the pore mobility of large molecular weight compounds and have been reported to be capable of more effective precursor removals under some conditions (1). These high-pore-volume characteristics are not available in most of the PACs typically used for taste and odor control in water treatment and may account for some of the ineffectiveness observed for precursor removal by these types of PAC (25).

In the application of PAC, several factors should be considered. As with other treatment phenomena for removing precursors, removal effectiveness is generally improved by lowering pH. In addition, a period of contact prior to coagulation can also be desirable since, once added, aluminum and iron coagulants can generate precipitates that obscure access to pores (25).

Time of contact is important for adsorption processes to progress towards maximum equilibrium uptake conditions. Contact in most rapid mix/flocculation basin trains is generally limited, thereby reducing the effectiveness of PAC in relation to its ultimate capacity. Approaches for overcoming this disadvantage have been proposed. These involve either an attachment of activated carbon to a media that is suspended in solution by an upflow process (Roberts-Haberer process) or an increase in the solids retention time by using fluidized bed or upflow blanket clarifier types of systems to allow the floc mass and PAC levels to accumulate in a sludge blanket (25, 47).

Another possibility for improving performance is to separate the adsorption process from the coagulation process. The adsorptive process would precede the coagulation stage in a separate contacting chamber that would provide adequate mixing and contact time before the carbon becomes fouled by coagulated floc. Slurry contacting systems, with PAC recycle, can be considered to allow for more complete use of adsorptive capacity.

EFFECT OF COAGULATION MODIFICATIONS FOR ORGANIC REMOVAL ON WATER TREATMENT RESIDUALS

Alteration of coagulation processes to increase removal of organic precursor compounds can require an increase in the coagulant dose. In some cases, this practice may result in substantial coagulant use as well as a considerable increase in sludge that must be handled and ultimately disposed. Moreover, increased dosages may change the character of waste solids by increasing the proportion of aluminum or ferric hydroxide precipitates relative to the clay content in a water. Because of the gelatinous nature of aluminum and ferric hydroxide precipitates, this can sometimes produce a sludge that is more difficult to dewater. The character of waste solids can also be changed by using alternative coagulants.

The effects of coagulant modifications on sludges need to be considered and incorporated into plans for altering coagulation processes. Where necessary, sludge facilities will need to be expanded or modified to accommodate the changes in sludge quantities and characteristics.

EVALUATION OF COAGULATION

One of the most fundamental tools for evaluating coagulation phenomena is the jar test, which is described in detail by Herbert E. Hudson, Jr. (20). This test allows for rapid screening of alternative coagulant combinations. Other tests include zeta potential and streaming current measurements that evaluate the charges on particle surfaces. Streaming current detectors are available as on-line monitoring devices, often providing useful plant performance information on a continuous basis. Hypothetically, the best coagulation condition under a charge neutralization concept would occur at a zero charge. However, several other phenomena come into play, and it is necessary to determine the optimum setting for each particular raw water. Optima for either charge determination technique can vary with water quality, which needs to be determined for each treatment situation. Seasonal variation in optimum coagulation dosage may also occur.

Particle counting is another technology for evaluating coagulation processes. This technology characterizes particles according to number and size, allowing assessment of the extent to which particle size is increased by coagulation. This information can be particularly valuable for direct filtration in which no sedimentation step is available.

In general, the following factors need to be considered in applying test procedures:

- The effect of chemical mixing should be taken into account in calibrating the test protocols to the performance of a full-scale plant. In particular, rate of dispersion of coagulant during the initial mix step can have important consequences for the effectiveness of some coagulation processes. Where necessary, test protocols for chemical addition, mixing, flocculation, and settling should be adjusted to simulate conditions in a full-scale plant as much as possible (20). In some situations, where performance at full scale is not equal to the jar tests, improvements to the full-scale mixing and/or flocculation processes might be indicated.
- Temperature effects need to be considered when temperature in the testing area is significantly different than in the full-scale plant. As has been discussed, temperature can significantly affect the chemical species formed by some coagulants, thereby affecting the outcome of the coagulation process.
- Low-turbidity (less than 5 NTU) waters are sometimes difficult to assess with jar tests. These waters do not always produce rapidly settling floc, so special care is required in evaluating results (32). Paper filters can be useful in determining the best coagulant and mixing combinations (see Chapter 13).

Conditions for optimum turbidity removal can be different from those required for optimum organics removal, which should be a consideration in evaluation of jar test results. Typically the best pH for turbidity removal may range from 6 to 7, whereas organic removal is best in the range of 5 to 6. This type of variation is illustrated by the jar test results in Figure 11–4 for a raw water located in central Virginia. Note that the pH region of lowest UV absorbance, which is used here as a surrogate for

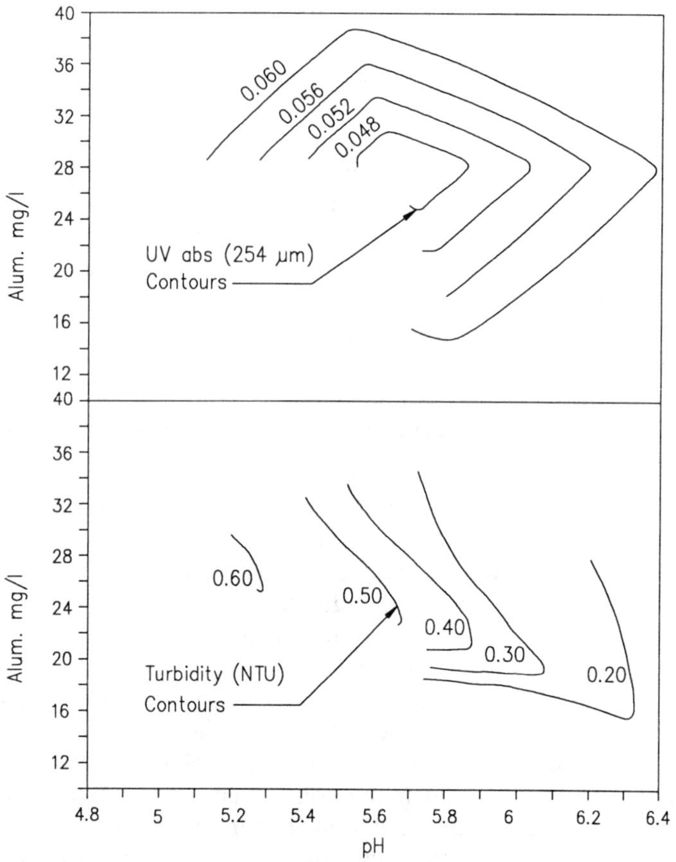

FIGURE 11–4. Effect of pH on alum coagulation for removal of UV absorbance and turbidity for a raw water in central Virginia.

naturally occurring organic materials of concern, lies in a range of 5.6 to 5.8, whereas settled water turbidity shows some improvement as pH is increased above this range. In this situation, plant treatment objectives required removal of both organics and turbidity, which ultimately resulted in operation in a pH region of 5.8 to 6.0, thereby creating a slight compromise between the two objectives. Jar test results confirmed plant experience with turbidity and organic removal in this particular situation. However, sedimentation and filtration may involve some complexities that are not always reflected by jar testing so that some caution should be exercised in test interpretation. In essence, testing provides an indication of coagulation phenomena, but adjustments may be needed for actual plant-operating conditions.

Some differences in optima for turbidity and organics removals also can be observed where zeta potential measurements are used for supplementing jar test evaluations. For example, optimal conditions for turbidity removal often occur at a slightly negative zeta potential, whereas optimal conditions for removal of organics often occur closer to the zero point of charge (32). These differences do not necessarily result in insurmountable obstacles, and a condition for accommodating both goals can normally be developed.

Research has provided a better understanding of the general phenomena associated with coagulation. Many of the coagulating species formed by the addition of aluminum and iron coagulants are intermediates that will at least partially disappear in time. In addition, their availability can be altered by the presence of other conditions, such as interactive anions like sulfates. Adding to this complexity is the varying effect of naturally occurring organic matter, which can react with aluminum and iron to further alter the distribution of chemical intermediates. Therefore, the testing of alternatives should be performed with some awareness of the potential for site-specific phenomena that may affect the selection of coagulation protocols.

During evaluation of the coagulation process, it should also be recognized that the addition of coagulants such as alum and ferric chloride affects the pH as a result of the acid properties of these chemicals. This can assist in reducing the pH to the slightly acid region in which both turbidity and organic removal are more favorable. However, in low alkalinity waters that are poorly buffered against this acidifying influence, it is frequent practice to add an alkaline supplement to avoid an excess depression of pH at the desired coagulant dosage. A reverse problem may occur where alum dose is inadequate to achieve the desired pH reduction such as with high-alkalinity waters that are buffered against change in pH. In these cases, it is possible to supplement the acidifying effect of coagulants with the addition of acid. This can reduce the coagulant dose that would otherwise be required for pH adjustment, also reducing the quantity of sludge that would be associated with the added dose. In any case, overdosing the coagulant to depress pH is poor practice. This can result in postflocculation in the distribution systems where an alkalinity supplement is added to increase the pH of the product water.

In short, the range of coagulation conditions can be greatly expanded by examining combinations of available acid and alkaline chemical additions, thereby providing more flexibility for optimizing the performance of the coagulation process. The addition of a separate pH-adjusting chemical may provide advantages in some cases, but could also add to process complexity. Addition of a separate pH adjustment must be considered based on its merits at each location. Many utilities use lime and caustic to increase pH for corrosion control, and this type of alkaline chemical is also frequently available for pH adjustment in the coagulation process. However, the addition of acids for achieving lower pH levels is an uncommon approach because these chemicals are not normally encountered in water treatment practice. While this may be an appropriate approach, it will require planning for the addition of a new chemical system with hazardous handling properties.

The characteristics of the optimum pH conditions for precursor removal are reported to depend on the nature of organic material to be removed. Where this material has a relatively homogeneous character, a more distinct optimum can be anticipated than in cases of heterogeneous character. In addition, low-alkalinity waters that are more sensitive to pH change with coagulant addition may have a sharper, more distinct optimum condition due to this sensitivity (32).

Regulations are placing more emphasis on limiting the aluminum residuals in drinking water. As more emphasis is placed on optimizing alum coagulation processes for precursor removal in the pH region of 5 to 6, there is more of a likelihood for increasing such aluminum residuals. The reason is that minimum aluminum solubility occurs between pH 6 and 6.5. As pH is increased or decreased outside of this range, solubility increases, resulting in increased levels of dissolved aluminum. This is undesirable from both operational and esthetic standpoints since excess aluminum residuals are susceptible to postprecipitation that can create deposits in pipelines and occasionally discolor water. In addition, aluminum residuals are also being discussed for possible more stringent regulation because of potential health-related concerns associated with Alzheimer's disease. Optimization of alum coagulation processes for precursor removals may, therefore, conflict with goals for minimizing aluminum residuals. Where optimization goals are considered important, some utilities may elect to consider a compromise pH that will allow low aluminum residuals, while still maintaining a relatively high degree of organic removal. Alternatives such as the iron coagulants or some of the polymerized aluminum coagulants that may be effective at a lower applied aluminum dosage also can be considered for reducing aluminum residual levels.

RAPID RATE FILTRATION MECHANISMS

Solids separation in rapid rate filtration depends on a combination of physical/chemical mechanisms. Two of the principal mechanisms are entrapment and attachment, depicted in Figure 11–5 (44).

With entrapment, the filter media acts like a sieve or a strainer. Coagulated particles carried to the filters are caught in pore openings that are

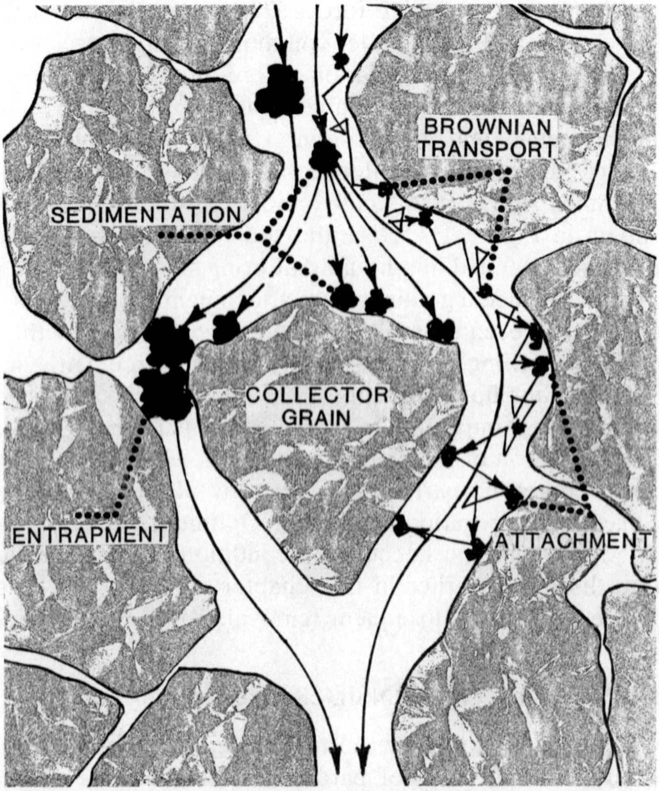

FIGURE 11–5. Principal mechanisms of solids separation shown schematically. (From Ref. 44. Reprinted from *Public Works Magazine* (June 1988), by permission.)

smaller than the size of the suspended particles and are physically removed. This separation process becomes progressive as the openings in the filter media are filled as particles are intercepted and stored. With this decrease in pore openings, smaller-sized particles are separated by entrapment.

In the attachment process, as flow passes through the filter media, suspended particles contact and attach to the surface of media grains. This particle attachment phenomenon has been attributed to van der Waals or other forces. However, chemical forces also can come into play as a consequence of coagulant chemicals added to condition particles. This results in additional interactions between floc particles as they accumulate in a filter. For the attachment mechanism to be effective, the suspended particles must be properly conditioned to achieve the appropriate combination of attractive forces. This typically means that negatively charged colloidal sized matter common in many source waters must be destabilized by proper coagulation before filtration.

Two transport mechanisms can affect particle removal by attachment: Brownian movement and interception. Under the interception mechanism, particles carried into the filters contact or intercept the media grains where attachment mechanisms cause them to adhere. Brownian movements, shown in Figure 11–5, are the somewhat erratic wanderings of small particles suspended in a liquid that bring such small-sized particles in contact with the media grains, where attachment forces can be exerted. Sedimentation represents another mechanism; particles with adequate size can achieve settling velocities that resist or overcome the interstitial velocity of the filter flow through. With this mechanism, particles also may be removed by simply settling onto the top surfaces of media grains.

With the exception of Brownian movements, all of these mechanisms improve with increased particle size, thereby placing additional importance on particle aggregation processes. Optimum aggregation requires appropriate rapid mix and flocculation conditions. Proper application of coagulation discussed earlier in this chapter will also help to optimize particle aggregation and subsequent removal in rapid rate filters.

PATHOGEN-CONTROL CONSIDERATIONS

Disease outbreaks due to waterborne pathogens such as *Giardia* have underscored the importance of particulate removal processes. *Giardia* and several other pathogens can be more resistant to the action of disinfectants, placing an increased emphasis on the need for particulate removal processes as a supplement to disinfection. Removal of waterborne pathogens can be more difficult under conditions that are not conducive to effective coagulation and filtration. These can include cold, low-turbidity, low-alkalinity waters, which have been cited as problematic for control of *Giardia* in particular.

Coagulation/Filter Ripening

Pilot plant studies (24) have indicated the need for proper coagulation to achieve high levels of removal of *Giardia* cysts during rapid rate filtration. These studies showed that high cyst removal efficiencies required achieving filtered water turbidities much lower than the prevailing standard of 1 NTU. Elevated levels of cysts were also observed during the initial ripening period, which occurs when a rapid rate filter is placed in service following backwash. Turbidity and cyst breakthrough during this period suggested the need for filter-to-waste or other provisions for reducing these effects.

Reliable first-stage solids removal in conventional treatment is essential where a high raw water turbidity is encountered. It is also appropriate to consider the use of more refined control measures for coagulant dosage and pH control since both parameters can have a significant influence on the effectiveness of coagulation and the subsequent filtration process. Coagulation control may include more rigorous use of jar testing as well as newer methods such as on-line monitoring using streaming current detectors or zeta potential measurements as previously discussed.

Because the filter ripening phase has a potential for high filtered water turbidity and pathogen breakthrough, phenomena associated with this period have become of interest in the development of comprehensive disinfection strategies. In this regard, a recent study of evaluations at two water treatment plants in Montana concluded that site-specific understanding of these profiles was important to control adverse effects during filter ripening (8). Although filter-to-waste has been a common filter ripening strategy, hydraulic surges associated with valve operation and other effects observed at the Montana study site resulted in undesirable breakthroughs in the transition from the filter-to-waste stage to normal filtration operation, thereby suggesting the need for additional precautionary measures in this situation. Chlorination of backwash water was recommended for maintaining disinfecting conditions in filters and backwash piping that would avoid the problems associated with an undisinfected remnant water that might otherwise remain in the filter following backwash. Use of polymers in backwash water was also recommended for accelerating the filter ripening process in order to shorten the duration of the turbidity and coliform peaks, thereby minimizing the time required for filter-to-waste. Care should be exercised if this latter approach is selected since excess polymer feed in this type of application can foul the filter media, resulting in mud-ball formation, premature buildup of head loss, and other problems.

Flow Surge Control

Breakthrough of *Giardia* cysts has been observed to coincide with conditions that are associated with turbidity breakthrough (24). Breakthroughs of this type occur at the end of a filter run and during short-term periods of suddenly increased filtration rates during a filter run. In some cases, significant levels of *Giardia* cysts have been observed during short-term events of hydraulic surging even though turbidity increased by only 0.05 to 0.1 NTU. Based on this observation, design for stable filter rates or for more gradual changes in such rates are a consideration for more reliable *Giardia* removal. This type of process sensitivity also influences the need for effective control of coagulation processes, chemical dosage, chemical mixing, and flocculation, all of which are essential for good filter performance.

Based on the findings of the importance of hydraulic stability, the following should be considered in the design and operation of rapid sand filters:

1. If filter to waste is included in the backwash cycle, the method for shifting from filter-to-waste wash cycle to filtration should minimize sudden changes in the filtration rate.
2. Rate controllers should be designed to minimize continuous hunting, which can cause continuous surges in filtration rate.
3. Rapid rate filters should not be used to produce finished water immediately after extended down periods or when bumping (flow surge) has occurred. Ideally, all filters should be kept in continuous operation with a master rate controller, adjusting gradually when plant output changes.
4. Where extended downtimes or significant hydraulic surges are encountered, consideration should be given to restarting with a filter ripening period until the filtered water turbidity is stabilized.

Evaluating Effectiveness of Rapid Rate Filtration

The most common measures of filtration performance have been product water turbidity, as an indicator of particulate content, and coliforms and heterotrophic plate count as standard bacterial indicators of microbial content. Interest in the use of particle counters has developed as a supplementary measure of filtration effectiveness. These devices are intended to give specific information on particle numbers by size category, whereas turbidity offers only a general indication of the total amount of particles.

Particle counters can evaluate particles over a general range of 0.4 to 200 μm, with specific range depending on the type of equipment (48). Measurements of interest can include the number of particles in the *Giardia* size range (8 to 12 μm). However, some limitations of particle counters must be understood in interpreting this type of data. In these devices, particles are measured as spheres, whereas most of the particles of interest do not have a spherical shape. One study (48) found that some particle-counting instruments categorized *Giardia* (8- to 12-μm size) as equivalent to 4-μm spheres and observed that the presence of *Giardia* would have been missed if channels were set to only include channels that encompassed 8- to 12-μm particles. This suggests that particle count data should not be interpreted too literally. If *Giardia*-sized particles are of particular interest, a broader range would have to considered to allow for deviations associated with nonspherical particles.

Another developing method for evaluating particles employs flow cytometry. This approach yields fluorescence information in addition to particle size categorization. Fluorescent labels have been used for identifying *Giardia* and *Cryptosporidium* cysts, and the availability of a fluorescence-sensing capability may yield benefits by providing more specific information on particle identity (49).

In addition to a potential role for identifying particles in a size range of interest, particle counters can also be considered for giving a general indication of filter performance. Used in this manner, a general measure of total particle content can often be evaluated. Some researchers have indicated that particle counts can yield better sensitivity than turbidity measurements (40). Note that this does not negate the value of turbidity for evaluating this phenomena, especially given the improved accuracy at low turbidity levels that can be obtained with newer ratio turbidimeters. However, it represents an alternative method for obtaining additional information on filter performance.

While particle counting can yield additional information about general filter performance, it does not characterize particles relative to microbial characteristics. One group of researchers has indicated that this approach cannot substitute for microbial counting (56). Evaluations have also suggested that total bacterial levels leaving a filter are not well indicated by turbidity or conventional microbial tests, such as coliform bacteria, and heterotrophic plate count (39). A microscopic total bacterial enumeration method has been suggested as an alternative. While this total bacterial enumeration is of interest, applicability as an indicator of specific microbial concerns remains to be established.

When rapid rate filtration processes are assessed and compared, care should be taken to sample filter effluent at the appropriate location. For example, the addition of posttreatment chemicals such as lime can frequently cause a slight increase in the turbidity of finished water. Turbidity and particle-counting measurements to determine filter performance should be made upstream of the addition point for posttreatment chemicals so that turbidity and particle counts from these additions will not interfere with analysis of filtered water quality, the true measure of filtration effectiveness.

SLOW SAND FILTRATION

A typical flow arrangement of the slow sand filter process is shown in Figure 11–1. The process train usually consists of the filter and a clearwell or treated water storage basin. Slow sand filtration is a passive filtration process subject to almost no control by the operator other than frequency of cleaning and duration of filter-to-waste during the ripening period. A major difference between this process and rapid rate filtration is the fact that the filtration step does not require the addition of chemical coagulants. As a consequence, slow sand filters use media of smaller effective size (0.15 to 0.40 mm vs. 0.45 to 1.30 mm) and have significantly lower filtration rates (0.016 to 0.16 gpm/sf vs. 2.0 to 8.0 gpm/sf). A typical effective size is 0.3 mm, and typical loading rates are in the range of 0.03 to 0.05 gpm/sf (55). There is less concern about maintaining low media uniformity coefficients with slow sand filters than with rapid sand filters. In fact, there may be an advantage to using a somewhat higher uniformity coefficient with slow sand filters that will allow greater intermixing of particles of different size to reduce the bed porosity.

Unlike conventional rapid rate filtration systems that can employ a sedimentation step prior to filters, slow sand filter systems do not have a capability for removing high concentrations of solids and can be blinded by high turbidity loads. As a result, these systems typically should not be applied for water with turbidity much in excess of 5 to 10 NTU. Where raw water of higher turbidity is anticipated, pretreatment processes might be used to reduce turbidity to acceptable levels prior to the slow sand filters. Such pretreatment to remove solids, however, should not include coagulation, which can produce particulate aggregations that will blind a slow sand filter.

A critical consideration for effective slow sand filter operation is the accumulation of a surface formation. This surface formation, called the *schmutzdecke*, consists of an accumulation of both inert deposits and biological material. Recent research has demonstrated that both the *schmutzdecke* and the biological growth within the sand bed have important roles in particulate removal, particularly at the beginning of a filter run (7).

Operation of slow sand filters requires two periodic tasks:

1. After head loss exceeds the design level (usually from 1 to 2 months) the *schmutzdecke* must be removed or scraped from the surface after draining the filter.
2. After successive scrapings have reduced the depth of sand in the filter to the lowest acceptable depth, sand must be replaced to restore the

filter media to its original design dimension. Alternatively, sand can be replaced to make up loss after each cleaning.

Until a new *schmutzdecke* can be established after resuming operation, the effectiveness of particulate removal will be reduced. It will also take time for biological growths to establish within the new sand layer, but this has much less impact on overall filtration effectiveness than the *schmutzdecke* accumulation.

Since slow sand filtration relies for the most part on biological mechanisms to facilitate treatment, this process may be effective for removal of biodegradable organic carbon as well as turbidity. While this attribute may be an added advantage, the lack of chemical removal mechanisms can limit its application for other goals such as reduction of color and removal of disinfection byproduct precursors. Process modifications such as use of preozonation may improve performance for such goals (53). Use of GAC as an alternative filter media may be another possible modification (42).

Recent studies have indicated the following performance by slow sand filters at typical design conditions (7, 33):

1. 99.0 percent removal of *Giardia* cysts with new sand (first time operation)
2. 100 percent removal (within detection limits) of *Giardia* cysts after development of *schmutzdecke*
3. 90 percent removal of coliform bacteria with new sand and no previous development of biological growth
4. 99.99 percent removal of coliforms after establishment of *schmutzdecke*
5. Reduction of coliform removal to 99.9 percent immediately after removal of *schmutzdecke*—restoration to 99.99 percent removal after a few days of operation

The above performance features need to be considered in the design of the alternative operation modes. For instance, when multiple slow sand filter units are available, it may be possible to pass the effluent from a newly cleaned unit to the other operating cells in a series arrangement until the *schmutzdecke* is established. In this manner, a high degree of removal of both coliform bacteria and *Giardia* cysts can be maintained. Alternatively, filter-to-waste can be practiced for the ripening period. In slow sand filter operation, a considerable amount of water would be wasted by filter-to-waste since several days or weeks may be required for ripening. In either case, flexibility for providing a filter ripening period will need to be made available by dividing the filter area into a workable number of cells.

PRECOAT FILTRATION

Precoat filtration was first introduced in 1942 using diatomaceous earth (DE) as a filter media. This process was adopted for U.S. Army field use in 1944 because it was effective for removal of *Entamoeba histolytica* cysts that were difficult to control by disinfecting agents. The precoat filter uses a disposable media approach, quite different in character from the more commonly used granular media filters. Two different materials are now used for precoat filtration: DE and perlite.

The precoat filtration process includes three individual steps. In the initial precoating step, a cake with a 3- to 5- mm thickness of powder-sized medium is applied to a porous support called a septum. A typical septum assembly may consist of a flat structural frame covered on both sides by woven stainless steel mesh or synthetic fabric. This leaflike assembly is attached to a pipe manifold for collection of filtered water. The precoat cake is formed by simply recirculating through the filter a flow into which the required amount of media has been introduced, which causes the slurried media to be deposited onto the filter septa. After this precoat deposit is developed, the second step is initiated by applying raw water for treatment. Solids contained in the raw water are separated on the surface of the cake and gradually accumulate to build up cake thickness.

Most raw water solids, especially those of organic origin, are compressible. As a consequence, the hydraulic force that holds the cake to the septum can compress the accumulated cake, thereby reducing its porosity. This condition can result in increased head loss across the filter cake and shortened filter runs. Therefore, a *body feed* of slurried media is normally added to the raw water feed stream, which, when deposited with the raw water solids, tends to maintain a matrix of the media to retain the porosity of the cake. When the accumulated cake ultimately reaches a thickness that results in a pressure drop equal to the maximum available head, the run must be terminated and the cake is flushed from the septa. A new run is then initiated, beginning with the precoat step.

The precoat filter is a particulate removal device that relies predominantly on an entrapment or straining mechanism for solids removal. Some smaller-sized solids also are removed by attachment mechanisms. However, without pretreatment, it is difficult to remove negatively charged, naturally occurring organic materials of colloidal size. In some cases, pretreatment of media with alum coagulant and/or PAC or ozonation of process water flow has overcome this limitation. Care, however, must be exercised with alum pretreatment to avoid excess dose conditions that will foul the media.

In certain situations, oxidizing the inlet flow will neutralize negatively charged colloidal particulates by breaking the bond of organics into inert matter. In a less beneficial manner, however, oxidation processes such as ozonation can also change the character of certain source water organic matter to a more biologically assimilable form as measured by biodegradable organic carbon (BDOC). These dissolved constituents are not removed and pass through the filter to the water distribution system. Where bacterial regrowth occurs in the distribution system, excess BDOC can exacerbate the situation since it serves as readily available food for such microorganisms.

A particular advantage of the precoat filtration process is the fact that a broad range of precoat media sizes are available to fit the particular treatment situation. Recent tests have shown the following removal performances for the most common grades of DE (7, 33):

- Practically 100 percent effectiveness in the removal of *Giardia* cysts
- Up to 99.8 percent removal of coliform bacteria
- Turbidity removals up to 99.9 percent
- Improvement in the reduction of both turbidity and coliform bacteria levels with the use of alum-coated media or preoxidation

Precoat filters are less effective in the removal of color. Where color is of organic origin, oxidation, especially with ozone, can be effective in improving color removal to acceptable levels.

In developing a baseline process employing the use of precoat filtration, the basic test program should include determination of the following:

1. The grade or size of media required to attain the established levels of turbidity and pathogen reduction
2. The possible need for pretreatment or media conditioning to improve color and colloidal particulate removals

If oxidation is required, further investigation will be necessary to determine if this will change the character of the product water quality in a manner that produces problems such as bacterial regrowth in the distribution system.

MISCELLANEOUS PARTICULATE REMOVAL PROCESSES

Other particulate removal processes include ultrafiltration membranes and cartridge filters. Ultrafiltration membranes have some similarities to reverse osmosis and nanofiltration processes. However, salt removal is not a specific goal; the focus is more on straining particulate matter. The objective of these membranes is to remove microbes by physical separation methods, reducing or eliminating the need for primary disinfection.

Cartridge filters use ceramic or polypropylene filter materials that are enclosed in a pressurized vessel or cartridge. They are available with a number of pore openings, with sizes in the range of 0.2 to 1.0 μm being typical for water treatment (32). Because of operational simplicity, this process has been applied in small system situations, particularly where *Giardia* has been a concern.

Pretreatment to limit solids loading can be important with membrane and cartridge filtration. Provisions must be made for cleaning accumulated solids from some cartridge filters. Some polypropylene cartridges, however, are disposable and are not cleaned.

MODIFICATION OF BASELINE TREATMENT SYSTEMS FOR BIODEGRADATION

Treatment modifications to achieve biodegradation are emerging as significant considerations for control of microbial growth in distribution systems. The concepts developed for the Choisy-le-Roi plant in Paris, France, illustrate a number of attributes of biodegradation systems (52). This plant contains a conventional rapid rate filtration train similar to that shown in Figure 11–1b. In addition, ozone is added both to the raw water and following the initial filtration step. A postfiltration GAC-contacting system has been added for biodegradation. The GAC system is followed by chlorination, allowing disinfection of the elevated microbial levels that are released from the biologically active media. Following a chlorine contact period, sodium bisulfite is added as a dechlorinating agent to precisely control the chlorine level in finished water to 0.5 mg/l.

The addition of ozone upstream of GAC enhances the removal of organic matter by biodegradation. The filters also are allowed to operate in the biological mode and achieve a first stage of biodegradation that includes ammonia removal by nitrification. The end result of these process combinations is significant reduction in ammonia as well as organic carbon, both of which exert chlorine demand. As a consequence of this reduction, the dose of chlorine required to maintain secondary disinfection has been significantly reduced. The reduction in chlorine dose rates reduces the opportunity for formation of chlorination byproducts. Furthermore, capability for maintaining a chlorine residual throughout the distribution system has been enhanced.

This particular process sequence demonstrates several objectives for biodegradation processes:

1. Reduction in BDOC (or AOC) to limit microbial growth in the distribution system
2. Removal of ammonia
3. Use of ozone with biological activated carbon for reducing TOC and associated disinfection byproduct precursor content
4. Reduction in chlorine demand, thereby limiting formation of disinfection byproducts and allowing a more stable residual to be maintained for secondary disinfection application

While the Choisy-le-Roi process sequence was selected to illustrate general attributes to consider for biodegradation processes, a number of other approaches are available. Moreover, process requirements will vary, depending on water quality. Other common biodegradation alternatives include rapid rate filters in which prechlorination is eliminated to allow microbial growth, and slow sand filtration processes (58), which are inherently biological in nature. Additional approaches include soil-aquifer storage, such as dune and bank filtration; fluidized bed methods; and aerated biological filters (45).

Biodegradation for removal of biodegradable organic carbon (BDOC) and other goals is a developing concept. As discussed in Chapter 2, BDOC (alternatively expressed in terms of an assimilable organic carbon (AOC) type of measurement) can serve as a food source for microbial growth in water distribution piping. While provision of a secondary disinfecting residual has been the traditional method for limiting microbial growth, this method has some limitations, as discussed in Chapter 2. As a result, BDOC removal is being implemented as an alternative approach by some European utilities. In many applications, BDOC removal can be considered as a supplement to secondary disinfection.

While BDOC occurs to a certain extent in raw source water, it can be increased by reactions between natural organic matter (NOM) and strong oxidants used as disinfecting agents (e.g., ozone, chlorine dioxide, and chlorine). As discussed in Chapter 7, ozone can have a particularly significant effect on BDOC. Chlorine dioxide disinfection also can result in significant increases in BDOC levels. Therefore, development of a treatment strategy for BDOC can be an important aspect of alternative disinfection strategies. Microbial growth can be a concern for conventionally chlorinated systems as well, and some utilities have evaluated methods for reducing the level of BDOC that occurs under these conditions (50).

BDOC removal by biodegradation typically requires a support media on which a biofilm can attach. Two general treatment approaches are commonly available:

1. *Biofilm attachment to conventional filter media.* Conventional filter media can provide a biofilm support if the applied water does not contain chlorine or other disinfecting residuals. In many cases, this can be accomplished by moving chlorination to a location downstream of filters. Although this approach can achieve a degree of biodegradation, the contact time and surface area available with many conventional filters may not be adequate for achieving the amount of BDOC removal desired. The acceptability of this approach, therefore, will depend on the required degree of removal. If this approach can achieve acceptable results, it normally is a more cost-effective method as compared with other alternatives.
2. *Biofilm attachment to activated carbon.* Activated carbon can provide a large surface area for biofilm attachment. General concepts for this type of process are presented in Chapter 10. GAC has been widely considered for biodegradation, and some suppliers have developed GAC media specifically for use in this process. In an alternative approach, at least one installation has evaluated the use of PAC as a support media in a sludge blanket clarification system that allows a buildup of PAC within the floc blanket (50).

Several options are available for using GAC, with selection based on the required level of biodegradation. Alternative methods involve either GAC filter absorber or separate postfilter GAC contacting methods. GAC filter absorber methods incorporate GAC as filter media that replace conventional sand or anthracite. In this approach, the GAC medium provides a filtration media as well as a support media for biodegradation. Although complete GAC replacement of conventional filter media is the common practice, partial replacement also has been evaluated. For example, one study has reported ammonia removal by nitrification, as well as BDOC removal using a system of replacing part of the media with GAC, thereby forming a dual media with GAC as the top layer (51).

Applicability of a GAC filter absorber approach can be limited by available empty bed contact time when GAC is being used to replace conventional filter media in an existing filter box. This limitation can be particularly severe for high rate filter configurations. In some cases, existing filter boxes can be modified with more compact underdrain arrangements that can expand the depth available for media. However, where adequate contact time cannot be provided, it may become necessary to apply GAC in a postcontactor or to construct new filters to reduce the filter loading rate. Because of the added cost for postcontactors as compared with filter adsorbers, pilot testing should be considered to determine which approach is necessary. Testing should consider the effects of temperature since biodegradation processes can be slower at lower temperatures.

Where contactor volume is not constrained by existing structural limitations, an empty bed contact time in the range of 10 minutes has been typical (52, 53). In general, research has indicated that rapid improvement in BDOC removal occurs as EBCT is increased up to this time period, with more limited improvement over longer periods (53). This type of breakpoint between rapidly removed and more refractory BDOC components can be explained by the fact that BDOC is heterogeneous in composition. Easily degraded components are more subject to degradation, while difficult components degrade more slowly (53, 54).

The effluent from biodegradation processes can exhibit elevated bacterial counts that may require a postdisinfection step. This step may be combined with the secondary disinfection step, with free chlorine or chloramines as the most likely agents. Alternately, as in the case of the Choisy-le-Roi plant, chlorine can be added for a period of disinfecting contact, followed by partial dechlorination (common dechlorinating agents include sulfur dioxide, sodium sulfite, and sodium thiosulfate) to precisely control the chlorine concentration in finished water.

As discussed in Chapter 10, some additional difficulties may be encountered with control of bacteria that may be attached to fine GAC particles that occur in the effluents from GAC beds. Therefore, postdisinfection of biodegradation processes requires special consideration. Results in treating one water indicated differences in disinfectants for achieving inactivation of bacteria that are found in the effluent following biodegradation. In this situation, a high level of disinfection was achieved in a few minutes with free chlorine, whereas one hour was required with chloramines (11). Where chloramines are desired as the secondary disinfecting agent, a period of contact with free chlorine may be considered to achieve a higher disinfecting effectiveness before the addition of ammonia to form chloramines. As discussed in Chapter 5, the acceptability of this approach will depend on the extent to which disinfection byproduct formation will increase as a consequence of the extended contact period with free chlorine. Free chlorine is not always superior to chloramines for disinfecting GAC fines (38), probably due to a high reactivity with GAC and an associated difficulty in fully penetrating these particles. Site specific evaluation, therefore, will be required.

While it appears that either filters containing conventional media or GAC can be converted for operation in a biological mode, this practice conflicts with previous practice, which has called for maintaining an applied disinfecting residual (20, 35). Problems such as mud-balling and slime clogging have been observed to increase in unchlorinated filters, particularly in situations where surface wash has not been supplied or where it is not effective. Conversion to biological filtration methods is, therefore, likely to place more emphasis on media-cleaning methods. Cleaning of the dual media interface by subsurface wash or air wash should be considered. Air wash is preferred for GAC filters. This cleaning method appears to be compatible with the biological approach to filter operation, since the air bubbles do not appear to excessively disrupt or damage the biological films that attach to the media. Some have also indicated that backwashing with chlorinated water does not appear to inhibit bacterial activity in the filters (28), while damage appears to have occurred in other cases (43). This indicates the effectiveness of this practice to be site specific.

While the use of biological methods in the filtration step may provide an economical means for removing BDOC, the effect on other water treatment goals should be considered. For example, in some plants, chlorination may be a key factor for maintaining an oxidized filter coating that is critical for achieving manganese removal, as discussed in Chapter 4. If this chlorine residual is eliminated or depleted, the manganese may revert to a soluble form in the water. Since conversion to biological filtration methods requires a chlorine-free environment, the use of alternative approaches for removal of manganese would need to be demonstrated before the suitability of biological filtration can be established in this situation. Possible biological mechanisms for manganese removal have been reported in some European plants, and it is possible that this type of removal mechanism could be used to replace chemical oxidation strategies (45, 46). The suitability of this approach is questioned because many utilities experience sporadic events of elevated manganese where colonization by manganese-oxidizing bacteria might not be consistent.

As another approach for control of manganese, alternative oxidizing chemicals can be used in place of chlorine. Some of these oxidants tend to rely on direct precipitation of manganese as opposed to adsorption of an oxidized filter coating that occurs with chlorine. While these methods can be effective, complexity is sometimes introduced due to a tendency of manganese to form small colloidal precipitates that can penetrate through a filter if not adequately coagulated. Also, a potential for overdosing exists in the case of ozone. When it occurs, ozone overdosing leads to the formation of soluble permanganate ions instead of a precipitated form of manganese that is susceptible to removal by sedimentation and filtration processes. Control of this problem is possible by controlling ozone dose to avoid overdosing. Note that the appropriate ozone dose may not be adequate for disinfection and other goals, requiring a separate ozone step that is specifically dedicated to optimized conditions for manganese oxidation; other ozone objectives would be achieved at different locations. As an alternative, GAC filter adsorbers can provide a possible multiple role of GAC: as a filter media, as a support media for biodegradation, and as a catalyst for permanganate removal (see Chapter 7). A culpability for permanganate removal would allow use of ozone in excess of the optimum required for manganese removal, thereby eliminating the need for a separate ozone step specifically for manganese removal. As indicated by these considerations, the concepts for manganese removal may require careful evaluation before converting filters for operation in a biodegradation mode.

COMPARISON OF BASELINE WATER TREATMENT PROCESSES

Some of the key attributes of alternative filtration and softening systems have been summarized in Table 11–1. While rapid rate filters are most commonly used for particulate removal, other processes such as slow sand filtration, precoat filtration, and cartridge filters have been widely applied to smaller systems because they can be less complex from a process control standpoint, thereby simplifying operating procedures. However, some alternative filtration methods may also have advantages in larger systems especially where cold, low-turbidity waters are encountered that are difficult to coagulate. As an example of this type of application, New York City is operating a demonstration plant to evaluate the use of precoat filtration for a planned 300 mgd facility.

On the other hand, coagulation in conventional rapid rate filtration systems is capable of higher levels of pathogen removal and may provide some advantage with respect to added safety for disinfection as compared to other particulate removal systems. It may be possible to deal with some of the cold water coagulation problems by use of alternative coagulants such as polyaluminum chloride. Coagulation processes typically offer the additional capability for removing color and organic precursors. Therefore, a complex set of considerations, including cost, affect the selection of process.

Because filtration processes can be vulnerable to rapid head loss buildup when high turbidity levels are encountered in raw waters, the type of source and susceptibility to high turbidity occurrences need to be considered. Alternatives to rapid sand filtration, such as precoat, slow sand, and membrane filters, are particularly vulnerable to flashy type water supplies. Where such potential exists, pretreatment methods such as roughing filters, infiltration galleries, and presedimentation basins may be needed to protect these processes from high solids loading conditions. The associated costs should be included when comparing processes. In considering pretreatment alternatives, compatibility with the filter process can be important. Water subjected to pretreatment using coagulation usually cannot be effectively applied to slow sand and can create problems with precoat filtration as well.

When alternatives to conventional rapid rate filtration processes are considered, it is important to recognize that relationships between filtered water turbidity and removal of pathogens are frequently not as strong as for the alternatives to rapid rate filters. For example, turbidity reduction for achieving effective removal of *Giardia* cysts becomes less critical in the case of both slow sand filters and precoat filters. In particular, while very high levels of turbidity removal appear to be necessary for rapid sand filters, precoat filters and slow sand can achieve desired levels of *Giardia* removal at turbidities greater than 1 NTU (8, 24). As a consequence, the pathogen-removal effectiveness of precoat and slow sand filters should not be compared to that for rapid rate filters on the basis of turbidity.

References

1. Anderson, M. C., R. C. Butler, F. J. Moldren, and B. H. Kornegay. 1981. Controlling trihalomethanes with powdered activated carbons. *JAWWA* 73: 432.
2. Amirtharajah, A., and K. M. A. Mills. 1982. Rapid-mix design for mechanisms of alum coagulation. *JAWWA* 74: 210–16.
3. Amirtharajah, A. 1981. Initial mixing. In AWWA preconference seminar *Coagulation: Back to the basics*, St. Louis, MO, June 1981.
4. AWWA Coagulation Committee. 1989. Committee report: Coagulation as an integrated water treatment process. *JAWWA* 81(10): 72–8.
5. Babcock, D. B., and P. C. Singer. 1979. Chlorination and coagulation of humic and fulvic acids. *JAWWA* 71: 149–52.
6. Baes, C. F., and R. E. Mesmer. 1976. *The hydrolysis of cations*. New York: John Wiley & Sons.
7. Bellamy, W. D., G. P. Silverman, and D. W. Hendricks. 1985. *Filtration of* Giardia *cysts and other substances:* Vol. 2, *Slow Sand Filtration*. EPA-600/52-85/026. Cincinnati, OH: U.S. Environmental Protection Agency.
8. Bucklin, K., and A. Amirtharajah. 1987. Analysis of filter-to-waste validity in water treatment. Paper presented at 1987 AWWA Conference, Kansas City, MO.
9. Chadik, P. A., and G. L. Amy. 1987. Molecular weight effects on THM control by coagulation and adsorption. *J. Environ. Eng. Div. ASCE* 113: 1234–48.
10. Collins, M. R., G. L. Amy, and P. H. King, 1985. Removal of organic matter in water treatment. *J. Environ. Eng. Div. ASCE* 111: 850–64.

11. Daniel, P., P. Meyerhofer, G. Lai, M. Lanier, J. March, and J. Beard. 1990. Using ozone to meet conflicting water quality goals. Presented at 1990 AWWA Conference, Cincinnati, OH, June 1990.
12. Dempsey, B. A., R. M. Ganho, and C. R. O'Melia. 1984. The coagulation of humic substances by means of aluminum salts. *JAWWA* 76(4): 141–50.
13. Dempsey, B. A. 1987. Chemistry of coagulants. In AWWA preconference seminar *Influence of coagulation on the selection, operation, and performance of water treatment facilities*, Kansas City, MO, June 1987.
14. Dempsey, B. A., L. Willnow, and P. Pageni. P. 1986. Temperature effects on coagulation processes using salts of aluminum. *Proceedings of 47th Annual Meeting of the International Water Conference,* October 1986.
15. Dentel, S. K., and J. M. Gossett. 1988. Mechanisms of coagulation with aluminum salts. *JAWWA* 80(4): 187–98.
16. Edzwald, J. K., W. C. Becker, and S. J. Tambin. 1987. Organics, polymers, and performance in direct filtration. *J. Environ. Eng. Div. ASCE* 113: 168–85.
17. Edzwald, J. K., W. C. Becker, and K. L. Wattier. 1985. Surrogate parameters for monitoring organic matter and THM precursors. *JAWWA* 77(4): 122–32.
18. Edzwald, J. K., and J. P. Malley. 1990. Removal of humic substances and algae by dissolved air flotation. EPA/600/S2-89-032. U.S. Environmental Protection Agency.
19. Hazen and Sawyer, P.C. 1989. Drinking water act evaluation. Prepared for Tamarac Utilities West, Tamarac, FL.
20. Hudson, H. E., Jr. 1981. *Water clarification: Practical design and evaluation.* New York: Van Nostrand Reinhold Company.
21. Hundt, T. R., and C. R. O'Melia. 1988. Aluminum-fulvic acid interactions. *JAWWA* 80(4): 176–86.
22. Hubel, R. E., and J. K. Edzwald. 1983. Removing trihalomethane precursors by coagulation. *JAWWA* 75: 527–31.
23. Liao, M. Y., and S. J. Randtke. 1985. Removing fulvic acid by lime softening. *JAWWA* 77(8): 78.
24. Logsdon, G. S., D. M. Symons, R. L. Goye, and M. M. Arozarena. 1981. Alternative filtration methods for removal of *Giardia* cysts and cyst models. *JAWWA* 73(2): 111–18.
25. Randtke, S. J. 1988. Organic contaminant removal by coagulation and related process combinations. *JAWWA* 80(5): 40–56.
26. Randtke, S. J., C. E. Thiel, M. Y. Liao, and C. N. Yamaya. 1982. Removing soluble organic contaminants by lime-softening. *JAWWA* 74: 192–202.
27. Reckhow, D. A., and P. C. Singer. 1984. The removal of organic halide precursors by preozonation and alum coagulation. *JAWWA* 76: 151–7.
28. Miltner, R. J., E. W. Rice, and A. A. Stevens. 1990. Pilot scale investigation of the formation and control of disinfection byproducts. Presented at 1990 AWWA Conference, Cincinnati, OH, June 1990.
29. Sinsabaugh, R. L., R. C. Hoehn, W. R. Knocke, and A. E. Linkins. 1986. Removal of dissolved organic carbon by coagulation with iron sulfate. *JAWWA* 78(5): 74–82.

30. Sinsabaugh, R. L., R. C. Hoehn, W. R. Knocke, and A. E. Linkins. 1986. Precursor size and organic halide formation rates in raw and coagulated surface waters. *J. Environ. Eng. Div. ASCE* 112: 139–53.
31. Thompson, J. C., and J. J. Ameno. 1987. Preventing the formation of trihalomethanes in Florida groundwater. *JAWWA* 79(1): 38–42.
32. U.S. EPA. 1990. *Technologies for upgrading existing or designing new drinking water treatment facilities*. EPA 625/4-89/023. Cincinnati, OH: U.S. Environmental Protection Agency, Office of Drinking Water.
33. U.S. EPA. 1990. *Guidance manual for compliance with the filtration and disinfection requirements for public drinking water systems using surface water sources*. EPA/68-01/6989. Washington, DC: U.S. Environmental Protection Agency, Office of Drinking Water.
34. Veenstra, J. N., and J. L. Schnoor. 1979. Seasonal variations in trihalomethane levels in an Iowa River water supply. *JAWWA* 71: 515–20.
35. White, G. C. 1986. *Handbook of chlorination*. New York: Van Nostrand Reinhold Company.
36. Young, V. S., and P. C. Singer. 1979. Chloroform formation in public water supplies: A case study. *JAWWA* 71: 87.
37. Zeta-Meter, Inc. 1988. Everything you want to know about coagulation and flocculation. . . Long Island City, NY.
38. McGuire, M. J., et al. 1989. *Optimization and economic evaluation of granular activated carbon for organic removal*. AWWA Research Foundation, Denver, CO.
39. Brazos, B. J. 1987. Total bacterial removals in a rapid sand filtration plant. 1987 specialty ASCE Conference: Environmental Engineering, Orlando, FL, July 1987.
40. Hergesheimer, E. E. et al. 1990. Pilot scale evaluation of filtration processes using particle counting. *Proceedings of Annual AWWA Water Quality Technology Conference* pp. 323–44, San Diego, CA, November 1990.
41. Laine, J. M., M. M. Clark, and J. Mallievaille. 1990. Ultrafiltration of lake water: Effect of pretreatment on the partitioning of organics, THMFP, and flux. *JAWWA* 82(12): 82–7.
42. Fox, K. R., R. J. Miltner, G. S. Logsdon, D. L. Dicks, and L. F. Drolet. 1984. Pilot plant studies of slow-rate filtration. *JAWWA* 76(12): 62–8.
43. Characklis, W. G. 1988. Bacterial regrowth in distribution systems. Report for AWWA Research Foundation, Denver, CO, January 1988.
44. Fulton, G. P. 1988. Contending with filter media problems. *Public Works* (June): 67–70.
45. Bouwer, E. J., and P. B. Crowe. 1988. Biological processes in drinking water treatment. *JAWWA* 80(9): 82–93.
46. Rittmann, B. E., and V. L. Snoeyink. 1984. Achieving biologically stable drinking water. *JAWWA* 76(10): 106–14.
47. Carlson, M. 1991. Disinfection byproducts: Precursor removal. AWWA Conference Seminar *Controlling disinfection byproducts: Utilities' experiences and future research needs*. 1991 AWWA Conference, Philadelphia, PA, June 1991.

48. Lewis, C. M., et al. 1990. Selecting and evaluating particle counters for discrete sample analysis. Proceedings of Annual AWWA Water Quality Technology Conference, pp. 363–86, San Diego, CA, November 1990.
49. Yentsch, C. M. 1990. Flow cytometry: Automated individual particle analysis for water quality. Proceedings of Annual AWWA Water Quality Technology Conference, pp. 345–62, San Diego, CA, November 1990.
50. LeChevallier, M. W., B. H. Olson, and G. A. McFeters. 1990. Assessing and controlling bacterial regrowth in distribution systems. Report for AWWA Research Foundation, Denver, CO, January 1990.
51. Bablon, G. P., C. Ventresque, and R. Ben Aim. 1988. Developing a sand-GAC filter to achieve high-rate biological filtration. *JAWWA* 80(12): 47–53.
52. Servais, P., et al. 1991. Microbial activity in GAC filters at the Choisy-le-Roi treatment plant. *JAWWA* 83: 62–8.
53. Bablon, G., et al. 1991. Practical application of ozone. In *Ozone in water treatment: Application and engineering,* Langlais, B., et al., eds. Chelsea, MI: Lewis Publishers, Inc.
54. Servais, P., A. Anzil, and C. Ventresque. 1989. Simple method for determination of biodegradable dissolved organic carbon in water. *Appl. Environ. Microbiol.* 55: 2732–4.
55. Cleasby, J. L., et al. 1984. *Effective filtration for small water supplies.* U.S. EPA 808837/01/0, NTIS No. PB84-181-905. Washington, DC: U.S. Environmental Protection Agency.
56. Brazos, B. J., and J. T. O'Connor. 1990. Seasonal effects on the generation of particle-associated bacteria during distribution. Proceedings of Annual AWWA Water Quality Technology Conference, pp. 1073–1102, San Diego, CA, November 1990.
57. Najm, I. N., et al. 1991. Using powdered activated carbon: A critical review. *JAWWA* 83(1): 65–76.
58. Schellart, J. A. 1986. Disinfection and bacterial regrowth: Some experiences of the Amsterdam water works before and after stopping the safety chlorination. *Water Supply* 4(3): 217–25.
59. Batchelor, B., and P. Yang. 1982. Technical note: Removing trihalomethane formation potential by coagulation with activated silica and cationic polymer. *JAWWA* 74(9): 494–6.

12

Improving Performance of Existing Baseline Facilities

The importance of the relationship between disinfection and baseline water treatment is discussed in Chapter 11. The principal requirements for baseline treatment and the credits that may be applied toward removal and inactivation of pathogens are found in the Surface Water Treatment Rule (SWTR). It would be safe to say that, at the time of the promulgation of the SWTR, most filtration plants in operation in the United States had been constructed when the maximum allowable treated drinking water turbidity was established at 5.0 NTU. Under changing regulations, these plants have more recently been required to maintain product water turbidity below 1.0 NTU.

The SWTR now establishes a filtered product water turbidity of 0.5 NTU for all plants using coagulation-based rapid rate filtration processes. Moreover, guidance criteria for the new regulations include stringent requirements for testing and rating existing chlorine contact facilities for detention time that may be applied toward the CT regulations. As a consequence of these criteria, many water systems will be faced with the need to improve existing treatment facilities and operating practices to comply with the new baseline treatment-disinfection regulations. This chapter concentrates on methods that may be considered to both modify existing operating practices and refurbish existing facilities to help meet these requirements.

SIGNIFICANT SWTR FEATURES

The SWTR requires that disinfection be included as part of the treatment of surface water for potable use. Overall, the SWTR requires a minimum

3 log removal/inactivation of *Giardia* cysts and a minimum of 4 log removal/inactivation of viruses, although greater removal levels are recommended for poor quality source water. The required removals are mandatory for surface water plants except those meeting specified characteristics for source water quality and very rigid disinfection CT requirements. The rule credits filtration in well-operated treatment systems with significant pathogen-removal capability, thereby making filtration an important component of an overall disinfection process.

In developing the guidance criteria for the SWTR, EPA assumed that removal or reduction of *Giardia* cysts and enteric viruses varies according to the type of filtration system as follows:

- Well-operated conventional treatment systems (coagulation with a preliminary solids removal step such as sedimentation and rapid rate filtration) that have been optimized for turbidity removal can be expected to achieve 2.5 log removal of *Giardia* cysts and 2.0 log removal of viruses.
- Well-operated slow sand filtration systems can be expected to achieve 2.0 log removal of *Giardia* cysts and 2.0 log removal of viruses.
- Well-operated diatomaceous earth and direct (rapid rate) filtration systems can be expected to achieve 2.0 log removal of *Giardia* cysts and 1.0 log removal of viruses.

SWTR regulations for performance of rapid sand filtration plants require a filtered water turbidity of 0.5 NTU or less for at least 95 percent of measurements. Because the relationships between turbidity and proper performance of slow sand and precoat filters are less extreme than those for rapid sand filters, a turbidity of 1.0 NTU or less is permitted for slow sand and diatomaceous earth (precoat) filtration plants on the same measurement basis.

In well-operated plants, filtered water levels of less than 0.1 to 0.2 NTU typically can be achieved; a past AWWA goal has been 0.1 NTU. Such operating results should be encouraged, especially for surface water supplies with turbidity levels of 1.5 or less. This type of goal also is important to maintain a cushion between normal operations and higher turbidity that might occur under worst-case operating conditions.

The SWTR and associated disinfection criteria emphasize the need for plants to optimize turbidity removal. As mentioned above, this may be difficult in many older filtration plants that have evolved, in both design and operation, around less stringent turbidity requirements of the past.

This chapter will concentrate on the more common rapid rate filter system problems. A brief review will be made of steps that can be adopted to improve the performance of precoat and slow sand filters. The intent is to cover not all functional problems that occur in contemporary water treatment plants, but rather the most common difficulties affecting product water quality, with emphasis on those that influence the ability to meet the standards of the SWTR.

RAPID RATE FILTRATION

Inhibiting Factors

Based on numerous plant rehabilitation project experiences, the following are considered to be the more common features that inhibit rapid rate filtration performance:

- Inadequate hydraulic design resulting in unequal flow distribution between parallel treatment units
- Short circuiting of flow through rapid mixing, flocculation, and settling units
- Poor maintenance of mechanical equipment, instrumentation and controls, and filter media
- Need for updated process control

These factors or faults may be grouped in two general categories: (1) operation and maintenance procedures or habits and (2) structural and mechanical faults resulting from poor design, design for less stringent water quality objectives, or wear due to inadequate maintenance.

In the evaluation of filtration performance made to determine the possible need for improvement measures, it is essential that operation and maintenance features be investigated first. In some plant situations, process faults or problems may occur primarily as a result of operation and maintenance oversights that have evolved in the climate of less stringent turbidity requirements that previously existed. Faulty or improper coagulation procedures may be practiced with the best of intentions and such practices may have gone undetected for extended periods. The promulgation of more stringent turbidity and filtration standards along with the attendant increased water quality monitoring requirements have changed this situation. It is now essential that many treatment plants adopt new procedures to realize the maximum treatment potential of available filtration facilities. After the operation and maintenance issues have been sorted out and resolved, the design or physical condition features can be more meaningfully investigated.

Although operation problems are more common in plants 20 years old or more, it is not unusual to find that many older plants produce excellent filtered water. In these cases, design problems that may have existed have been corrected and a good maintenance program is in effect. Most importantly, in the well-run older plants, the operating staff knows and understands the principal influencing features and idiosyncracies of the facilities and process under their control. The staff also knows how to respond to changes in source water quality.

It is also not unusual to find newer facilities, perhaps in operation less than 10 years, where operation and maintenance procedures are not as yet fully established. In such plants, erratic treatment performance may still continue to occur as procedures are being developed.

There is no doubt that seasoned, well-motivated operators are an important element in a water treatment system. As drinking water quality requirements become more stringent and the implications of maintaining such requirements become more sophisticated, there will be more demand on operator skills, training, and overall background experience.

Chemical Feed Difficulties

Chemical feed is the one area of drinking water treatment where the judgment of the plant operating staff will have the most impact on successful filtration performance. Chemical feed is related to the type of chemical, the rate of feed, and the point of application in the process train. It is one area in treatment plant operation where errors in process can most easily be corrected. Despite the fact that the greatest control over process performance can be exercised in chemical feed, it is probably the most error-prone aspect in drinking water treatment operation.

Coagulation is the most critical feature of chemical feed to affect rapid rate filtration. In terms of total volume or weight of chemical used annually, alum is by far the most common coagulant used. Alkaline chemicals such as lime, caustic soda, or soda ash, used for adjusting pH during coagulation and for subsequent stabilization of the finished water product, rank second in volume used. The unique features of alum (or other coagulants) and the alkaline chemicals are probably the roots of the principal chemical feed problems found in water treatment practice today. Coagulation concepts as they apply to rapid rate filtration are discussed in Chapter 11.

Coagulation

In general, some simple but essential rules must be observed for successful coagulation and subsequent filtration to occur:

1. Sufficient coagulant must be added to either neutralize the negatively charged raw water particles, provide a hydroxide precipitate for a

sweep floc mechanism, or some combination of the two mechanisms. Some of the newer coagulant preparations, such as polyaluminum chloride and some polyelectrolytes, focus more on charge neutralization, whereas older approaches such as alum, ferric chloride, and ferric sulfate can involve either mechanism.

2. Control of pH during coagulation is extremely important. For example, many aluminum-based coagulants, such as alum, exhibit an optimum pH for turbidity removal in a region between 6.0 and 7.0. A slightly lower pH might be selected as a compromise condition that will allow somewhat higher removals of the naturally occurring organic matter that is associated with both color and the formation potential for disinfection byproducts. Similar considerations may be associated with other types of coagulants as well.
3. Proper procedures should be observed in the handling and feed of coagulant chemicals. For example, alum must not be diluted below a concentration of 1.0 percent prior to mixing in the process flow. Otherwise, its effectiveness can be reduced by preflocculation in the solution vessels. Alum is most effectively utilized when it is dispersed rapidly throughout the process water. Casual blending results in wasted alum.

Many coagulants, such as alum, ferric chloride, and ferric sulfate, are naturally acidic and can significantly reduce the pH of the process flow. The greater the dosage of these coagulants, the more the pH and alkalinity of the process water will be reduced. In situations that involve treating water with a low natural alkalinity, the consequence of alum addition might be to reduce the pH below the desired range for coagulation unless an alkalinity supplement is used. Conversely, with highly alkaline waters, an acid addition might be considered to achieve the desired pH for optimum coagulation.

Supplementary Alkalinity

Alkaline (base) chemicals are used principally to increase alkalinity during the coagulation process. Alkalinity supplements may also be used to adjust the final pH for stabilizing or reducing the corrosivity of the product water. In such cases stabilization may require a separate alkali addition step since the optimum pH for coagulation (typically 6.0 to 7.0) is often less than the pH required for stabilizing finished water.

Depending on availability, lime is often the least costly alkalinity supplement. By comparison, the cost of the alternative, caustic soda (sodium hydroxide), can be about three times that of lime in many locales. Lime has the added advantage of providing additional calcium to the product water for further corrosion protection. The presence of calcium also can have an enhancing effect on coagulation under some circumstances.

Available as a solution, caustic soda has some advantages with respect to handling. Use of caustic, however, will increase the content of sodium in the product water, which may be a disadvantage. Sodium as a constituent may be of concern because of its potential adverse impact on the health of consumers with hypertension conditions. This disadvantage is somewhat site specific and depends on the actual caustic soda additions necessary to achieve the desired results and on the amount of sodium present in the source water.

A significant problem in the use of lime arises from the clinkers or unreacted solids that remain after reaction, especially when lime is added downstream of filters for the final pH adjustment step in finished water. The unreacted solids can be carried out in the product water and may accumulate in storage tanks and pipelines. When stirred by hydraulic action in the distribution system, the unsightly solids can be evident in water drawn from the tap by the consumer. This problem does not exist when lime is used to supplement alkalinity to enhance the alum reaction in coagulation. Any untreated lime particulates will become enmeshed in the floc and will be removed in subsequent settling or filtration. However, the addition of lime downstream of filtration is difficult to avoid in many instances where the optimum pH for coagulation is lower than the desired pH in the finished water. Excess pH prior to filtration can weaken floc and create problems with excess aluminum residual as a result of dissolution reactions. Consideration should also be given to the influence of the final pH adjustment location on disinfection by chlorine and ozone, since a higher pH requires higher disinfecting doses for a given contact time.

Principal Chemical Feed Problems

The primary rules for effective alum coagulation comprise the essential aspects for successful operation of rapid filtration processes. There are, of course, additional requirements such as thorough mixing and energy input that also are important for the generation of the necessary floc characteristics. Most mixing and energy input problems that cause poor coagulation and flocculation are related to physical facility deficiencies rather than control of operation. Physical facility problems and corrections are discussed later. It is essential in operation, however, to conduct both bench-scale and full-scale tests to determine the most advantageous combinations of coagulant feed rate along with mixing and flocculation energy input.

Typical Chemical Coagulation Problems

It is practically impossible to accomplish effective alum coagulation and flocculation if any of the primary rules discussed before are severely violated or neglected. Frequently, established plant operating procedures may tend to neglect one rule while maintaining other essential conditions. There is also a tendency to "bend" the rules to avoid problems elsewhere. The principal problems are, therefore, related mostly to misplaced priorities.

Some common misplaced priority situations inherent in drinking water filtration plant operation and the problems that ensue are illustrated in the following case situations.

Case 1: Excess Alum

An excess amount of alum is added over that required for charge neutralization and hydroxide generation in order to reduce pH to the optimum range for flocculation. As a result, unreacted alum can be carried through to the finished water. Excess aluminum is undesirable for health reasons. In addition, if pH adjustment is practiced for corrosion control, postflocculation can occur in the distribution system from a reaction of excess alum and the added alkali. Such particulates can accumulate and eventually reach the consumer. To correct this situation, alum should be used in sufficient amounts to accomplish the desired neutralization and generation of the hydroxide precipitate. Instead of excess alum, addition of sulfuric or hydrochloric acid should be considered with waters of high alkalinity to achieve the optimum pH for coagulation. In all cases, pH should be maintained in the range of least aluminum solubility (typically 6 to 7) throughout the coagulation/filtration processes.

Case 2: Excess Alkalinity

To avoid the problem with lime clinkers in the final product or to avoid the use of more expensive sodium compounds to supplement alkalinity, lime is sometimes added with alum at the beginning of the process to produce and maintain the desired final pH for corrosion control. Clinkers can then be removed in settling and filtration. At the elevated pH levels that are typical of finished water, however, poor flocculation can result, which inhibits removal of particulates in settling, in filtration, or in both removal steps. Vulnerability to filter breakthrough and elevated aluminum residuals will also exist. Two-stage pH adjustment should be considered so that the pH in the first stage can be optimized for coagulation. In the second stage, which should be located downstream of filtration, pH adjustment can then be optimized for finished water goals with increased operational attention to the clinker problem. Alternatives to lime addition include the following: (1) limit the need for elevated pH in finished water by using corrosion inhibitors that are effective at a lower pH, (2) use caustic soda in place of lime as a low solid content, poststabilization pH-adjusting chemical and accept its disadvantages (i.e., cost and increased sodium), or (3) where possible, evaluate use of a substitute coagulant such as the iron salts, ferric chloride and ferrous sulfate, or polyaluminum chloride. All may work effectively above pH 7.0. Functional and economical analyses will have to be conducted to determine which is the best method for coagulation and pH control.

Case 3: Insufficient Alum
Alum is added in sufficient amount to naturally low pH waters to produce pH in the desired 6.0 to 7.0 coagulation range. The amount added is, however, insufficient for coagulation. With inadequate coagulation, poor settling and/or filtration will result, with a tendency for solids carryover and turbidity breakthrough. Where raw water colloidal color may exist, color may also be carried over into the finished water. To correct this situation, sufficient alum should be added for coagulation along with the addition of an alkaline chemical to adjust the pH to the range desired for effective coagulation and filtration. As an alternative, polyaluminum chloride or other coagulants that are normally used at lower dosage rates, requiring less alkalinity for reaction, may be used to reduce the extent of pH reduction due to coagulant addition.

Case 4: Insufficient Alkalinity
Source water alkalinity is sufficient to provide alum reaction requirements for long term dry weather flow, but intensive rainfall can produce spikes in source water color and turbidity and/or the rapid runoff that can dilute the source water alkalinity. These changes can result in insufficient natural alkalinity to complete the alum reaction. This can cause poor coagulation or postflocculation (after filtration) as the posttreatment pH-adjustment chemicals react with the unreacted alum that is carried through. It is essential in such borderline alkalinity situations that source water quality be monitored to alert the plant operating staff to supplement alkalinity in response to this condition.

Other Chemical Feed Practices

While the more critical problems experienced in chemical feed are related primarily to the addition of coagulants, other chemicals can have an effect. For example, prechlorination of incoming raw water was a common practice in the past. The general preference was to chlorinate in two steps: at the inlet to the plant and at the filter outlet. In addition to disinfection, chlorination tends to inhibit the proliferation of biological growths and, in many instances, appears to enhance coagulation. In the reaction with certain raw water organics, an oxidant such as chlorine may alter the composition in a manner that is beneficial to coagulation.

To reduce the level of disinfection byproduct (DBP) formation, many plants have discontinued prechlorination. As a consequence, some of the benefits have been lost. In some cases, the need for higher coagulant dosage has resulted. In other plants, biological growths have proliferated in filter media.

Where prechlorination cannot be employed because of the DBP potential, substitute oxidants such as potassium permanganate should be tested. In some plants, ozonation may be beneficial. While ozone equipment is relatively expensive, the multipurpose benefits that could result in reducing coagulant and postchlorine demands may make ozonation more economically attractive. At present, such consideration is more practical for larger-capacity applications because of the relative economy of scale.

Filter Media, Design, and Maintenance

The filter media is the central component of the filtration process; all other features are ancillary and are oriented to maintaining the filter media in proper condition. Proper design and maintenance of filter media are therefore essential for effective filtration. In the earlier period of development, most granular filters were fitted with sand media. Later, ground anthracite was used in place of sand. With a much lower density, anthracite could be expanded using lower backwash rates than required for sand. After World War II, both sand and anthracite were used together in dual and multiple media arrangements. In more recent times, activated carbon, with a lighter density than anthracite, has been adopted for filter media in some locations.

Physical Characteristics

Media grain size, distribution, and shape will define the size of flow passages through a filter. In general, with relatively uniformly sized media, the larger the media size, the larger the flow passages through the media. Media grain size is defined by the percentage (by weight) of media particles passing through the mesh of a particular standard sieve. Following are the two principal media size definitions:

- Effective size—The sieve size or size opening that will permit 10 percent by weight of a sample of media to pass through

- Uniformity coefficient—The ratio of sieve sizes that will permit passage of 60 percent (by weight) and 10 percent (by weight) of a media sample, respectively

A high uniformity coefficient indicates media with a broad range of grain sizes, whereas a low uniformity coefficient indicates media of more uniform size. The ideal uniformity coefficient of 1.0, though impossible to accomplish, would indicate media with all grains of the same size.

Media may also be classified as rough, like crushed anthracite, to smooth, like river and sea sand. A smaller effective-sized round media must be used to achieve the same solids separation as achieved in rough-shaped media. However, the head loss of flow through rough-shaped media is greater than that for a similar-sized smooth-grain alternative.

Over time, filter media is subject to wear due principally to the hydraulic agitation produced in backwash. Some controversy exists over the importance of such wear. The media photographs discussed later in reviewing certain case histories, however, definitely show rounding off of rough grains where media is left in place for extended periods of time.

Friability is the measure of the relative crushability of a particular granular material and is an indication of its durability. It is important to note that two somewhat different measures are applied for assessing particle durability. Hardness is the more common measure and is used as an indication of the resistance of a surface to abrasion. Friability, on the other hand, is a measure of the susceptibility of a material to fracture and breakage. While many materials with good hardness properties are not friable, some hard materials can be brittle and subject to breakage. It is, therefore, important to consider measures of both types of characteristics. The relative friability of materials used for filter media is as follows:

- Garnet sand—hardest, least friable
- Sand—hard, resistant to wear
- Anthracite—softer, vulnerable to both wear and fracture
- Activated carbon—softest, least resistant to wear and fracture

Wear of media may not only round off the shape of the grains (concern for hardness), but may also break down the grains into smaller-sized particles (concern for friability). A particularly vulnerable situation exists where sand is used in combination with activated carbon media. With sufficient mix at the interface, the hard sand can break down the softer activated carbon. As a consequence, the activated carbon selected for this type of application should have reasonably low friability or this dual media arrangement should be avoided. The potential for wear in the intermix also exists where sand and anthracite are used in a dual media arrangement, but to a lesser extent. It would also be important to use an anthracite media with a low friability with this arrangement.

Where multiple media is used, the size and density features of the media are important to avoid wear. This relationship should be such that the extent or depth of mix at the interface is minimized. For the most part, this is influenced more by the uniformity coefficient (discussed below) and the percentage of fines in the sand media.

Filtration Process Influences

Filter media serve not only to remove or separate solids, but also to store the separated solids until backwash is required. The essential feature of filter design is the selection of a media arrangement with the effective size and uniformity coefficient features that will promote effective solids separation and, at the same time, provide sufficient particulate storage to permit reasonable operating periods between backwashings. Effective size and uniformity coefficients will also influence the separation of media during the backwash cycle.

Uniformity Influence

In the evaluation of the performance of single media filters or the performance of individual layers in multiple media arrangements, the uniformity coefficient is critical. A high uniformity coefficient may adversely affect media separation and storage as well as media wear. The higher proportion of finer grains in such media will fill in the media interstices and reduce overall porosity. Where a significant amount of media fines migrate to the top of the layer due to backwashing action, more solids will be intercepted at this layer, thereby preventing filtration with depth. With this condition, the full depth of the media cannot be effectively used for either particulate separation or storage. Shorter filter runs and a greater tendency for turbidity breakthrough are consequences of this type of condition.

In backwash expansion of filter media, the smaller-sized grains expand more or rise higher than the larger-sized portion at a fixed backwash upflow rate. Where the dual media arrangement (anthracite over sand) is employed, sand grains that are too small may rise into the anthracite layer above. These smaller grains will fill between anthracite voids and reduce porosity. The sand grains also may abrade and wear down the softer anthracite during backwashing. This wear action will further reduce the anthracite porosity and the attendant solids storage capability.

The uniformity coefficient of media installed in a filter is basically controlled by specification and cost. A reputable supplier will furnish media with the uniformity coefficient required. The lower the uniformity coefficient, however, the more media must be wasted in sieving procedures by the supplier. Hence, the cost will be higher.

The uniformity coefficient may be improved significantly beyond that originally supplied by skimming the top layer during installation. In this procedure, usually a 10 percent excess of media (by depth) is installed. The installed layer is then subjected to a number of successive backwash operations to both clean and stratify the media. After slowly reducing the backwash rate to allow a stratification in which the fines rise to the top, the filter is drained, and the finer media is skimmed from the surface to produce the depth required. In many situations, skimming the fines can produce the desired uniformity coefficient at a lower cost than sieving by the supplier. With the more sophisticated filter operation used today, uniformity coefficients as low 1.3 can be attained, but cost is often a consideration. A decision must be made for the needs of each particular situation.

Effective Size

As mentioned, selection of the proper effective-sized media is probably the most critical step in the design of dual or multiple media arrangements. With dual and multiple media, the relative sizes of the different media layers will influence the intermix that occurs during backwashing. The media selected for the different layers should have similar expansion characteristics for the same backwash rates to minimize intermixing. For some media, it is especially important that the lower, finer-sized media layers do not expand significantly into the upper, coarse layer to reduce porosity and cause abrasion. Therefore, effective sizes for these media layers must be compatible and cannot be selected independently. In part, the abrasion problem results from the fact that the friability of anthracite is not always specified, leaving it susceptible to abrasion if an anthracite with high friability is supplied. This problem can be reduced by specifying friability. Some proprietary mixed media preparations work well with intermixing, presumably with a sufficiently durable anthracite layer.

There is little research that will permit selection with confidence of different layers of media with matching backwash expansion characteristics. For some time, the standard anthracite/sand dual media has consisted of an anthracite-sand combination with effective sizes of approximately 1.0 mm and 0.5 mm, respectively. This combination has enough intermix problems in dual and multiple media installations to suggest that it might not be suitable. Recently some have had better success with an anthracite/sand combination of 0.85 mm and 0.50 mm, respectively. This tends to compensate for variations in density of anthracite that can be encountered and ensures good separation during backwash expansion.

While this media can work well for many applications, the smaller anthracite may blind with appreciable algae content and a slight increase in both anthracite and sand sizes may be considered. Skimming off the fines becomes more important with the finer anthracite.

For decades, single media with effective sizes ranging from 0.45 to 0.70 mm provided successful filter performance for media up to 30 inches in depth. In more recent times, single media with an effective size from around 1.0 to 2.0 mm and sometimes larger have been advantageously applied in deep bed arrangements (48 inches or more) in many drinking water filter installations. Where activated carbon media has been used in deep bed arrangements, effective sizes of up to 1.25 mm have worked well depending on the particular solids removal requirements.

Choice of the type and size of media to use for a particular filter installation will be limited by both the solids removal and the backwash rate requirements. For similar media expansion rates, larger media, as well as more dense media, will require higher backwash rates. It may not be practical, therefore, to use sand media of 1.0 mm in a deep bed filter arrangement that relies on hydraulic backwash. Backwash rates required to attain 30 percent expansion would be over 30 gpm/sf. Lighter anthracite and activated carbon media might be considered for these larger media sized applications. Alternatively, air/water backwash approaches that do not require full bed expansion can be considered.

Media Case Histories

Samples of filter media obtained from suppliers and from operating filter plants help to illustrate some of the common and uncommon problems encountered in filter plants. All of the operating plant samples evaluated in case history reviews were skimmed from the top surface of the filters. In the illustrations, existing media is shown alongside samples of new media of the type and size originally specified.

Improper Size

A basic problem in many granular filter installations is incorrectly sized media where the media from the supplier simply does not meet specification. Figure 12–1 is an enlargement of two samples of sand media. The specification for both samples of sand called for an effective size of 0.45 mm. It is obvious that the grain size of the sand media actually supplied on the right is noticeably larger. The same is true of the two anthracite media samples shown in Figure 12–2. Specifications for both samples called for an effective size of 1.0. Again, the grain size of the media installed (center) is noticeably larger. In both figures the samples with the smaller-sized grains of each pair are closest to that specified.

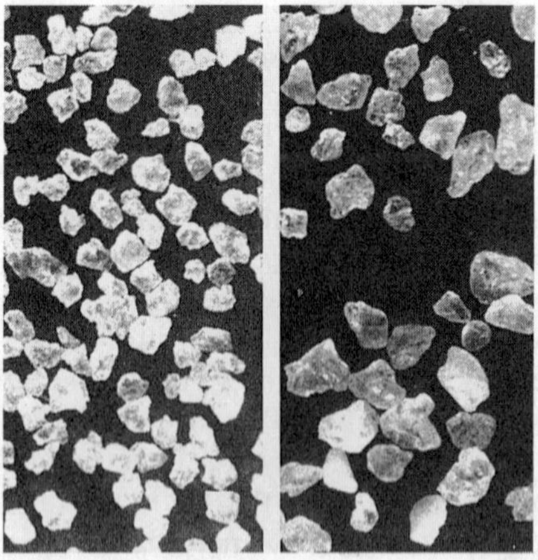

FIGURE 12–1. Comparison of two samples of new sand media. (From Ref. 3. Reprinted from *Public Works Magazine* (June 1988), by permission.)

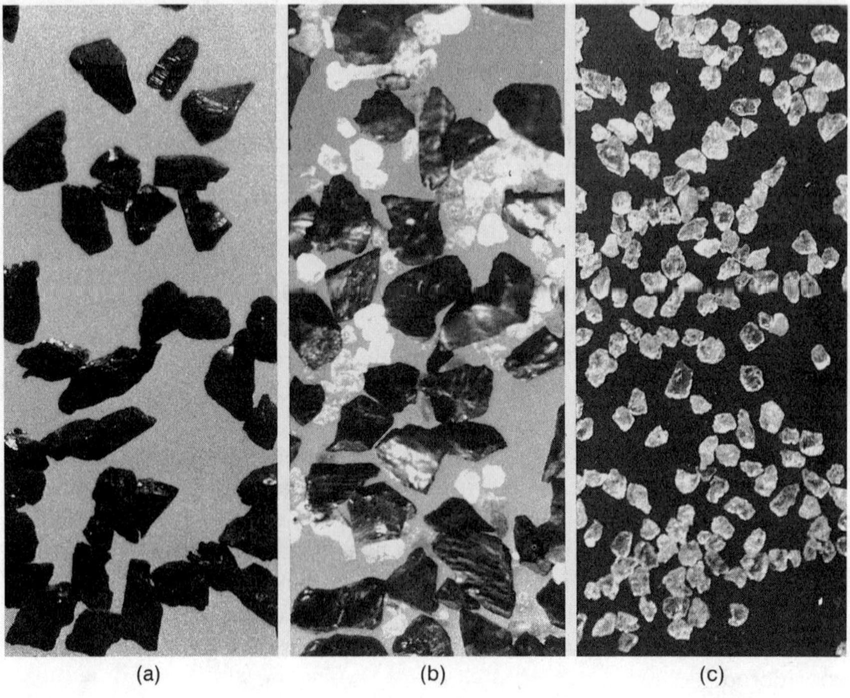

FIGURE 12–2. Poor anthracite-sand media match: (a) effective size—1.0 mm; (b) filter sample; (c) effective size—0.45 mm. (From Ref. 3. Reprinted from *Public Works Magazine* (June 1988), by permission.)

Poor Dual Media Match

Installation of correct media size, discussed above, is especially critical in dual media or multimedia arrangements. In backwashing, the media is expanded. As discussed before, if the different media do not expand at close to the same rate in backwashing, it is possible for the media to mix. The hard silica sand can wear down the friable anthracite material, and the small sand grains may fill in a significant layer of voids in the anthracite strata. This will tend to reduce the solids storage capacity of the anthracite media and reduce the length of filter runs.

The center panel of Figure 12–2 shows media skimmed from the top of a dual media filter. This media had been in place for about a year. As shown, sand from the lower 10-inch layer penetrated completely through the 20 inches of anthracite due to the backwashing action. The media shown on either side show the approximate size of the sand and anthracite media that should have been furnished. It appears that the sand size is close to specification. The anthracite media size is, however, noticeably larger. If this is the case, the anthracite expansion during backwash would be less than intended, permitting sand with a higher rate of expansion to rise through the top layer of media.

Another cause of excessive media mixing would be too high a uniformity coefficient for the lower sand layer. A high uniformity coefficient will indicate a higher percentage of finer-sized media grains. The finer fraction of sand media will rise highest when the bed is expanded with a consistent upflow rate.

Slime Growth/Single Media Wear

In many filter plants, halting the practice of prechlorination to reduce the trihalomethane formation potential has created new problems. Slime growths previously inhibited by chlorine will proliferate in the media. Progressive slime growth ultimately clogs media and prevents effective filtration. At such time, it is necessary to remove the filter from service to clean away the growths in place by means of superchlorination or caustic washing. The filters are filled with superchlorinated or caustic solutions on a batch basis. After sufficient time has elapsed to permit destruction and separation of the slime coating, the filter is backwashed several times before returning to service. Improved filter wash procedures also should be considered for this type of filter operation; either improved surface wash or conversion to air scour methods to improve agitation could be considered.

The left panel of Figure 12–3 shows sand media that has been slime coated for a period of several months. This particular sample was

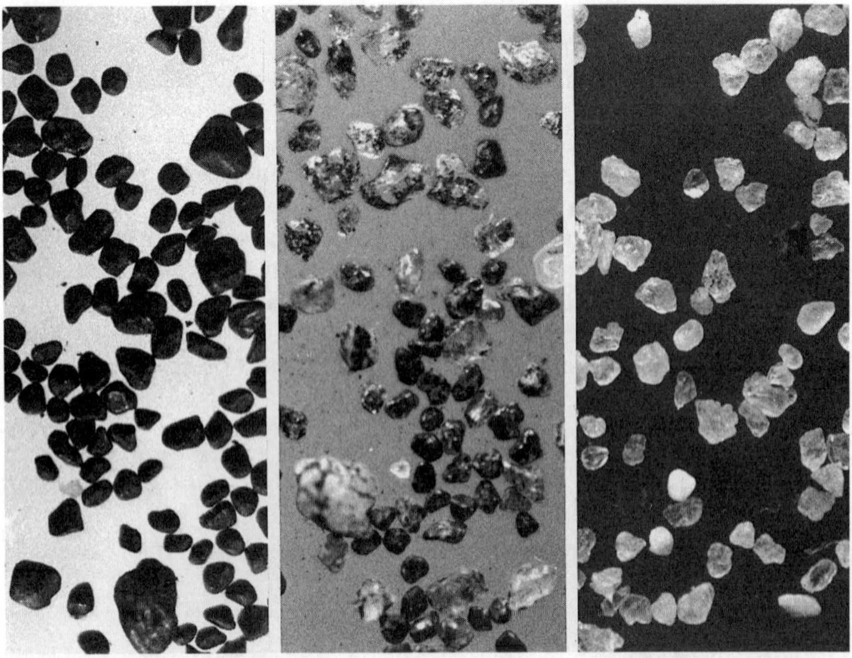

(a) (b) (c)

FIGURE 12–3. Example of slime-coated media before and after caustic cleaning: (a) filter sample; (b) caustic cleaned; (c) new media. (From Ref. 3. Reprinted from *Public Works Magazine* (June 1988), by permission.)

skimmed from the top of a single media filter. The right panel of the figure shows the media as first installed; the center panel shows the media sample after caustic cleaning. It is obvious that the cleaning process is very effective. The slime growth has been almost completely removed. Just a little staining remains on the sand media after cleaning.

The caustic-cleaned sand media in Figure 12–3 exhibits another somewhat common filter problem. This particular media was first installed more than 10 years ago. In this somewhat long period of service, the media was topped off from time to time with additional media to replace that lost in backwashing. Comparison with the new media on the right shows the over-10-year-old media to be somewhat worn. No sharp edges remain. In addition, there are a significant number of larger-sized media grains in the cleaned sample. Over the years, the finer fraction of sand has been washed out so that the effective size of the media bed has increased.

Since the sample has been skimmed from the top of the bed, it may be expected that the lower media exhibits an even higher effective size. This media bed probably should have been replaced after about 7 years of use.

Caked Media/Anthracite Media Breakdown

The left panel of Figure 12–4 shows a magnification of a sample taken from the top surface of a dual media filter. This media has been in continuous service for almost 20 years. At first glance, the sample exhibits characteristics of media that has remained too long in service. Compared to the new anthracite media to the right, the media sample grains appear to have rounded or worn edges and the uniformity coefficient is obviously high. The grain size spread (smallest to largest) must be considered to be unusual.

The caustic-cleaned media in the center panel discloses an entirely different story. The largest-sized grain particles are anthracite; the

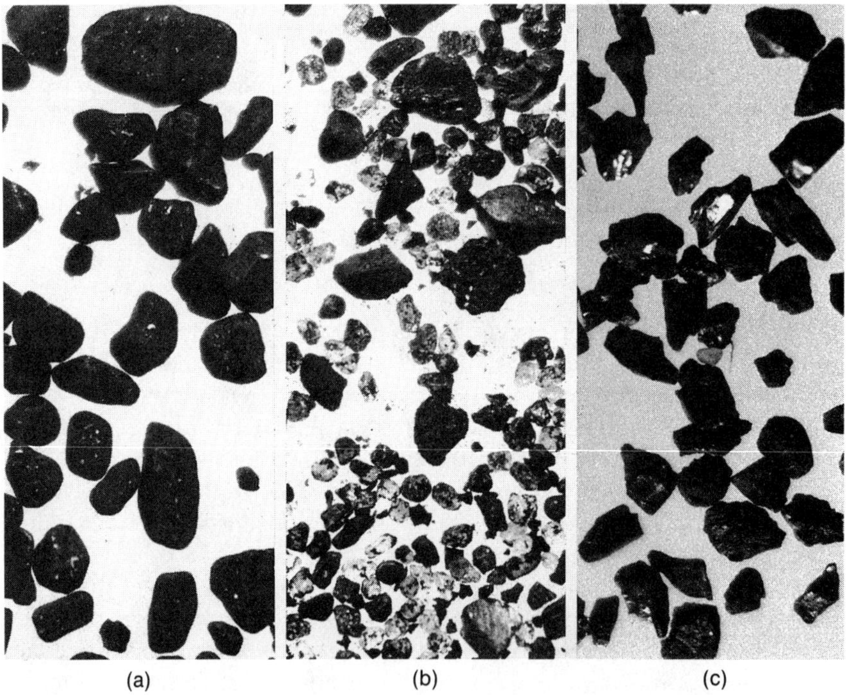

FIGURE 12–4. Caked media showing anthracite breakdown: (a) filter sample; (b) caustic cleaned; (c) new anthracite. (From Ref. 3. Reprinted from *Public Works Magazine* (June 1988), by permission.)

smaller grains are mostly sand. Moreover, a significant amount of dust-sized matter is evident. The media probably reached this condition over the years due to several parallel actions:

- Due to a poor size match, sand expanded into the anthracite layer and progressively broke down the anthracite grains.
- Inadequate backwashing resulted in caking of the media grains.
- Alum floc coalesced the worn media into larger-sized particles.
- Powdered carbon, used frequently in this plant, was also mixed and blended into the coalesced media particles.

The uniformity coefficient of the coalesced anthracite-sand-powdered carbon media increased to a point where effective filter performance must be doubtful at best. On the other hand, if this media were to be caustic-cleaned in place, a significant portion of media would be flushed out after the first backwash. Cleaning would literally have destroyed the media bed.

Figure 12–4 illustrates an unusual combination of media problems. In this case, the media caking tended to extend the media life. In more typical circumstances, media caking, caused by inadequate backwashing, starts with individual media grains, but eventually develops into mud-balls or caked areas of the filter. In most instances, the mud balls and caked areas will accumulate below the top surface of the filter bed so that the condition can go unnoticed for long periods of time. In short, the need for adequate filter washing to maintain the condition of filter media cannot be overemphasized.

Filter-Operating Deficiencies

Relative filter operation performance is measured in terms of product water quality and length of filter runs between backwashing. Practically all filtration of drinking water is accomplished on a batch-type basis. Solids are removed from the flow and stored in the filter media until clogging increases the hydraulic head loss to the maximum available or until the storage ability of the media is exceeded and the accumulated particulates begin to break through. Solids breakthrough has traditionally been defined as a rise in product turbidity above a target level. The filter must be cleaned or backwashed when one of these conditions occurs, thereby permitting start of another batch run. In a properly performing filter, maximum head loss is attained before breakthrough occurs, as shown in Figure 12–5. In fact, where breakthrough occurs prior to maximum head loss, a problem may be indicated. Frequently, this can result from inadequate chemical conditioning in the coagulation process.

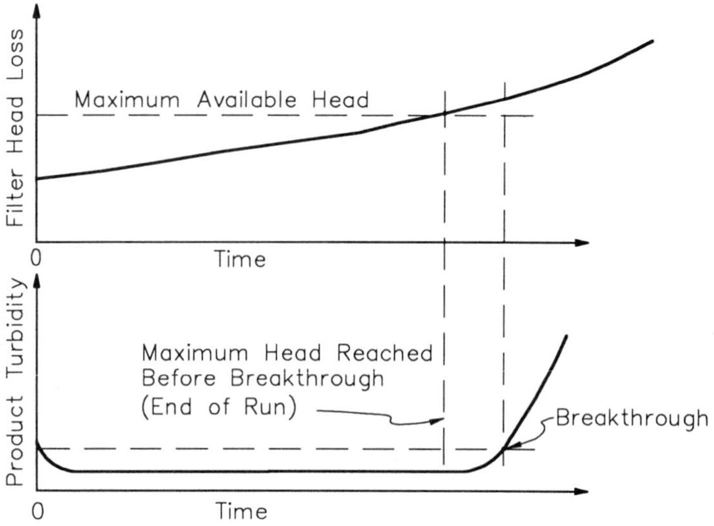

FIGURE 12–5. Head loss and turbidity breakthrough vs. time in ideal filter. (From Ref. 1. Reprinted by permission of International Ozone Association.)

In addition to the coagulation features discussed above, aspects of filtration that may be controlled in operation include the following:

- Rate of flow to the filter (except for declining rate filters)
- Backwash rate of flow
- Method and degree of media cleaning by either hydraulic or air scouring methods
- Extent of time for both the backwash and scouring (air or hydraulic wash) cycles
- Transition procedures between the backwash and the filtration modes (discussed in Chapter 11)
- Length of run

Instrumentation that should be provided to individual filters to monitor effective operation includes measurement of rate of flow and loss of head along with continuous monitoring turbidimeters to indicate variations in effluent turbidity.

A significant design-related problem that can occur in many plants is the air binding of filter media. This condition occurs at localized points of flow restriction or high head loss in beds that are not designed or operated with an adequate depth of submergence. High velocity of flow created by the restrictions create negative head conditions or a vacuum at these locations. The vacuum then causes gases to be drawn out of solution, which accumulate in the media, causing a blinding condition that disrupts the filtration process. This problem is a common design-related consideration, and is discussed in Reference 4, as well as other general water and wastewater design texts.

Other air-related problems can occur if air enters backwash piping by being drawn into the pump suction or through faulty pipe joints. This can cause sudden increases in turbulence during backwash, resulting in disruption of gravel layers and loss of media. Design and operation of backwash systems should incorporate features to minimize this type of problem.

The principal media problems that develop in filter plants are due to improper operation procedures or poor habits related to the condition of the media. Mud-balls or media caking can exist that may not be noticeable to the operator even though the surface of the media may be exposed in backwashing. This condition develops slowly as media grains are coated or as large volumes of media are literally cemented together by the gelatinous hydroxides produced in coagulation.

A secondary, although important problem, may develop where the filter backwash is not adjusted for changes in water temperature to compensate for the differences in the resulting water viscosity. This latter situation, discussed below, may be particularly critical where process water temperatures can vary from 80°F down to or close to freezing.

Backwash Adequacy

Adequate cleaning during backwash is imperative to maintain media condition. The reversed backwash upflow must expand the media sufficiently and should provide enough flow to flush out the collected particulate solids. After the media is sufficiently expanded, a declining rate of backwash flow should be used to stratify the media into relative grades of finer to larger grains, top to bottom.

Except for ungraded filters such as some of the monomedia—deep bed type—the quantity of water required to properly expand and stratify a media bed backwash generally dictates the upper limits of backwash flow rates. In fact, too high backwash flow rates can reduce the opportunity for particle interactions, thereby reducing the cleaning effect. Experience has shown that, with few exceptions, supplementary scouring action is necessary to ensure adequate scrubbing during backwash. Such supplementary action may be achieved by air scour or hydraulic surface wash methods. Although air scour alternatives should be considered for use in new filter design, hydraulic surface wash units using rotating arms with nozzles attached to a rotating pipe are the most common units encountered in older filters. These devices direct flow outward and downward, first against the drained surface of quiescent media, then through the media expanded by the backwash flow. The jet action of the nozzles causes the surface wash unit to rotate.

Other hydraulic backwash devices include fixed jet systems that do not rotate. While less common, fixed jet systems may provide superior performance for interface wash in dual media filters. Such systems can be activated without full fluidization of a dual media filter, allowing a high degree of particle interaction. Conversely, rotating arm systems require full fluidization for providing subsurface scour at the dual media interface.

Where filter bottoms are replaced in existing plants, it would be possible to install bottoms equipped to furnish an air scour as an alternative to surface wash. This method of supplementary media scour will permit modifying the media wash sequence where scour occurs at a relatively low backwash rate followed by a period of higher upflow to both remove loosened particles and then a gradually reduced rate to restratify the media. An alternative to underdrain replacement is systems that place the air piping in the gravel layer.

Media condition deteriorates when the alum floc is not thoroughly removed because of insufficient agitation provided by the backwash flow and the supplementary surface or air scour action. Depending on the type and extent of deficiency, the following can occur:

- Caking of individual media particles resulting in enlarged media size and a change from a characteristic sharp-edged form to a more rounded shape.
- Formation of mud-balls where media and attached floc will tend to agglomerate
- Caking of media, where large areas of the media will literally cement in sheet form

The most severe consequence of the mud-ball and caked media conditions are restricted flow area for both filtration and backwash cycles. With more concentrated flow through limited filter surface area, negative head conditions can be generated during filtration to release air and bind the filter. Concentrated flows will also occur during backwash, causing volcanoes where the media erupts. The general result is a no-win situation. Backwash flows must then be reduced, which only compounds the problem, resulting in further media deterioration. Negative head and erupted media will require a reduction in the filter application rate. In severe cases, with considerable caked areas, media may be carried over to waste, even at reduced backwash rates.

Media Restoration

To resolve filter problems, it is important to ascertain first whether the basic causes are improper operating routines or inadequate facilities. Caked media may be restored by filling the filter with caustic solution of sufficient concentration (less than 20 percent to protect concrete) to dissolve the entrained and attached aluminum hydroxide. Sometimes it helps to agitate the media with an air wand to facilitate more complete dissolving. A wand can be made of a length of 1-inch-diameter copper pipe, sealed at one end as shown in Figure 12–6. Spaced holes 1/16 to 1/8 inches in size are drilled in the sides of the pipe to the depth of the granular media. Compressed air is supplied by hose to the open end of the pipe as it is moved through the media. After the hydroxide has been consumed in reactions, the spent caustic can be drained to waste. Care must be exercised during this procedure to avoid disturbing the gravel support layer.

Where caking is not severe, or is restricted to dead areas not covered by rotating surface wash units, use of the air wand on a routine basis may help to maintain adequate media condition. After the media is restored to its original condition as much as possible, tests may be conducted to determine whether conventional backwash rates of 12 to 18 gpm/sf can be used. It also will be important to know whether surface or air scour flows

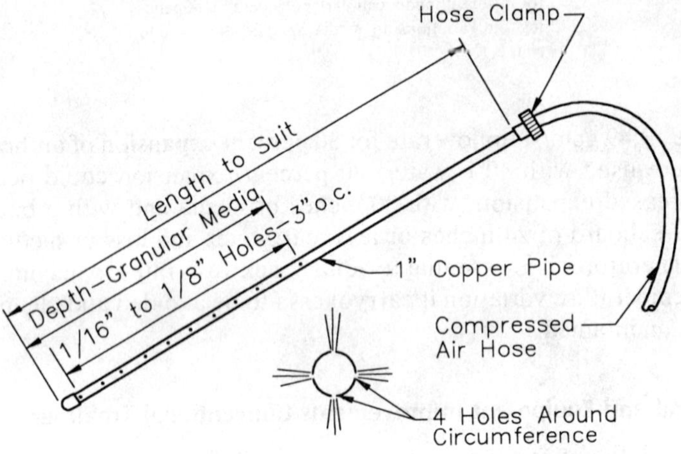

FIGURE 12–6. Air wand details.

are adequate. If media carryover occurs with clean media conditions or if caking of media continues to develop despite adequate backwash rates, the basic problem can be attributed to the media or to erratic backwash facilities. Adequate clearance between the top of the expanded media and bottom of troughs should also be checked.

Cold Water Operations

In many plants, severe problems will exist because adjustments are not made for cold water operating conditions. Water at 40°F is more dense and has a higher viscosity than water at 70°F. Media particles, therefore, may be expanded to the same extent using lower upflow rates at lower backwash water temperatures. The upflow rate required for 30 percent expansion of single media sand and anthracite media (both 0.60 mm in size) would be approximately as follows for different water temperatures:

Water Temperature (°F)	Upflow Rate[a] (gpm/sf)	
	Sand	Anthracite
40	11.73	7.58
50	14.77	9.55
60	17.82	11.52
70	20.86	13.49

[a] Example to show relative rates. The upflow rates for different media can vary considerably depending on variations in media specific gravity and shape.

If the 13.49 gpm/sf upflow rate for 30 percent expansion of anthracite at 70°F were used with 40°F water, 80 percent expansion could occur. At this increased expansion, with 30 inches of media and with a backwash trough freeboard of 24 inches or less, carryover and loss of media could occur. Therefore, it is essential to adjust backwash rates to accommodate water temperature variation if carryover is to be avoided and clean media is to be maintained.

Structural and Equipment Improvements/Conventional Treatment

Until a relatively few years ago, the so-called conventional treatment train was almost the universal arrangement for granular filtration of drinking water. The conventional process arrangement comprises two stages of solids removal (settling and filtration) with separate facilities for each step of process. In most such plants, pretreatment chemicals are added at a single point—usually in the mixing basin at the head of the plant. Most of the state standards of 25 years ago for drinking water treatment included conventional treatment design criteria similar to the following:

Chemical mixing: 30 sec detention
Flocculation: 45 min detention
Settling: 4 hr detention
Filter rate: 2 to 3 gpm/sf
Chlorination: 30 min detention

The standards also included other design details, such as the length-to-width ratios in settling tanks, the type and depth of filter media, and other structural and mechanical features. An almost universal standard for filter media, for instance, was 30 inches of single media, sand or anthracite. These standards greatly influenced the size of the principal components. Several of the process units designed under today's regulations could have, perhaps, half or less than half the volumes or areas required for component design under the older standards. This size factor can influence or produce the problems in many older-design water treatment plants.

It is likely that the supposedly conservative design standards of 25 years ago were promulgated to compensate for the possibility of less vigilant staff operating procedures that developed during a time when no nationwide drinking water standards existed. At the time, it seemed natural to assume that more complete chemical mixing or more complete settling would occur with greater detention in the respective chambers or basins. In fact, however, the emphasis on larger-sized basins resulting from such standards produced less attention to many of the features that actually cause short circuiting of flow. Short circuiting can occur where flow concentrated in a pipe or channel is released to the expanded or open volume of tanks or basins, or where flow exiting from such volume passes over or through restricted passages. High-velocity currents in which most of the flow is condensed or concentrated are established. Short circuiting may also be caused by the density currents generated by temperature stratification in large basins. Not only will short circuiting reduce detention and its fundamental benefits, but the uneven flow patterns that are established tend to diminish the ability of mixing and settling basins to perform as intended.

The net result of short circuiting is a solids carryover that can overload filters, shorten filter runs, and increase breakthrough of turbidity. It is possible that many of the short circuiting and other problems in older design plants can be corrected with somewhat simple, inexpensive additions or alterations that control inlet and outlet conditions as well as flow patterns through the basins.

Flash Mixing

The more common flash mixers found in water treatment plants are concrete tanks, square in horizontal cross section, usually fitted with vertical shaft impellers. The primary purpose of flash mixing is to thoroughly disperse chemicals in the incoming water flow for reaction. In some instances, granular or powdered materials like clay and activated carbon are added for physical-chemical actions. Since most chemical reactions in flash mixing are instantaneous, flash mixing is deficient when the chemicals added are not thoroughly contacted with the incoming water flow within the mixing chamber.

Three important features of flash mixer design are as follows:

- Circulation capacity
- Point of chemical introduction
- Detention time

Since the chemical reactions associated with alum are practically instantaneous, detention time is important only because, with circulation of flow in the chamber, opportunity is offered for more thorough mixing of the chemical or chemicals. Low detention time is not a usual problem in most flash mixer installations unless a plant capacity has been uprated significantly without addition to this part of the process line. Most problems exist because the chemicals are introduced at locations where thorough dispersion in the water flow is not possible. This problem is further aggravated when the mixer does not have sufficient horsepower or the impeller does not have the characteristics necessary to maintain reasonable recirculation within the flash mix chamber.

Figure 12–7 shows the recirculation patterns in mix chambers fitted with propeller and straight-bladed impeller, each with and without vertical baffles. The flow patterns shown in this figure indicate that improvement in circulation in general and chemical dispersion in particular could result with the following:

- Addition of baffles
- Moving chemical injection as close to the eye of the impeller as possible

When measures to improve an existing flash mixer chamber action are considered, these two somewhat simple changes should first be made. Change in impeller arrangement can also improve mixing action. As

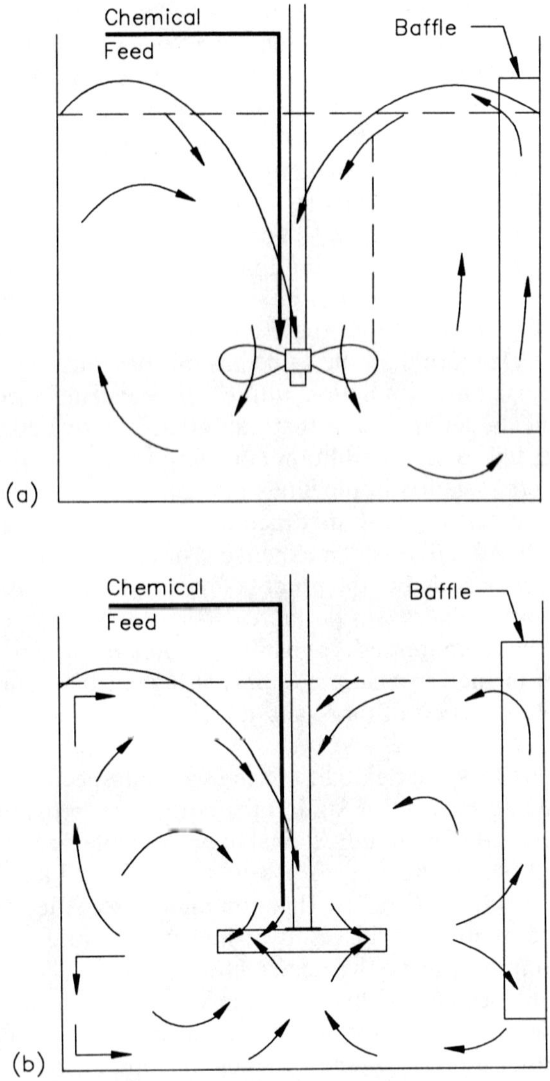

FIGURE 12–7. Circulation patterns in flash mix chambers with and without baffles. (From Ref. 2. Reprinted from *Public Works Magazine* (July/Aug. 1987), by permission.)

shown in Figure 12–7, a change from propeller to an alternative type of impeller might improve mixing action. The straight-bladed impeller shown here tends to intensify mixing in comparison to the smoother, more regular circulation pattern of the axial-flow propeller. If the available horsepower of an existing flash mixer is not totally used by a single impeller, the addition of a second impeller to the shaft may be considered. Double impellers are usually more advantageous where the water depth–to–width or –diameter ratio is 2 : 1 or more.

Where major alteration or addition to existing flash mix facilities is required, a series arrangement of mixing chambers should be considered. It is generally recognized that the effective detention time of two mixer basins in series is more than the same basins operating in parallel. Where polymers are used in conjunction with other coagulants, sequential addition of chemicals, an approach that can often improve coagulation, can easily be adapted to series addition configurations.

Static mixers installed in pipelines may also be considered to supplement or replace existing flash mix facilities. In-line static mixer additions are particularly effective and inexpensive in applications where certain chemicals must be added to the process flow in sequence. Experience has shown that static mixers can be more efficient than flash mix chambers because of the compressed, dynamic mixing environment provided. Static mixers in the same service apply a higher mixing intensity or G factor for a short period of time, and the emphasis is on rapid dispersion of chemical.

Static mixers lack the flexibility of the variable speed mechanical mixers. Since mixing energy for static mixers must be provided by the hydraulic flow rate, the minimum allowable or available hydraulic flow must be considered before electing to use a static mixer. Inadequate mixing would result if flow falls below this minimum rate. Adequate and more than adequate mixing would result at higher flow rates, but additional energy is required to drive the higher flow at a higher head loss through the fixed mixer. Because of this hydraulic head requirement, static mixers are generally more suitable for installation in existing plant inlet and outlet works where more head may be available for operation.

Other mixing devices can be considered for new installations. These include turbine mix devices placed across a narrow opening, in-line mechanical mixers placed in pipelines, and pump injection mixers that use multiple nozzle arrangements to inject the coagulant into a process stream. Each of these approaches deviates from the older concept of providing contact time during mixing; the focus of these alternatives is instantaneous dispersion. Each approach has advantages and disadvantages that need to be evaluated for the particular application.

Flocculation

Following are the two most common problems with flocculation facilities in existing water plants:

- Short circuiting of the process flow through flocculator basins
- Lack of flexibility in energy input applied by mechanical paddles or agitators

The average of 30 to 45 minutes of nominal detention time provided in most filtration plants is usually adequate for flocculation. Short circuiting, however, will reduce the time available for floc formation and the opportunity for floc conditioning. The energy applied by the moving paddles enhances floc contact for buildup in particle size and helps to densify the built-up floc.

In trouble-shooting or endeavoring to improve treatment plant flocculation conditions, the first emphasis must be on the elimination or reduction of short circuiting. There are many causes of short circuiting in flocculation basins. Most depend on the type of equipment and baffles installed. In general, the worst operation situations exist where flow through the basin is longitudinal, parallel to the axis of the paddle drive shaft—usually where end-around baffles have been installed. Openings must be provided through the baffles for the flocculator drive shaft. Since water flow driven by the head differential (inlet to outlet) usually seeks the most direct path, flow in these basins is substantially along the axis of the drive shafts, passing through the openings in the baffles. Figure 12–8 shows how such a short-circuiting condition was successfully corrected. The wood baffles were extended to separate the flocculator into three individual sections. Circular steel baffles were attached to the flocculator drive shaft on each side of the fixed wood baffles. The shaft openings were enlarged. As can be seen in this figure, the former short circuiting was eliminated by the changes in flow direction imposed by the new rotating baffles.

In general, flocculation chambers should be arranged in series for best performance. To inhibit short circuiting, baffling or the flow path provided from inlet to outlet should result in a mazelike pattern to force radical changes in flow direction. Flow movement should fill as much of the volume of the flocculation basin as possible. Flocculation flow patterns may involve art more than science, where baffle or flow improvements for each situation must be developed on a rational basis.

Floc condition may also be enhanced where energy input is tapered from high to low from inlet to outlet. In the three-section flocculator shown in Figure 12–8, the highest energy would be applied by paddles in the first compartment and decreased in the subsequent two steps. This

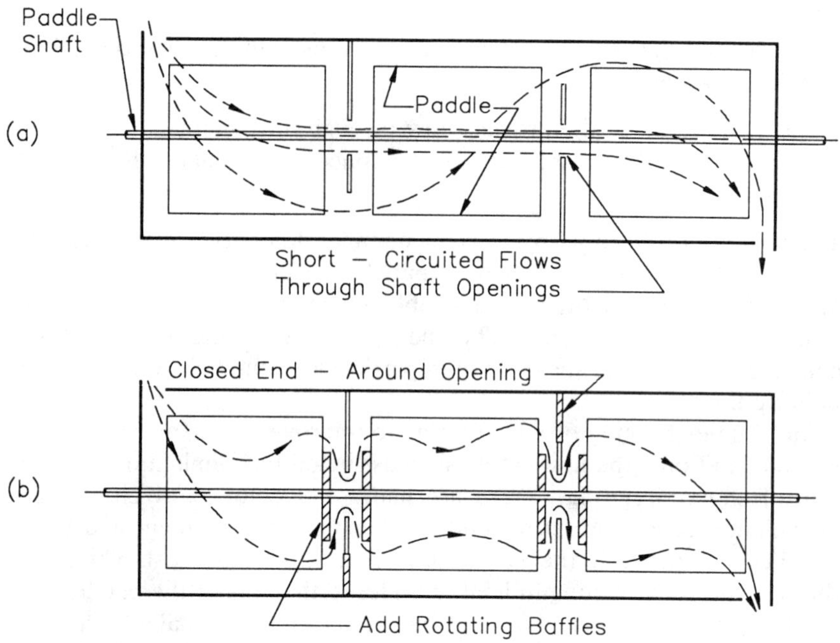

FIGURE 12–8. Flocculator modifications correct short circuiting. (From Ref. 2. Reprinted from *Public Works Magazine* (July/Aug. 1987), by permission.)

provides a high energy to initially form floc in the first compartment, followed by energy inputs in subsequent compartments that are decreased to avoid shear of floc as it grows in size. In this particular situation, where a single drive shaft serves all three compartments, energy can be varied only by the surface area provided by the paddles. More energy is imparted where the paddle area is greatest. Where separate drives are available, energy input can be varied by adjusting speed of paddle rotation in each compartment.

Two common problems experienced with flocculator drives are horizontal shafts with leaking stuffing boxes where shafts pass through tank walls and worn sheaves on variable speed drives. Flocculator drives are most often installed in enclosed, below-ground chambers, where they are unfortunately "out of sight, out of mind." Stuffing box leaks may be repaired with replacement of glands or with the use of improved packing material. Adjustable-speed drives that use tapered sheaves or pulleys, with a belt connection between motor and output shaft, tend to wear prematurely unless the position of the pulleys is changed from time to time. Left in a fixed position, the belt edges will tend to wear grooves in the pulleys. This situation is also aggravated if belts and pulleys are not cleaned on a regular basis.

Where flocculator equipment must be replaced, consideration should be given to vertical units where all drives and gears are located above the water level. The fact that the mechanical units are visible and have easy access from the top of the tanks ensures improved maintenance. In side-by-side installations, the vertical shaft, variable speed flocculator units have been shown to outperform the horizontal shaft alternatives in most cases.

Sedimentation

Short circuiting of through-flow is the basic cause of inadequate solids removal performance in most older, large volume settling tank systems in operation today. Short circuiting results from a combination of design faults, including uneven distribution of inlet flow, the length to width ratios, unusually large basin volume, and inadequate effluent weirs or launders in terms of length and surface area of the tank.

While the calculated average detention time in many of the old-design basins is on the order of 4 hours, short circuiting will reduce actual detention of a considerable portion of the water flow to significantly less than half this time. Short circuiting generally produces carryover of floc that will reduce the length of run (time) of the filters that follow. This reduction in filter run is probably caused more by the character of the floc than by the additional solids load imposed.

A well-performing settling system should remove 85 to 90 percent or more of the particulate solids in the entering flow. If actual removals are less than 85 percent, poor control or distribution of flow probably exists. With lack of good flow control or distribution, settling basin operation can be very sensitive. The least change in conditions such as water temperature or the solids concentration in the inlet flow can cause erratic behavior where surges can result in carryover.

The larger volume and surface areas of the older-design tanks will offer opportunity for partial improvement measures. In order of priority of benefits that may result, the following are the principal partial improvement or alteration measures that may be considered:

- Retrofit of a new effluent collector launder system
- Structural modification of the existing settling tank inlet arrangement and/or the addition of baffles to accomplish more even distribution
- Installation of baffles in the body of the basin, between inlet and outlet, to inhibit short circuiting or to redistribute the flow

The principal difficulty with structural modifications to improve performance of larger-sized basins is the fact that any extensive addition of baffles or dividing walls to help control flow direction can interfere with the sludge removal operations.

There is no question that well-designed effluent modifications will accomplish the most improvement in solids removal performance for the cost. Figure 12–9 shows a relatively inexpensive launder system design. Borrowing from the technology developed for high-rate solids contact clarifiers, this arrangement uses plastic pipe 6 to 10 inches in diameter. Orifice openings are drilled in the bottom at a spacing to ensure uniform collection of flow along the length of each launder. The pipe launders are connected to the end-of-tank effluent channel system. The most costly portion of this type of installation will be the structural support to hold the launders. Many older tanks have a strut and walkway system between sidewalls that will facilitate installation of the plastic pipe launders with minor structural support modifications.

Settling tank inlet flow arrangements vary considerably. A general design feature can, however, be suggested to improve inlet flow distribution. It has been found that multiple orifice or port baffles can be very effective in converting a high-velocity concentrated flow to a relatively uniform flow pattern. The baffle breaks up the continuity of the inlet flow. Flow through the orifices or ports is then reestablished primarily as a result of

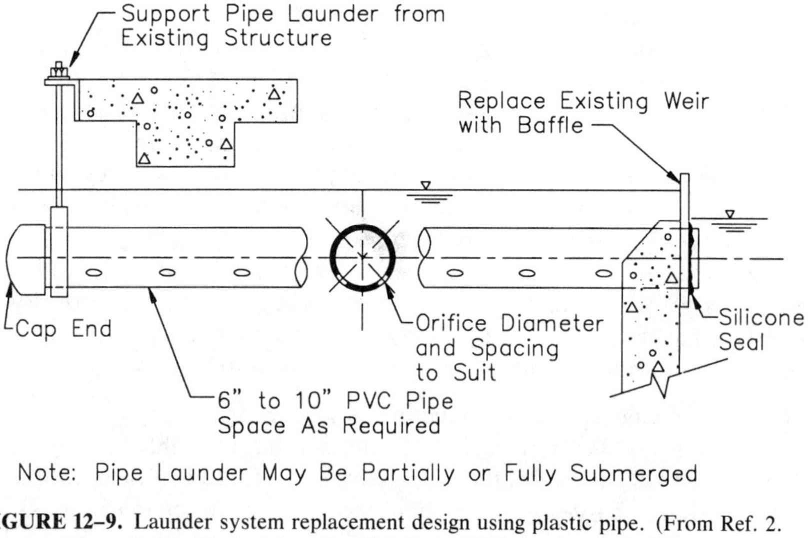

FIGURE 12–9. Launder system replacement design using plastic pipe. (From Ref. 2. Reprinted from *Public Works Magazine* (July/Aug. 1987), by permission.)

the difference in static head on either side of the baffle. Figure 12–10 shows this type of modification as applied to a situation where existing flow enters the settling tank through openings in the bottom of a transverse inlet channel. In this type of design, short circuiting is inherent because most of the flow tends to enter the tank through the openings at the end of the channel. When flow is established in a transverse channel, the established flow momentum will cause most of the flow to exit into the tank at the extreme end close to one sidewall. With flow entering one end of a transverse channel, such entry causes flow to hug one sidewall. If flow enters in the middle of the inlet channel, the flow tends to divide and the major portion of the flow will exit at both ends of the channel. This entry causes flow to hug both tank sidewalls. Figure 12–10 shows a possible solution where a ported channel can be constructed just below the existing inlet channel. Here, more uniform flow distribution is established by the static head above the ports or orifice openings. Structural design of the ported wall addition should take into account the force applied by the entering flow.

Modification to the center or main body of existing settling tanks is more difficult because of the diversity of tank designs and, in some installations, the need to avoid interference with sludge-removal operations or

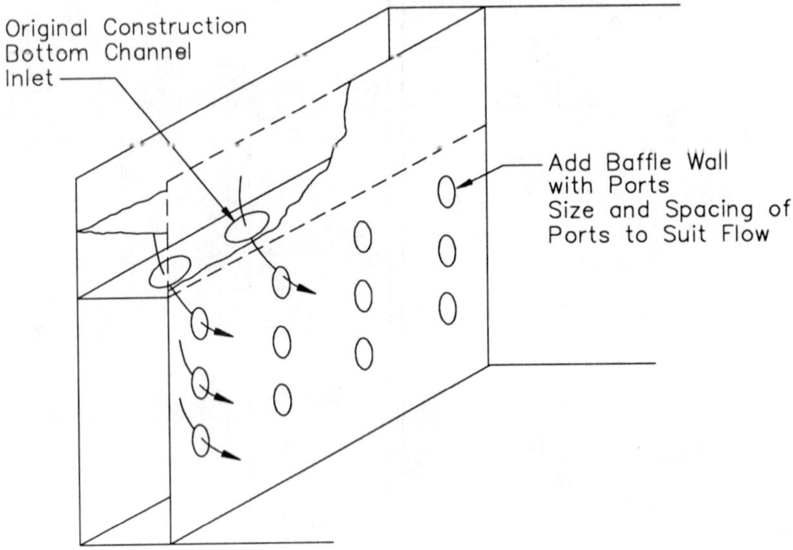

FIGURE 12–10. Ported baffle inlet for settling tank. (From Ref. 2. Reprinted from *Public Works Magazine* (July/Aug. 1987), by permission.)

equipment. In general, the only feasible way to contend with short circuiting in this part of the tank is with the installation of vertical baffles. The feasibility of baffle improvements will depend entirely upon the arrangement of the present tank structure. If existing strut and walkway arrangements facilitate installation, then baffles may be considered. If the tank is completely open, with no cross-structural supports, baffles might not be as economically feasible because of the added cost of structural support.

In general, the purpose of the baffles would be to interrupt and redirect short-circuited flow. Since design is so subjective, actual tests in the problem tank or tanks are necessary to develop a meaningful baffle arrangement. The use of flexible or roll plastic is an inexpensive solution that appears to be most helpful in reducing short circuiting. In testing, the many variations of length, width, and position of the plastic baffles often must be tried before an acceptable solution is discovered or developed. Heavy plastic sheeting is used extensively in the construction industry. Figure 12–11 shows how the plastic baffle works. A double layer is used by folding the plastic sheet back. A metal pipe or rod can be used to weigh the plastic sheet down on the bottom. Width of baffle is controlled by

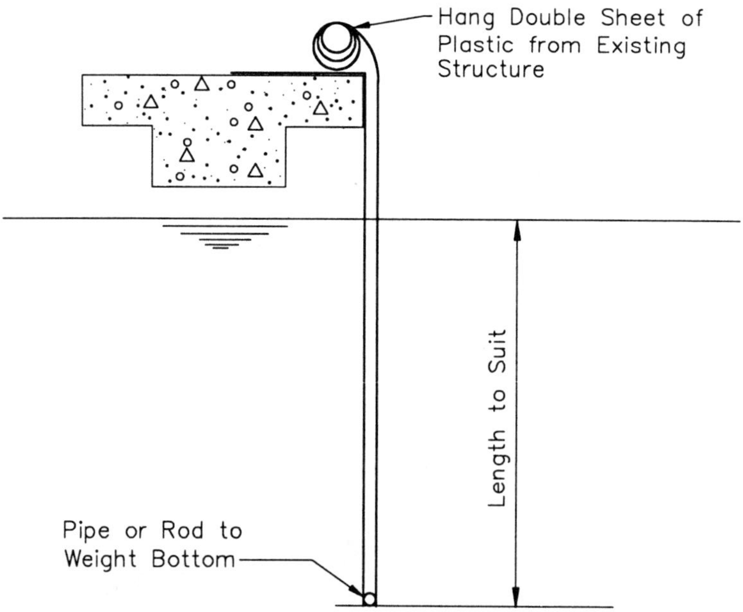

FIGURE 12–11. Weighted plastic sheeting facilitates tests of baffle arrangements that redirect short-circuited flow in a settling tank. (From Ref. 2. Reprinted from *Public Works Magazine* (July/Aug. 1987), by permission.)

cutting the plastic to size or by using multiple sections. Depth of baffle can readily be adjusted from the top by raising and lowering one side of the double plastic sheet. After tests determine the feasibility of baffles, final installations can be constructed of marine plywood, stainless steel webbing, or, if properly designed, plastic sheeting. Some commercial adaptations of the plastic baffles may be available in many locales.

Filtration

Media problems that may be encountered in rapid rate filter operation were discussed earlier. The more common problems related to the physical condition of drinking water filters include the following:

- Media that is of an improper type or size or that from years of use has become caked or worn
- Backwash systems that do not provide sufficient flow or that do not permit adequate control of flow rate to minimize surging
- Surface wash systems that do not provide uniform or complete coverage of the top surface or that, because of inadequate design, become clogged with media
- Rate control—either improperly designed systems or poorly maintained systems that do not provide adequate control of flow in relation to plant process flow variations

The wear and caking of media and the need for replacement were discussed earlier. In many plants, filter performance can also be significantly improved by the replacement of single media with dual or multiple media. Figure 12–12 shows the head loss characteristics for both types of arrangements for 30 inches of media depth. In the case of the single media, much of the solids interception is closer to the top of media. In fact, to avoid solids breakthrough, it is almost necessary in single media

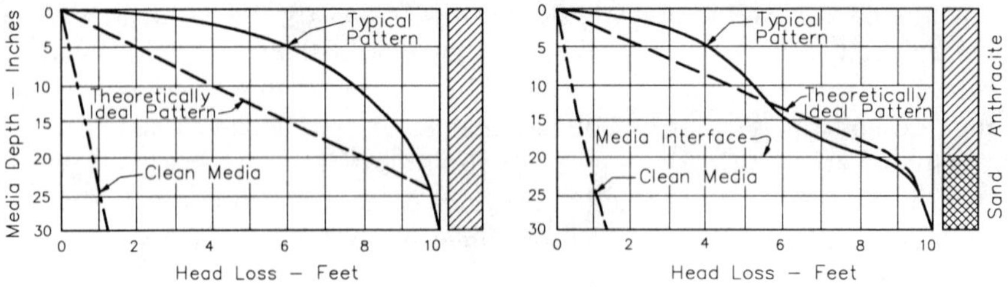

FIGURE 12–12. Typical end of run head loss patterns for single-media (left) and dual-media filters. (From Ref. 2. Reprinted from *Public Works Magazine* (July/Aug. 1987), by permission.)

design to somewhat inhibit media penetration. With the dual media arrangement, and the same total depth, in-depth solids penetration occurs with more available storage. The smaller-sized, tighter media of the bottom layer provides breakthrough protection as it intercepts the finer particulates that may pass through the upper layer.

Where breakthrough is a chronic problem, after all efforts for improvements through chemical conditioning have been exhausted, consideration often must be given to a change to a smaller-sized, tighter media, or, if space is available, a deeper media. Because of the somewhat shallow design of filters in the older plants, the alternative of greater depth, single media to inhibit breakthrough often cannot be considered. Design would be limited to media depths ranging, for the most part, from 24 to 30 inches.

While the maximum rate may never be used, backwash facilities should be designed to provide backwash rates up to 20 gpm/sf. Media expansion requirements for proper stratification of different layers in multimedia configurations dictate higher backwash rates than those required for older, single media filters where lower backwash rates can be acceptable. It may, therefore, be necessary to modify existing pipe and valve systems or to replace backwash pumps with higher capacity units, or both, to provide the higher rate in upgraded filters. In addition, greater separation may be required between the top of media and filter troughs to accommodate the greater degree of media expansion. This distance may be constrained in older, single media filters, and possible modifications may need to be considered.

Many backwash flow controls, because of poor design or poor maintenance, do not permit smooth transition of flow. Erratic flow, surging in particular, can result in nonuniform backwashing and carryover of media. Many plants still employ balance beam-type backwash flow controllers. These do not permit a two-stage backwash control where flow in the first and last stages of backwash is at half the middle stage rate of flow. Where existing backwash facilities do not perform properly, the controls should be replaced with systems that permit simple adjustment of backwash flow rate, either on a manual or automatic basis. The venturi portion of existing rate-control systems can be retained if it has sufficient rated capacity.

Unless properly maintained, the rotating-type surface wash devices can, in time, become clogged with sand. In addition to periodic maintenance to remove sand, the performance of rotating surface wash units often can be improved by replacement of the nozzles with those that incorporate a check-valve flap design. Special attention also should be given to the end nozzles that are intended to provide sprays that reach out to the dead areas not covered by the circular wash pattern. Sometimes adding nozzles to provide more flow in this direction will improve washing in the dead areas. Replacement of larger units with smaller-diameter rotating wash units or with units of a different design is sometimes necessary to improve area coverage. Simply increasing the supply pressure of surface wash can be detrimental. Rather than improving washing, the increased flow rate may upset the media.

Another area of flow concern is the filter rate master control system provided in many plants to (1) enhance uniform distribution of flow to a battery of filters and (2) ensure that the maximum set rate is not exceeded. The second function is almost always accomplished. Flow through the filter will not exceed that rate set on the effluent rate of flow controller. Unless a master controller is provided that will reset each individual filter control, when total flow to a battery of filters is less than the total of the settings on the individual filter rate controllers, the control valves on all or most filters will tend to go to the full open position. With most valves full open, the filter battery is not operating on a rate control basis. It is operating rather in the declining or variable rate mode. In effect, when the valves are full open, no flow control exists. Actual rate of flow through each filter in a battery will then be determined by the resistance provided by the media and the solids in media storage. The controller will tend to limit flow up to the maximum set point only through filters with clean or relatively clean media.

That this variable rate or modified variable rate mode exists in so many filtration systems is most interesting in light of the controversy between proponents of variable and controlled rate methods of filter operation. In part, selection of the method of operation to use is influenced by the number of filters in a plant. Where six or more filters exist, variable rate filtration can be considered. With proper scheduling of backwash, the filters will range, in regard to degree of clogging, from clean to ready to be backwashed. With six units, an adequate number would be available for declining rate control, even with one filter out of service for maintenance. With five units or less in a battery, the controlled rate mode is desirable if a relatively uniform rate of flow to the consumer is to be maintained. Otherwise the removal of one filter for backwashing will result in a significant increase in the filter rate of the other filters. Therefore, where filter rate control systems are inadequate because of design or condition, replacement should be made for plants or filter batteries numbering five or less filters. In such replacement, a master controller should be added, where the set rate for each filter is adjusted in proportion to the plant inlet flow.

Where six or more filters exist in a battery, variable rate operation would be an adequate mode of operation that could be accomplished at greatly reduced cost. In modifying an existing plant for variable rate filter operation, only the venturi and the control valve or device need to be retained. The control device is placed in the partially open position which will limit the maximum rate of flow that can pass through a clean filter. The venturi would be retained to measure and record flow through each filter. All other elements of the rate control system can be discarded.

COLD LIME SOFTENING

Most of the problems encountered in the operation of cold lime softening plants may be considered to be similar to those reviewed before for rapid rate filtration. The problems inherent in the design and operation of chemical feed, chemical mix, settling, and filtration facilities would be essentially the same for rapid rate filtration and cold lime softening plants. Some differences occur in flash mixing and flocculation systems due to phenomena associated with formation of a precipitate. For example, detention time in mixing can provide more time for initial precipitate formation prior to flocculation. Also, solids recycling is often beneficial during flocculation due to the fact that previously formed particulates can enhance the precipitation process. This has led to use of solids contact clarifiers that provide for internal recycling. Process-specific issues or factors that must be considered in any program to improve treatment performance and product water quality in cold lime treatment of drinking water are as follows:

1. Sufficient lime (and other alkalinity supplements) must be added to the flow to raise the pH to levels that maximize removal of the calcium and magnesium precipitates produced. Polymers may be added to improve solids removal efficiencies.
2. Proper control must be exerted over recycle systems in solids contact–type processes. Otherwise solids carryover may occur. Some solids contact devices, especially those that fail to provide a physical separation to contain the recirculating zone, are particularly sensitive to solids carryover.
3. Adequate recarbonation must be provided before filtration and disinfection to reduce pH to a level that minimizes subsequent scaling of downstream system elements and filter media and generally to enhance the effectiveness of disinfection.
4. Appropriate hydraulic loadings to achieve settling must be used.

In any trouble-shooting procedure where product water quality is not up to standard, it probably would be desirable to start the investigations with a check of the above process-specific features. This would be followed by a review of the problems related to the common deficiencies encountered in rapid rate filtration plants discussed in this chapter.

SLOW SAND FILTRATION

The most significant feature of slow sand filtration is that it is a passive process, subject to few operator decisions. Sand used for media is smaller in effective size than that used for rapid rate alternatives. This smaller size inhibits in-depth penetration of the separated solids, which mostly accumulate in a thin layer on top of the sand bed. This layer, called the *schmutzdecke*, is composed of inert particulates as well as living and dead microorganisms and macroorganisms, and is the dominant filter medium.

Assuming that an adequately sized sand medium has been installed (see Chapter 11), the basic operator responsibilities are as follows:

1. Maintaining the filter flow application rates within an acceptable range. A typical range is 0.03 to 0.05 gpm/sf, as discussed in Chapter 11.
2. Scraping or removing the *schmutzdecke* when the accumulation of solids results in maximum available head loss.
3. Addition of replacement or reconditioned media to maintain minimum media depth.
4. To meet present-day standards, filter-to-waste of the initial flow passed through the filter after cleaning until a new *schmutzdecke* becomes established.

Similar to any filtration process, the two measures of greatest interest for slow sand filter performance are filtered water quality and length of filter run. In addition to a change in media size, the only corrections or adjustments available to improve water quality or filter run efficiency would be related to the basic features of operation listed above. Deterioration of filtered water quality may require a change to a smaller-sized media, to a lower filter rate, or to the time of filter-to-waste until the *schmutzdecke* can be established. Consideration can also be given to use of a media with a somewhat higher uniformity coefficient to promote a degree of media intermix, thereby reducing bed porosity. Unless it affects finished water quality, it might be possible to improve the rate of filter production by increasing the rate of flow application, by increasing the media size, or by both measures.

PRECOAT FILTRATION

Significant Features

Many of the basic mechanisms involved in the separation of particulates in the flow through porous media are essentially the same for precoat filtration and rapid rate filtration using granular media, but with different emphasis. Beyond these fundamental features, however, the similarities between these two modes of filtration cease.

In precoat filtration, a powderlike media is used once, disposed of, and replaced after each filter run. The rapid rate filter employs granular media that remain in the filter until it is literally worn out in time periods of from 5 to 10 years. In rapid rate filtration, process control is exerted by conditioning the source water solids through coagulation to increase the size and susceptibility of source water solids to filtration. Conversely, coagulant addition is not used in precoat filtration; it is the media size that is varied to match source water solids characteristics.

Perhaps the most distinctive features of precoat filtration are the several options available to enable adjustment in operation to meet or compensate for changing conditions of source water quality and the solids carried in suspension. The more significant features of precoat filtration that may affect operation in general and filtered water quality in particular are discussed below.

Precoat Filter Septa

The first step in precoat filtration is to form a layer of precoat over the septum, which is basically a woven wire or synthetic fabric. Flow is horizontal; the hydraulic force of the flow through the septum holds the accumulated precoat cake, powdered diatomaceous earth (or perlite), to the fabric. Precoating is accomplished by circulating a suspension of diatomaceous earth through the filter until the whole filtering area has relatively uniform coverage to a depth of about 1/16 to 1/8 inch (2 to 4 mm).

Openings in the septum fabric are actually larger than the precoat media particles. The built-up media literally bridges the openings in the septum so that the media, not the cloth, accomplishes the solids separation. It is only necessary that the fabric septa characteristics permit adequate bridging of the precoat.

Maintaining Porosity, Body Feed

After the precoat step is completed, recirculation is phased out and the process flow is introduced to the filter. The primary mechanism for solids separation in this type filtration is entrapment or straining. Without further adjustment the precoat would quickly become obstructed by the finer solid matter removed from the liquid. As the separated solids accumulate in a built-up cake, porosity will be further reduced to result in shortened filter runs. As porosity is reduced, the applied hydraulic head must be increased to maintain a constant filter flow rate.

Some solids, particularly those of organic origin, have compressible features. As the accumulated cake increases in depth, the increased force of applied pressure required to maintain the filter rate will tend to compress the cake and further reduce porosity. To compensate for this effect, a body feed, usually a slurry of the same material used for precoat, is added to the incoming flow to maintain or improve porosity. Body feed is added in proportions amounting to several magnitudes of the source water solids content. The body feed acts as a matrix in which the separated source water solids are distributed throughout the accumulating cake. At the appropriate ratio of body feed to suspended solids (usually expressed as turbidity), the filter runs can be extended to achieve more cost-effective operation.

Hydraulic Control

The nature of precoat filtration is such that a continuous, uninterrupted flow is required at all times to hold the precoat and accumulated cake to the septa. Changes may be made in applied flow, but not on a sudden basis. For instance, for average drinking water treatment conditions, precoat is usually applied at a rate of about 1.0 gpm/sf of septa area. After recirculation, the process flow may be introduced at application rates of from 1.0 to 3.0 gpm/sf. As long as such changes in rate are accomplished slowly, the precoat will remain intact. If at any time, the flow through the filter is halted, even for a few seconds, the cake may separate from the septa to end the run. Sudden surges in both flow and pressure will disturb the cake and its filtering integrity.

Septa Conditions

While the precoat filter septa usually do not have significant impact on solids separation, certain source water characteristics may be the cause of blinding of the septum. Unstable iron or manganese in solution, for instance, can deposit and build up on the strands of the woven septa cloth. In time, the pores in the septum can be filled, inhibiting both flow and the deposit of precoat. Certain organic constituents and media-conditioning materials like alum can produce the same blinding effect. Any blinding that inhibits precoating must be removed by cleaning or by replacement of the septum cloth in accordance with the filter manufacturer's instructions. In order to inhibit or slow down blinding, it is absolutely essential that the filter septa be thoroughly cleaned by hydraulic means at the end of each filter run.

Pretreatment Options

Pretreatment with coagulation is an essential feature of effective rapid rate filtration. Pretreatment is an option in precoat filtration, used principally to enhance the removal of solids in the colloidal size ranges that are associated with color levels or with bacteria and viruses.

Colloids of natural origin usually found in source water supplies have negative charge characteristics and may be small enough to pass through precoat filters without conditioning to neutralize the particles. Unless neutralized, a substantial number of these particulates can pass through the media and the accumulated cake. Two basic pretreatment methods may be employed to neutralize and condition these particles as follows:

1. Alum conditioning—where both precoat and body feed media slurry are conditioned with alum to impart a positive charge to the media. The negative colloidal particles can then attach to the positively charged media. Care must be exercised, since alum tends to shorten filter runs.
2. Ozonation—where the ozone is believed to destroy the bond between the color or other inert matter and the organics that form the colloidal particle, thereby effecting depolarization. The depolarized solids then may be separated by attachment to the media.

In almost all situations where pretreatment is used for drinking water applications, the intent is not necessarily to improve the solids removal or turbidity reduction, but rather to enhance removal of particular constituents like color or viruses that would otherwise pass through the media. Colloid-sized particulates usually constitute a minute fraction of the overall suspended solids content, but can be a significant part of other raw water features like color and microorganisms.

Correcting Principal Operation Deficiencies

Most deficiencies in precoat filtration are related to incorrect operations. The basic problems that result most often are manifested as an inability to adequately precoat the filter or as poor filter performances in terms of product water quality or operating efficiency. Discussion of the principal problems encountered in precoat filtration of drinking water is, therefore, divided into the precoat and filter cycle components of operation.

Precoating

The first group of common precoating problems is related to increased pressure on the inlet side of the filter during this phase of operation. This increase may have occurred gradually over an extended period or may be a sudden, unexpected occurrence. Checks and corrective steps should be taken in the following order:

1. Verify accuracy of pressure-sensing equipment.
2. Check filter housing (pressure-type unit) for possible air binding—the venting equipment may not be functioning properly.
3. Check precoat material—a finer grade than normal may have been used.
4. Check precoat recirculation rate—reduce if higher-than-normal flow rate has been used.
5. Check filter septa for blinding: (1) first thoroughly sluice and/or backwash the septa; (2) thoroughly flush and rinse filter piping; (3) if above cleaning is not effective, remove filter from service, check for blinded areas and use chemical cleaning recommended by manufacturer for filter septa cloth as required.

The second group of problems is related to poor clarity of the recirculated flow after the recycle period (usually about 15 minutes). The check procedure should start with an investigation of the external features first and then proceed to an inspection of the characteristics of the precoat pattern itself as follows:

1. Insufficient amount of precoat material used to prepare the slurry.
2. Finer grade of precoat material used than septa is designed to handle—precoat media cannot bridge openings.
3. Precoat slurry is too dilute—prepared slurry concentration should be between 12 and 15 percent by weight. Concentration of the slurry in the recycle flow volume is normally between 0.6 and 1.0 percent; if below 0.3 percent, the media particles may not effectively bridge septa openings.
4. Precoat slurry is added to recycle at too low rate—must be introduced in a time period of from 1 to 2 minutes.
5. The filter and/or connected piping are subjected to excessive vibration (from nearby mechanical equipment) and/or flow surges cause some of the precoat to be dislodged from screens.
6. Recycle rate is too low—some of the precoat material introduced does not reach the filter leaves (septum) and settles to bottom of filter—increase recirculation rate.

7. Precoat is eroded by flow—reduce flow down to as low as 1.0 gpm/sf application rate—check filter inlet baffles for possible generation of excessive turbulence.
8. Tops of filter septum are not precoated—precoat flow is too low (see 6 above) and/or filter volume was not sufficiently filled prior to introduction of precoat slurry.
9. Check filter septa and frames for holes and defective seals.
10. Check for worn gaskets in the connection between filter leaf discharge and discharge manifold.

Filtration Cycle

The two fundamental measures of filter operating performance are product water quality and length of filter run. Solids removal and product water must meet the established limitations of turbidity and color. Filter run length affects labor and material utilization. Shorter filter runs require more labor as well as more precoat material and more water for cleaning the filter at the end of run. Filtration problems, causes, and resolutions are, therefore, discussed in reference to product quality and efficiency of operation.

Several of the problems that produce unsatisfactory filtrate quality are similar to those that create poor clarity in the precoating cycle. Careful surveillance of the precoat phase of operation and the clarity of the recycle at the end of precoat will avoid similar problems in filtration. The more significant causes of filtrate quality problems are as follows:

1. Improper match of media to source water solids removal needs—too coarse media will not intercept sufficient particulates—too fine media may not provide a uniform precoat on openings of selected septa and allow bleed of both filter and source water solids into filtrate.
2. Vibrations and/or hydraulic flow and pressure shocks imposed on the filter or the filter piping systems, which, if severe, can cause a breakdown of bridged precoat allowing solids (precoat and source water) to bleed into filtrate.
3. Equipment damage, wear and tear—without corrective maintenance, holes or tears in a septum, loss of filter area from fouled (blinded) septa, worn or damaged O-ring and other types of gasket seals and damaged or improperly designed inlet baffles can all upset the integrity of precoat and accumulated cake to allow bleed of particulate solids into the filtrate.
4. Incomplete venting of air from the filter vessel, which results in erratic precoat and cake accumulation at the air-water interface in the septa.
5. Adequate turbidity removals but breakthrough of color and coliform

organisms—increase in colloidal content of source water supply that requires pretreatment to improve removals of colloid-sized matter.

Shortened filter runs may be the result of either improper filter operation procedure or the lack of recognition of changes in source water quality that may require adjustment of such procedures. The principal causes of shortened filter runs are as follows:

1. Filtration rate inadvertently increased as a result of operator error or inaccurate flow controls.
2. Increase in source water solids—increase body feed to restore laminar (straight line) pressure vs. time relationship.
3. Breakdown of filter media in size gradation as a result of excessive handling in pipeline flow and in storage mixing—discard batch and restore with new material.
4. Filter screen fouling (see 5 in the previous list).

GENERAL APPROACH FOR UPGRADING PERFORMANCE OF BASELINE PROCESSES

It has not been possible to cite in one chapter all possible problems that may be encountered in operating baseline treatment processes. Each plant will have its own specific set of problems. The information presented herein illustrates the more common problems and the type of rationale needed to discover and to resolve the particular difficulties.

In all cases, filtered water quality or clarity should be continuously monitored in operation through the use of turbidimeters. Establishing the accuracy of the measurements is an important preliminary consideration. These measurements should be checked periodically in the laboratory using separate instruments. Sample lines as well as continuous monitoring instruments may be prone to deposits of slimes and biological growths, which, if dislodged or located on the optical devices, can yield false turbidity and color readings. When unsatisfactory water quality measurements occur, the first check made should be of the monitoring instruments and the sampling system. If such checks do not disclose any deficiencies, other features should be investigated.

Most studies of plant rehabilitation needs have indicated that significant improvements are possible with relatively minor modification of facilities. In fact, unless major uprating in capacity is required, simple adjustment of chemical feed procedures and rehabilitation of filter media may be all that would be required in many plants to make it possible to maintain less than 0.5 NTU product water turbidity. Therefore, to avoid unnecessary cost and efforts, it would be essential to accomplish all nonstructural or nonmechanical water treatment improvements as a first step. The two principal treatment features that would be included in the first step are (1) chemical feed program and (2) filter media effectiveness.

Chemical Feed Adjustment

Chemical feed changes are the most simple to accomplish. In addition to the type of chemicals used and the respective feed rates, adjustments in the location of chemical introduction to the process stream should be investigated. Where more than one chemical is used, the sequence of chemical introduction may be important. The five features of chemical feed that are most important in water treatment are as follows:

1. Introduction of undesired contaminants or byproducts (i.e., aluminum residuals when using alum, some organic compounds of concern when using polymers, and impurities that may occur as contaminants of commercial chemicals)
2. Rate of feed
3. pH maintained for reaction
4. Sequence of multiple chemical feed
5. Need for alternative chemicals

The chemical feed investigations should be conducted in the above order. Changes in type of chemicals employed in treatment should be accomplished only after the first four features have been checked and corrected. A change in chemical type would be indicated where unwanted byproducts may be generated or where other improvements might be accomplished, such as optimized flocculation or reduced formation of waste solids.

Media Refurbishment

No matter what type of filter is used, the filter media size or its relative porosity must be suitable for the service intended. Media inadequacy may simply be a result of poor selection for the particular service. Poor filtration could also occur due to media wear or media fouling that results from caking (by coagulated solids) or biological growths. Inadequate filter wash procedures also could contribute to poor performance. Where fouling is suspected, the initial step in granular filter investigation, therefore, would be to thoroughly clean the media using strong caustic or chlorine solutions. After such cleaning and after upgrading the chemical feed program, the adequacy of the media match to the service required may be established. If media change is indicated because of wear or size inadequacy, such replacement must be accomplished before proceeding with the subsequent physical structure studies.

Structural and Mechanical Improvements

As discussed above, the more common physical design problems evident in existing rapid rate filtration plants are as follows:

1. Chemical mixing—inappropriate mixing and configuration of mixing facilities for rapid dispersion
2. Flocculation—inappropriate mixing pattern, short circuiting
3. Settling tanks—short circuiting
4. Chlorine contact chambers—short circuiting
5. Filters—inadequate distance between

It is obvious that short circuiting with its resultant effect on detention time is a problem that is common to several elements of the conventional arrangement of rapid rate filtration. Energy input in chemical mixing and flocculation would be the second most common problem that should be investigated in both the conventional and direct modes of rapid rate filtration.

References

1. Richard, Y., and P. Blue. 1978. Ozone pretreatment of drinking water. I.O.I. Ozone Technology Symposium, Los Angeles, CA, May 1978.
2. Fulton, G. P. 1987. Upgrading filtration to meet pending standards. *Public Works,* July 1987, pp. 55–58, and August 1987, pp. 68–72.
3. Fulton, G. P. 1988. Contending with filter media problems. *Public Works* (June): 67–70, 110.
4. Hudson, H. E. 1981. *Water clarification processes: Practical design and evaluation.* New York: Van Nostrand Reinhold Company.

13

Evaluating and Planning Disinfection Systems

GENERAL EVALUATION AND PLANNING CONCEPTS

Evaluation and planning of disinfection systems involves consideration of a number of water treatment process interrelationships not recognized in previous design practice. Planning should take into account the integration of new disinfection concepts into a baseline treatment train in a manner that maintains all treatment objectives. Within this treatment train, the overall disinfection strategy will frequently involve multiple treatment steps so that the relationships between these steps need to be considered. For example, the EPA Surface Water Treatment Rule has placed emphasis on the use of filtration processes for removing pathogens in a role that supplements the microbial inactivation achieved by disinfectants. With such emphasis, the level of disinfection required of chemical agents is influenced by the level of removal credit achieved by filtration. In this manner, the removal capabilities of filtration provide an additional barrier against pathogens that can provide some safety when problems occur in the chemical disinfecting steps.

Interactions that affect other treatment goals can be a significant consideration when making evaluations of alternative disinfection approaches. These often can be subtle and not clearly identified upon initial examination. For example, as discussed in Chapter 4, changes in chlorination practice may reduce the capability for manganese removal and alter the capability of the process to control iron, sulfides, color, tastes and odors, and nuisance growths within a treatment plant and its pipeline systems. In another example, the use of chloramines to achieve benefits such as reduced THM formation may result in concerns for biological nitrification as discussed in Chapter 5. Coagulation and filtration processes can also be affected both positively and negatively by the oxidizing properties of different disinfectants. It is therefore essential that the full range of outcomes of a disinfection strategy be considered to ensure success.

Depending on treatment conditions, each chemical disinfectant produces characteristic byproducts. While the levels of some undesirable byproducts may be reduced by changing disinfectants, the levels of other byproducts or the generation of new byproducts may be increased with such change. These effects need to be considered to determine whether additional treatment methods will be required when existing processes do not provide the desired level of byproduct control. Notable examples are the possible incorporation of biodegradation processes to remove increased levels of biodegradable organic carbon that may be formed with ozone (see Chapter 7) and the need for processes to remove excess levels of chlorine dioxide residuals following its application as a primary disinfectant (see Chapter 6).

Except for extremely high-quality sources of supply, the treatment system for a surface water treatment application will typically include a filtration process for particulate reduction, along with various combinations of disinfectants or disinfectant application. Other chemicals may also be added either to support filtration processes or to achieve some additional goals such as corrosion control and fluoridation. Because of the somewhat complicated cause-and-effect situations that usually result from different arrangements of chemical additions, an evaluation or test program should consider the effects of a broad range of possible relationships between various processes and treatment objectives.

BASIC ALTERNATIVES

Controlling or limiting the formation of disinfection byproducts while maintaining effective disinfection are important components to include in any disinfection evaluation. General strategies for achieving these goals are as follows:

1. Provide effective baseline treatment to remove pathogens and reduce the dependency on disinfectants (see Chapter 11).
2. Select a disinfectant (or combination of disinfectants) to minimize undesired byproduct levels while providing acceptable microbial quality and, where relevant, oxidation characteristics for nondisinfection goals. Disinfectant alternatives include chlorine (Chapter 4), chloramines (Chapter 5), chlorine dioxide (Chapter 6), ozone (Chapter

7), and ultraviolet radiation (Chapter 9). Although limited, potassium permanganate also has a disinfecting capacity (Chapter 8); it is used most often for its oxidation properties to obtain nondisinfection goals.
3. To limit possible byproduct formation, reduce the concentrations of precursor organics in the water prior to the addition of disinfectants. Precursor removal methods can include coagulation (Chapter 11), oxidation by chlorine dioxide (Chapter 6), the use of ozone (Chapter 7) or potassium permanganate (Chapter 8), adsorption by activated carbon (Chapter 10), and removal by membrane processes (Chapter 9).
4. Apply disinfectants and subsequently remove undesired disinfectant byproducts that may be formed. Applicable processes include adsorption by GAC and PAC (Chapter 10) and air stripping of volatile organics (Chapter 9).
5. Combinations of various of the above strategies.

Microbial goals to be maintained under each strategy will be governed by compliance with CT criteria. In fact, constraints associated with these criteria can have an effect on overall disinfection/disinfection byproduct strategy. As an example, if time T can be improved or increased by treatment plant modification or addition, a lower C is required, and the disinfectant feed rate to achieve a specified CT can be reduced. Steps that reduce disinfectant demand can also reduce required disinfectant additions for meeting these criteria. It is likely that such types of modifications can not only reduce byproduct formation, but also the overall cost of disinfection.

When contending with disinfection byproduct criteria, selection of applicable processes or process combinations will depend on the level of reduction of disinfection byproducts required. Where moderate levels of reduction are necessary, lower cost alternatives may be adequate. These approaches may include precursor removal by coagulation or other baseline process means (Chapter 11). Supplemental precursor removal can sometimes be accomplished at relatively reasonable cost through use of powdered activated carbon adsorption (Chapter 10) and by the addition of potassium permanaganate (Chapter 8). Modified chlorination practices, in which ammonia is added to form chloramines following a period of primary disinfection contact with free chlorine, may be a lower-cost alternative that can reduce disinfection byproduct formation by limiting contact time with free chlorine (Chapter 5). Because of the lower cost, these types of process applications often represent the first level of process modification for consideration. In some cases, combinations of these process modifications can reduce disinfection byproducts to lower levels than can be achieved by each of these processes individually.

Where greater levels of reduction in disinfection byproducts must be achieved, it may become necessary to consider more costly options. These can include chlorine dioxide (Chapter 6) and ozone (Chapter 7) as alternative primary disinfectants to replace free chlorine (Chapter 4). Ultraviolet radiation also is a primary disinfecting alternative that may become applicable for groundwaters in which *Giardia* is not a concern (Chapter 9). Note that while these three alternatives are applicable for primary disinfection, they do not provide a secondary disinfecting residual. This will require either free chlorine or chloramines (unless criteria limiting chlorine dioxide residuals become less restrictive and allow its use as a secondary disinfectant).

In some cases, alternative disinfecting agents, particularly ozone, function as oxidizing agents to reduce precursor content and chlorine demand to levels that result in limited formation of chlorination byproducts. Biodegradation processes (Chapters 2 and 11) have been used to further augment these reductions. Whenever these reductions are still not adequate for meeting disinfection byproduct goals with the use of free chlorine, conversion to secondary disinfection with chloramines may become necessary. This type of secondary disinfection application requires consideration of the need for prior contact time with free chlorine. Where biodegradation processes are employed upstream of the secondary disinfection step, a period of free chlorine contact may provide better disinfection of residual microorganisms leaving such processes (Chapter 2), although the use of chloramines may be better in situations where bacteria are attached to GAC fines (Chapter 11).

Other processes are available for attaining disinfection objectives in special situations. For example, some membrane systems (Chapter 9) can achieve extremely high levels of precursor removal. These systems may be used where such removals are a major consideration, especially where these systems can be applied for other treatment goals such as softening and desalting. Air stripping systems (Chapter 9), useful in the removal of volatile disinfection byproducts, can be especially applicable where these systems are already in place for removing synthetic volatiles. Since many byproducts of concern may not be sufficiently volatile for efficient stripping to take place, use of air stripping may be limited for this purpose alone.

GAC (Chapter 10) has the potential for removing either precursors or byproducts, although low adsorptive capacity may adversely affect its economic viability in many locations. In general, more success has been reported in precursor removal, and it is possible for adsorptive removals to be supplemented by biodegradation processes that can occur naturally in GAC beds. Further removal can be achieved by ozone addition both to convert the precursor material to more readily biodegradable material and to enhance the biological environment in the GAC media (Chapter 7). In addition, new adsorption ion exchange approaches now the subject of research may merit consideration as an alternative to GAC in the future.

Important in the selection of alternatives for control of disinfection byproducts is the ability to control not only gross measurement of byproducts such as total THMs and TOX, but also some specific byproducts as well. In this regard, there is growing interest in the effect of bromide on the formation of specific THM compounds (chloroform, dichlorobromomethane, and bromoform). Since health effect evaluations suggest that dichlorobromomethane may be a stronger carcinogen than other THMs, formation of dichlorobromomethane and the other brominated THMs can be a significant consideration when bromide is present. Care should also be exercised where bromate, another byproduct of health concern, can be formed through disinfectant oxidation, especially when ozone is used.

Many of the strategies that reduce the formation of total THMs can have much less of an effect on reducing the formation of dichlorobromomethane and other brominated THMs. Studies have shown that brominated THMs become an increasingly significant proportion of the total THM content as precursor levels are reduced and, therefore, are not as readily affected by precursor removal strategies (3). These types of effects should be considered in evaluations of methods for reducing byproduct formation. The formation of brominated byproducts is related to the initial bromide level and some benefits could be achieved if bromide could be removed. However, bromide is relatively soluble and not readily removed by conventional treatment methods.

COMPONENTS OF A DISINFECTION EVALUATION PROGRAM

While specific process variables and needs will differ for individual drinking water treatment situations, evaluation of the following general characteristics would be common in the development of most disinfection test programs:

1. Source water quality variations including those that affect both disinfection byproduct formation and disinfectant demand
2. Physical characteristics of treatment facilities
3. Baseline treatment process interactions with disinfection
4. Disinfectant/oxidant alternatives
5. Supplemental precursor removal alternatives
6. Distribution system microbial characteristics
7. Possible conflicting goals or new problems associated with alternatives

Source Water Quality Variations

Except for certain groundwater supplies, water quality from most sources will exhibit significant variations throughout the year. Features such as temperature, rainfall, and sunlight vary seasonally to influence chemical and biological phenomena. River and watershed sources may also react to storms where sudden increases in runoff or stream flow will cause changes in suspended and dissolved constituents.

In any disinfection test program, investigations should include worst-case or close-to-worst-case situations. Worst-case situations may require significant modification of routine operating protocol to compensate for changes. Typically, variations in source water content will affect the chemical demand for coagulants and disinfectants, as well as the disinfection byproduct formation potential. Unless the complete range of source water quality conditions is considered, design criteria may prove to be inadequate to cope with extreme conditions. In the case of the current regulations for THMs, the standards are based on running averages over four consecutive quarters. While this may reduce the impact of the most extreme conditions on compliance, the effects of variations on the running average still should be considered.

The types of variations that can be encountered are illustrated in Figure 13–1, which shows trends for TOC, THM-formation potential, and TOX-formation potential in a source water that supplies Thornton, Colorado (7). Note that seasonal variations shown for this source are significant and that the magnitude of variation also can change from one year to the next. Therefore, the whole picture does not begin to develop until some of the worst-case periods are evaluated. More complete understanding of trends will gradually improve as more data are compiled over time. Frequently, data available for these parameters are not as extensive as shown in Figure 13–1, and judgments are necessary to select the appropriate degree of adjustment to allow for possible worst-case conditions.

Another important consideration is the variability of characteristics that affect disinfectant properties. Long-term operating records of existing treatment plants often provide historical information on variations in chlorine usage. Other information can also provide a valuable basis for evaluating potential process performance. For example, ammonia and organic nitrogen, which can significantly affect chlorine and chloramine chemistry, can show considerable variability as demonstrated by the total Kjeldahl nitrogen data shown in Figure 13–2.

Other significant factors that can influence the process demand for disinfecting agents are oxidant-demanding forms of several inorganic constituents such as iron, manganese, and sulfide. The stability of a disinfec-

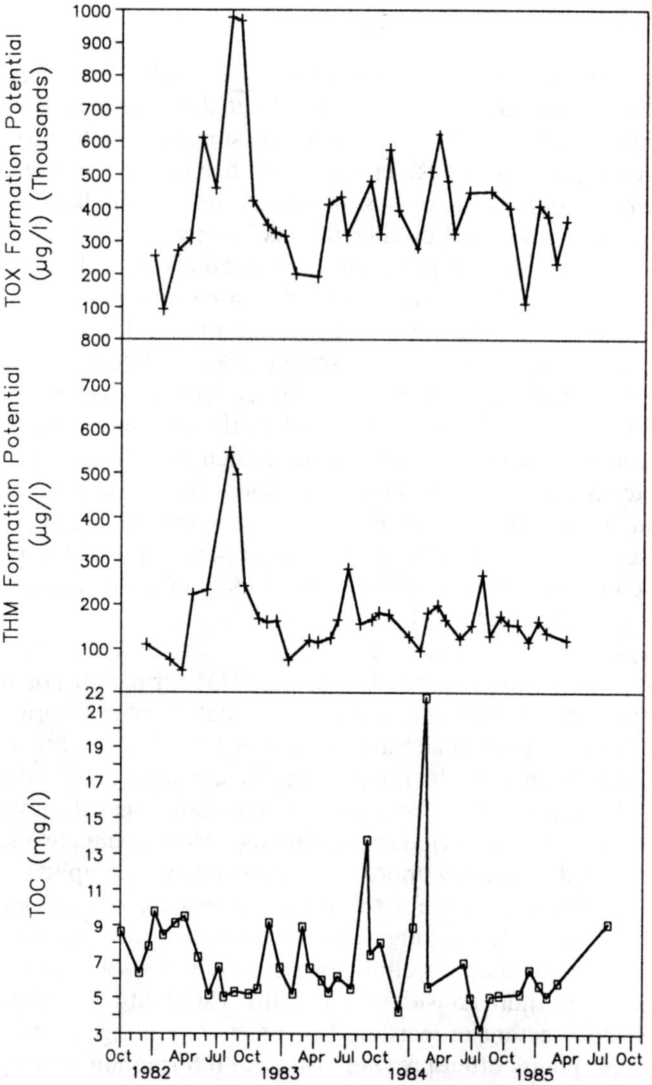

FIGURE 13–1. Seasonal variations in TOC, THM formation potential for Gravel Lakes, Thornton, Colorado. (From Ref. 7, with permission of U.S. EPA.)

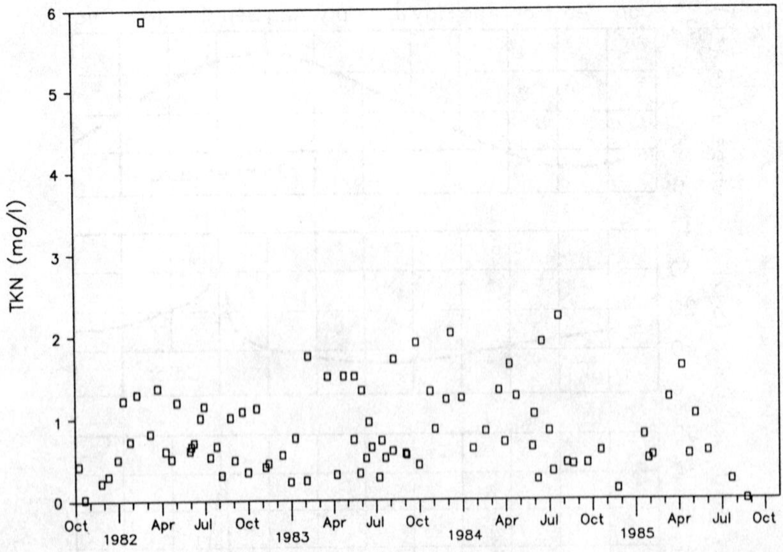

FIGURE 13–2. Total Kjeldahl nitrogen concentration in the Standley Lake, Thornton, Colorado. (From Ref. 7, with permission of U.S. EPA.)

tant is also affected by seasonal variations in temperature. This is often found in records that show greater problems in maintaining disinfecting residuals in distribution systems during the summer period. Many utilities require higher disinfectant dose rates during this warm weather period to maintain the minimum residual. As the summer also is often the time of greatest availability of precursors, source water conditions in this season can be extremely critical for evaluation of disinfection performance.

Since the reactivity of disinfectants can vary widely with pH, this is another important parameter to characterize when assessing disinfectant demand. In the case of free chlorine, a decrease in pH may enhance primary disinfection in the water treatment plant. However, decreased finished water pH may be somewhat detrimental to the capability for maintaining residuals to meet secondary disinfection goals because of the more rapid dissipation of residual that occurs. The end result may be an increased chlorine demand for meeting secondary disinfection goals.

Data shown in Figure 13–3 are typical of commonly available historical records. These data show the variations in water temperature, color and turbidity for a water supply covering a single year. Trends are obvious for this particular reservoir supply. As water temperature increases, color

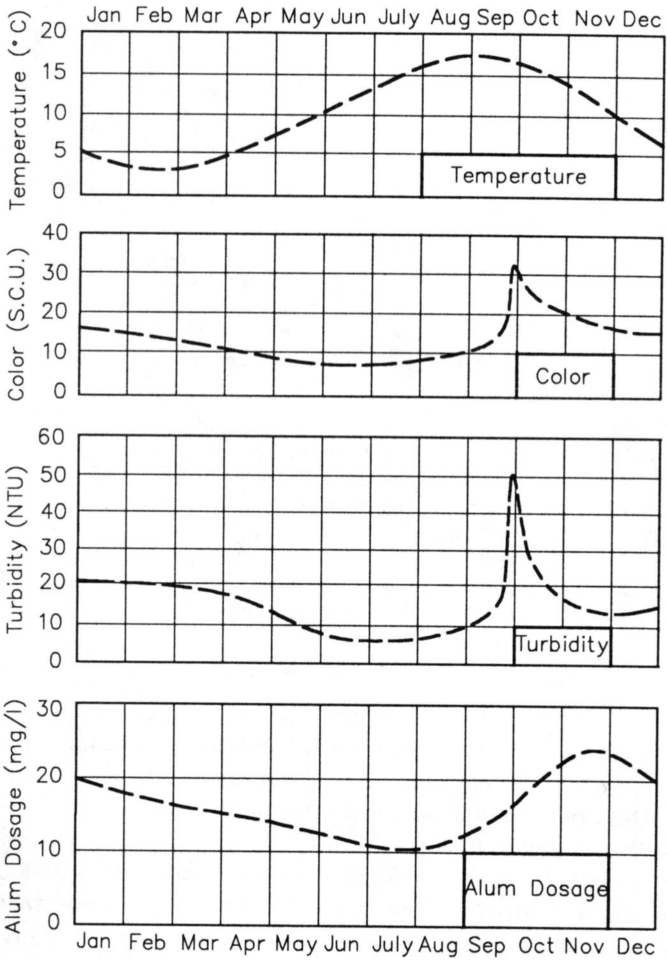

FIGURE 13–3. Croton Lake supply seasonal parameter variations—1975.

and turbidity tend to increase. For this source, a significant increase in color and turbidity occurs in late summer, followed by a turnover event just after the maximum temperature is reached, which lasts for a matter of weeks. It is interesting to note that alum requirements for coagulation increased and decreased with changes in color and turbidity for this supply. Because organic content is typically indicated by color, the associated formation potential of disinfection byproducts also exhibits a similar general trend, although some differences in color composition may alter the relationship somewhat. This type of variation can be important, and a test program to evaluate conditions that can be expected should begin with a review of historical water quality data.

Because these analyses were not widely used until the 1980s, there will be limited historical data for organics TOC, TOX, THMs, THMFP. As a result, other indicators such as color and turbidity will usually have to be investigated as indicators of long-term past organic trends. For certain supply sources, correlations between these surrogates and the organic precursor content may be developed during testing to assist the evaluations. Where such correlations are reasonably consistent for the specific supply situation, these surrogate data may be used to assess possible extremes. However, direct correlation between surrogate constituents and organic parameters of direct concern may not always be possible. For such situations, however, use of a surrogate parameter may still provide some indication of source water quality under worst-case conditions. A factor of safety could then be selected to account for lack of direct correlation.

The annual water quality variations shown in Figure 13–3 are common for many reservoir sources, but deviations from these patterns shown can be expected. Actually, there have been other years where the trend for this particular source has been significantly different from that shown in the figure. In some years, high rates of rainfall and runoff after droughts have caused peak color and turbidity conditions in the spring of the year. Reservoir turnover generates peaks in the late summer-fall period. In other years, the right combination of temperature, sunlight, and nutrients has resulted in the proliferation of unusual algae blooms, which affected water quality over an extended season. Drought conditions have also produced atypical water quality. Therefore, where possible, source water quality conditions should be reviewed over a number of years to establish the relationship between extreme source water quality conditions and the water quality used in the test program. As a minimum, evaluations should examine key general parameters, such as temperature and pH, that influence disinfectant and disinfection byproduct characteristics.

Physical Attributes of Baseline Treatment Train

Typically, most water treatment plants provide two basic physical features that are important for disinfection: mixing and detention.

Mixing

For maximum effectiveness, disinfectants should be mixed and thoroughly dispersed in the process flow at the point of feed. Field investigations can be conducted for existing plant design situations to determine whether the disinfectant is uniformly dispersed. With multiple treatment trains, it is important that thorough mixing occurs before flow splitting. In existing plant situations, if other chemicals or disinfectants are being fed at the location in the process train under consideration, one simple approach would be to analyze a group of downstream samples to determine whether the chemical content (or reaction content) is consistent over time and not erratic.

For evaluating new chemical feed locations in an existing treatment train, surrogate tracer chemicals can be fed to the water flow stream with the same downstream analysis procedure. This method might also be used to evaluate performance of alternative diffusers and different locations of chemical feed for optimum dispersion and mixing conditions. Fluoride and sodium chloride have been used effectively as tracers. Where fluoride addition is part of an existing water treatment program, it is sometimes possible to shift the point of feed temporarily during the tests. However, care must be taken to avoid the possible disruption of filter performance if this section of the plant is to be exposed to high levels of fluoride. Fluoride can react to some extent with other water treatment chemicals, so these possible effects may need to be considered.

For new designs, mixing and detention concepts can be based on published recommendations that include documents such as the *Guidance Manual for Compliance with the Filtration and Disinfection Requirements for Public Water Systems Using Surface Water Sources* by the EPA (4), *Handbook of Chlorination* by George C. White (6), and the AWWA/ASCE book on *Water Treatment Plant Design* (5).

In-Plant Detention

Tracer tests are a common method used to characterize in-plant detention times. In conducting these tests, coordination with plant staff is required to select times and conditions necessary for testing on a schedule that will not interfere with plant operations. Tracer tests required to demonstrate contact times for CT criteria are detailed in Appendix C of the EPA *Guidance Manual* (4) and are also discussed in *Water Clarification Processes* by Herbert E. Hudson, Jr. (1).

EPA criteria indicate that, where possible, tracer studies should be carried out throughout the flow range expected at the plant (4). The maximum flow tested should be at a level of at least 91 percent of the highest flow to be experienced at each point in the plant. Other recommended test flow ranges should represent average flow, one below average flow, and one in between the maximum flow and the average flow. It is possible that flow splitting ratios and flow distribution in treatment plant basins will vary with changing flow rates. If only one tracer test is to be performed, it is recommended that the flow be greater than 91 percent of the highest flow expected. The detention time determined by that test can be used for determining or estimating the remaining detention times, which are assumed to be inversely proportional to the flow in the measured run. Tracer tests should be run under constant flow conditions; otherwise complexities are introduced into evaluations of data. Where some variation in flow is necessary to maintain plant function during testing, it is recommended that tests be conducted when levels are falling rather than rising. This results in a more conservative estimate.

One tracer test can be run for a group of processes in series, but it is often more advantageous to run individual tracer tests for each process to take advantage of higher concentrations in the earlier stages. As a compromise, the tracer chemical can be added at the most upstream point and concentrations read at each point to be included in the computation. Except for measuring mixing effectiveness before flow splitting, it is not necessary to run tests through two identical units or trains operated in parallel.

The first major decision for a tracer test is selection of the tracer material and the quantity to be used. Background levels of some tracer compounds may occur in a particular raw water, and these effects need to be considered in making these decisions. The more popular tracers used in the past have been sodium chloride and fluoride. A dye, rhodamine-WT, is also allowed, but rhodamine-B is not recommended by EPA (4). For continuous feed tests, sodium chloride doses are usually on the order of 20 mg/l; fluoride in concentrations, 1 to 2 mg/l. (At least one state regulatory agency is recommending 3 to 4 mg of fluoride/l during the test to improve accuracy.) The choice of tracer can depend upon the extent to which background concentrations might obscure test results. If fluoride is used, allowances should be made for possible fluoride loss due to reactions with other water treatment chemicals. In particular, fluoride losses can occur due to adsorption onto chemical flocs in coagulation and filtration processes.

Tracers are added either in a *step-dose* fashion, where the tracer is continuously fed until the outlet concentration approaches the feed concentration, or in a *slug-dose* fashion, where all of the tracer is added in one slug and detention time characteristics are determined based on the degree to which this initial slug spreads upon passage through facilities being tested. Normally, the step-dose method is a more desirable technique, but if feeding equipment is not available, the slug-dose method is used. The tracer concentrations are measured until the chemical approaches equilibrium in the step-dose method or until nearly all the chemical has passed in the slug-dose method. Selection of the sampling time intervals depends on the detention time to be tested. For short detention times, sample intervals would be correspondingly short since the tracer will pass through the basin quite rapidly. However, longer intervals are more appropriate for larger volumes, which may require testing over several hours. For step-dose methods, detention time characteristics can be determined from a plot of $C_m - C_B/C_0$ (dimensionless) vs. t (time), where C_m is the measured concentration, C_B is the background concentration, and C_0 is the concentration added. This graphic plot gives a direct indication of the percent of flow exiting at a given time. EPA criteria specify that contact time for CT be based on the time when the curve passes 10 percent. In other words, 10 percent of the flow exits by this time, while 90 percent of flow is retained for a longer period. The time when 10 percent of the flow has exited may be determined from the graphic plot as the time where the dimensionless parameter is equal to 0.10. Note that this time, designated as T_{10}, is often much less than the theoretical contact time computed based on flow and volume. Slug-dose methods require additional mathematical manipulation to develop detention time requirements. These methods are described in the EPA guidance criteria (4).

When carrying out ozone contact tank tests, either air or oxygen can be used in place of ozone if degradation of the tracer is a problem. Also, EPA has developed specific guidance information for evaluating CT in ozone contactors, as discussed in Chapter 7. For flocculation tanks, several tests might be performed in which the mixers are run at varying mixing intensities over the range expected in actual operation.

Distribution System Detention

Evaluation of detention in the distribution system is important for several reasons.

- *In-pipe retention time to the first customer can augment time available for CT credit for primary disinfection.* Care must be exercised in defining "first customer" since the water treatment plant is often considered to be that first customer. In some cases, this limitation can be overcome by providing a small separate contact volume for the plant potable water system, thereby gaining credit in the distribution mains for time to the next customer connection. Unlike basins and tankage found in treatment plants, pipelines do not exhibit significant short circuiting, and it is possible to directly compute available time without performing tracer studies.

- *Areas of prolonged storage or dead ends in the distribution system may represent problems with undesirably long detention times that can both deplete disinfection residuals and increase the opportunity to form disinfection byproducts.*

Baseline Treatment Process Uses for Disinfection Goals

In many treatment systems, evaluation of interactions with baseline treatment processes is a fundamental consideration in the development of a complete disinfection program. Baseline processes can strongly influence disinfection approaches in two major areas:

- A reduction in the level of microbial contaminants can be achieved by baseline particulate removal processes, thereby augmenting the disinfection process and providing an additional barrier to the intrusion of pathogens.
- A reduction in the level of organic material can be achieved, thereby reducing the precursor content available for reaction with disinfectants. These processes also can reduce disinfectant demands, permitting more stable residuals at lower dosages. This yields benefits for disinfection as well as for disinfection byproduct goals.

The credits of several baseline processes for removal of microbial contaminants are illustrated by the following log removal criteria (4):

	Log Removal Credits	
Baseline Treatment	*Giardia*	Viruses
Conventional	2.5	2.0
Slow sand filtration	2.0	1.0
Direct filtration	2.0	2.0
DE filtration	2.0	1.0

These values assume a well-operated plant, from a reasonably good source of supply, which may mean that improvements in plant operation first have to be completed in the baseline processes, as described in Chapter 12.

Conventional treatment is defined by the guidance manual as a two-stage solids removal process that achieves some reduction in the cyst and virus content in a first-stage process such as coagulation and sedimentation, followed by filtration as the second solids removal stage. All other baseline particulate removal processes involve single stage separation in which the entire separated solids loading must be held in the media—hence the lower removal and inactivation credit available for these processes. In any comparison of alternative water treatment processes, incorporation of the appropriate log removal credits would be the first step in the development of integrated disinfection procedures since disinfecting agents would be required to provide the additional log removals to yield the total 3.0 and 4.0 levels required for *Giardia* and viruses, respectively. While the lower viral removal credits for several of the processes result in a requirement of 2 log or greater inactivation, the adjusted CT for *Giardia* can still be more restrictive for the use of chlorine and chlorine dioxide. On the other hand, adjusted CT for viruses can be more restrictive for using chloramines and ozone under some conditions.

The capability of various baseline processes for achieving reductions in organic precursor content can affect baseline process selection in some situations. Coagulation processes that are involved in conventional and direct filtration approaches have a capability for achieving significant reductions in precursors. In some cases, conventional processes may have some advantages over direct filtration by allowing flexibility for higher coagulant doses for improved precursor removal. Slow sand filters have less flexibility for precursor removal, although some process modifications using ozone or GAC can be considered, as discussed in Chapter 11. Precoat filtration processes generally offer less opportunity for precursor reduction. However, developing technologies for precoat filtration give promise for precursor and byproduct removal using preozonation and resin substitution for precoat material. Certain membrane processes are applicable for reducing precursor content, and very high levels of removal can be achieved where conditions merit this type of process.

Each situation should be evaluated to determine viable baseline processes or process modifications. The benefits of pathogen and precursor removal capabilities should then be determined based on site-specific conditions and needs. These capabilities can then be incorporated into a comprehensive evaluation of the full range of treatment goals for the alternative baseline processes.

Where an existing baseline system is in place, consideration might be given to alternative systems that yield greater advantages for pathogen and precursor removal. However, this can be quite costly, and such a decision should be reached only after a comprehensive review of all factors that relate to treatment. Many treatment trains have been developed over a number of years of operation based on considerable experience in dealing with site-specific problems, so some caution should be exercised before making changes. Such background development may include several generations of valuable operator experience that may not always be apparent at first glance.

Disinfection Alternatives

Inactivation Goals

The critical aspects of planning a disinfection program involve methods required to achieve both primary and secondary disinfection goals. These goals are somewhat different in character, and it is important to make distinctions in the disinfecting attributes required for each.

Primary Disinfection

The goal of primary disinfection is to provide a barrier at the water treatment plant to prevent the introduction of waterborne pathogens into the distribution system. The present regulatory trend is to judge disinfecting effectiveness by the CT criteria, which combines the effect of disinfectant concentration, *C*, and time of contact, *T*, into a single term.

Secondary Disinfection

The goals of secondary disinfection are to prevent subsequent growth of microbes in the distribution system and to provide a degree of protection in the event of contamination by cross-connection.

The key to accomplishing an effective primary disinfection strategy is the capability for applying an adequate concentration for the time required to achieve the CT. This capability will be determined by the volume of the pertinent plant components and critical retention time characteristics, such as T_{10}. Where the available T_{10} is low, disinfectant concentration must be higher to meet the CT criteria. Where basin configurations result in a high level of short circuiting, the total volume and resulting average retention time for the major portion of the flow may be quite high as compared with T_{10}. This may result in longer periods of contact between a disinfectant and the bulk of the flow. This type of condition, therefore, can have the undesired effects not only of requiring a higher disinfectant concentration, but also of extending the contact time with the bulk of the plant flow. The combination of these conditions tends to exacerbate potential problems with the increased formation of disinfection byproducts. The extent of concern for these conditions will vary depending on the type of disinfectant and the quantity of precursors present and the levels to which disinfection byproducts must be reduced. Where necessary, contacting conditions can be improved by providing internal baffling to increase detention in existing basins or by the installation of separate contacting facilities designed for efficient flow retention characteristics.

The predominant choices for primary disinfection are free chlorine, chlorine dioxide, and ozone. Ultraviolet radiation and potassium permanganate might be considered under certain circumstances, while chloramine use for these goals may be limited by low disinfecting capabilities for both *Giardia* and viruses. The principal features of each of these disinfecting agents are summarized in Tables 2–2 and 13–1.

The choice of primary disinfecting agents will be affected by the types of pathogen categories that need to be addressed. For instance, while both *Giardia* and viruses are concerns in most surface waters, *Giardia* may not be a concern in many groundwater supplies. This may allow consideration of disinfecting technologies such as ultraviolet radiation, which are considered to be effective for viruses but not *Giardia*. High mineral content in many groundwaters, however, may produce scaling of ultraviolet lamps that could interfere with ultraviolet radiation. Where applicable, pilot studies should be considered to determine the potential for such scaling.

Disinfectants applied to achieve secondary disinfecting goals must have a capability to maintain a residual for the much longer periods involved in the transport of water through distribution system piping and

TABLE 13–1. Principal Features of Alternative Disinfectants

Free Chlorine

Method of Delivery/Formation

- Typically delivered as a compressed gas or as a granular or solution form of hypochlorite.

Disinfection Properties

- Effective primary disinfectant for all pathogen categories. Disinfecting capability is lower as pH increases.
- Provides a relatively stable residual for secondary disinfection. Stability improves as reactivity is reduced by increased pH.

Oxidation Properties/Nondisinfection Uses

- Direct oxidation of iron relatively rapid at normal pH range of 6 to 8.
- Direct oxidation of manganese slow below pH 8, but chlorine is effective in maintaining an oxidized coating on filter media that removes manganese by adsorption.
- Oxidant for sulfides.
- Effective for oxidation of color.
- Selective effectiveness for removing taste and odor compounds. However, some compounds, notably phenols, react to produce more severe tastes and odors.
- Can be an effective biocide to limit nuisance biological growths in raw water pipelines and in water treatment plants. Continuous addition can be required to be effective for control of zebra mussels and Asiatic clams in raw water pipelines (11, 12).

TABLE 13–1. *(Continued)*

Disinfection Byproducts and Disinfectant Residuals

- Forms THMs and a wide variety of other halogenated byproducts.
- THM formation increases while total formation of halogenated byproducts decreases with increased pH.
- The presence of bromide ions will increase THM formation, but not necessarily overall halogenated byproduct formation.
- In general, THMs can represent about half and haloacetic acid about a quarter of the halogenated byproducts formed, but specific proportions may vary on a site-specific basis. The relative carcinogenicity of specific byproducts could be radically different from the relative concentrations and caution should be taken not to place too much emphasis on THMs.

Chloramines

Method of Delivery/Formation

- Formed on-site by reactions between chlorine and ammonia. Control of chlorine to ammonia ratio is critical.

Disinfection Properties

- Weak primary disinfectant for *Giardia* and viruses.
- Provides a relatively stable residual for secondary disinfection.
- Sequence of adding chlorine vs. ammonia is site and goal specific.
- Presence of organic nitrogen may result in formation of organic chloramines, which may not be effective disinfectants.

Oxidation Properties/Nondisinfection Uses

- Not effective oxidant for iron and manganese.
- Not effective oxidant for sulfides.
- Not effective oxidant for color.
- Applicable to avoid some taste and odor conditions that occur due to reaction of free chlorine with substances found in some source waters. Not effective for oxidizing existing taste and odor compounds.
- Can be an effective biocide to limit nuisance biological growths in raw water pipelines and in water treatment plants.

Disinfection Byproducts and Disinfectant Residuals

- Chloramine residuals may be toxic in excess quantities. Warnings may also be required for specific situations: e.g., chloramines can be fatal for dialysis patients. Warnings are also required for aquarium owners.
- Byproduct formation is influenced by the sequence of chlorine and ammonia addition. Lowest byproduct formation occurs with preformed chloramines.
- Presence of organic nitrogen can result in the formation of *N*-chloroorganics.
- Less known about specific byproducts than those of free chlorine. THM formation is minimal, but other halogenated organics appear to be formed. Formation of aldehyde odor–related compounds has been reported in the presence of certain amino acids. Measures of mutagenic activity have typically been lower for chloramine byproducts than for chlorine byproducts. However, the opposite trend has sometimes been observed. Epidemiologic study has suggested lower incidence of bladder cancer when chloramines are used, as compared with free chlorine.

(continued)

TABLE 13–1. *(Continued)*

Chlorine Dioxide

Method of Delivery/Formation

- Typically formed on site by reactions between sodium chlorite and chlorine. Generation reaction requires precise control to minimize impurities.

Disinfection Properties

- Strong primary disinfectant for all pathogen categories. Does not readily react with ammonia, which does not cause a chlorine dioxide demand. This contrasts with high demand of ammonia for free chlorine. However, sulfides, organics, iron, and manganese can exert significant chlorine dioxide demands, and the relative demand as compared with free chlorine is site specific.
- Capable of providing a stable residual for secondary disinfection. Dosage limitations to address health concerns, however, restrict allowable dosages below levels required for reliable residuals.

Oxidation Properties/Nondisinfection Uses

- Direct oxidation of iron.
- Direct oxidation of manganese. However, small colloidal precipitate may be formed that can penetrate filtration processes. This may require use in conjunction with a coagulant that will agglomerate the precipitate into particles of a filterable size.
- Oxidation of sulfides.
- Can be effective for removal of color.
- Can be effective for oxidation of a wide range of taste and odor compounds, including some that are a problem with free chlorine. These include phenols.
- Can be an effective biocide to limit nuisance biological growths in raw water pipelines and in water treatment plants. Applicability will be dictated by chlorine dioxide demand; high demand will dictate an excess dosage to provide a biocidal residual.

Disinfection Byproducts and Disinfectant Residuals

- Significant health concern for excess residual levels of chlorine dioxide and its degradation products, chlorate and chlorite. Oxidation/disinfection reactions initially lead to the formation of chlorite as the primary degradation product; chloride represents most of the remaining chlorine component of chlorine dioxide. Further degradation of chlorite can lead to the formation of chlorate over time, a reaction that can be accelerated in the presence of sunlight. To resolve residual concerns, consideration may be given to methods for removing chlorine dioxide residuals after a period of contact for primary disinfection.
- THM formation is typically limited. Can occur to an extent in the presence of bromide, but this type of formation is less than that occurring with ozone due to the need for light to catalyze the reaction. THM formation can also occur if excess chlorine is used to generate chlorine dioxide. This effect might be reduced by adding ammonia to react with any excess chlorine.
- Overall formation of halogenated byproducts is low. However, a number of nonhalogenated byproducts may be formed, including carboxylic acids, aldehydes, and quinones. Formation of bromide-related halogenated organics is often lower than occurs with ozone.
- A limited degree of chlorine dioxide off-gassing can occur at some taps, resulting in reactions with some organics in carpets and other household vapors to create objectionable odors as a byproduct.

TABLE 13–1. *(Continued)*

Ozone

Method of Delivery/Formation

- Generated on-site by passing air or oxygen through equipment which provides an electrical discharge.
- Requires special contacting basins to dissolve in water. Contacting basins are covered and the off-gas is collected for treatment in ozone destruction systems.
- Air preparation systems that produce high quality air and adequate cooling systems are critical design considerations. These affect efficiency of operation and protect ozone generation equipment from damage.
- Molecular ozone can react directly or form a hydroxyl radical, which then becomes a reactive agent with some oxidation properties that differ from those of molecular ozone.

Disinfection Properties

- Effective primary disinfectant for all pathogen categories. Disinfecting capability at a given residual not significantly affected by pH. However, residuals dissipate more rapidly as pH is increased, thereby causing some degradation of ozone disinfection at higher pH levels.
- Not suitable for secondary disinfection due to rapid degradation of residual.

Oxidation Properties/Nondisinfection Uses

- Can react directly or be modified by reactions that form hydroxyl radicals.
- Important to understand that pH can have a significant effect on ozone oxidation characteristics due to increased formation of hydroxyl radicals with increased pH. Specific hydroxyl radical–based applications use hydrogen peroxide and UV light as agents to intentionally induce radical formation. Improves performance for some goals, but can diminish performance for others; beneficial use is site specific. Presence of carbonate and bicarbonate ions can diminish the effectiveness of hydroxyl radical processes and are a consideration in developing dosage requirements and assessing applicability.
- Direct oxidation of iron.
- Direct oxidation of manganese. Soluble permanganate or small colloidal precipitates may be formed that can penetrate filtration processes. Depending on filtration conditions, ozonation may have to be followed by coagulation to agglomerate colloids or by methods for removing permanganate. Hydroxyl radical–based applications can be less effective for manganese removal, requiring higher doses.
- Effective for oxidation of color. Hydroxyl radical–based applications can be less effective for color removal.
- Selectively effective for taste and odor compounds by direct reaction. Conversion to hydroxyl radical–based applications can yield significant improvements in effectiveness for some difficult compounds including MIB and geosmin.
- Limited effectiveness as a biocide for control of nuisance growths due to rapid loss of residual.
- Can provide enhanced coagulation that can substantially reduce coagulant dosages at some locations.

Disinfection Byproducts and Disinfectant Residuals

- Does not form THMs and other halogenated byproducts directly; indirect formation may occur when bromide is present.

(continued)

TABLE 13–1. *(Continued)*

- A number of nonhalogenated byproducts are formed, including aldehydes, epoxides, and peroxides. Bromate and iodate formation are also significant concerns when bromide and iodide are present.
- A high level of BDOC formation can occur with the addition of ozone and can increase the need for adding treatment processes for BDOC removal.
- Can cause fruity tastes and odors at small doses in the presence of some compounds.
- Can reduce THM formation under some conditions, while increasing THM formation under others. Requires site-specific evaluation.
- Mutagenic activity formed by ozonation is typically less than that formed by free chlorine. Higher mutagenic activity may occur in application of ozone at pretreatment locations as compared to downstream points of addition.

Potassium Permanganate

Method of Delivery/Formation

- Delivered as potassium permanganate cystals.

Disinfection Properties

- Moderate disinfecting capability for viruses.
- Not suitable for secondary disinfection due to rapid degradation of residual.

Oxidation Properties/Nondisinfection Uses

- Direct oxidation of iron.
- Direct oxidation of manganese; can also enhance deposition of manganese on filter media. Action is improved by addition of potassium permanganate prior to coagulants, allowing coagulation to agglomerate precipitates into particles of filterable size.
- Capable of some taste and odor reduction.

Disinfection Byproducts and Disinfectant Residuals

- Limited formation of byproducts; formation of some oxidation byproducts is possible.
- Can achieve some reduction in THM formation potential in some cases where used to reduce chlorine demand or by direct reaction with some natural organic matter.

Ultraviolet Radiation

Method of Delivery/Formation

- Radiation is produced by ultraviolet lamps.
- Scaling conditions produced by water hardness may coat lamp surfaces and interfere with radiation. Effectiveness of cleaning needs to be evaluated.

Disinfection Properties

- Effective primary disinfectant for viruses. Not effective for *Giardia*. May have application where water source does not have a *Giardia* risk. Possible application for groundwater.
- Not suitable for secondary disinfection due to lack of residual.

Oxidation Properties/Nondisinfection Uses

- Most nondisinfection applications are limited. Can interact with ozone to produce a hydroxyl radical–based approach.

Disinfection Byproducts and Disinfectant Residuals

- Byproducts not an issue. Some photochemical interactions might be possible. No residuals are formed.

storage. Only two chlorine-based disinfecting agents, free chlorine and chloramines, can provide reliable residuals required to meet secondary disinfection goals for most waters. Another possibility, chlorine dioxide, also has a capability for providing a lasting disinfecting residual, but concerns for health effects associated with residuals are likely to limit its use as a secondary disinfectant.

Byproduct Objectives

A major consideration in evaluating disinfection alternatives is the effect on the formation of disinfection byproducts. Early evaluations focused on elimination of byproducts associated with free chlorine, most notably the trihalomethanes. However, a broader perspective is currently necessary, so it is important to consider the characteristic of byproducts formed by each alternative disinfecting agent. As previously discussed, the outcome of using an alternative to free chlorine is the possibility of the formation of different byproducts, not simply of the elimination of more familiar byproducts. It is essential that the comparative health concerns of the respective byproducts be considered. As discussed in Chapter 3, understanding of these health concerns is influenced by limitations on both the analytical methods for identifying and characterizing byproducts as well as on the methodology and lack of data needed for assessing the health effects of byproducts once they have been identified. Therefore, there is a significant potential for growth in the basic scientific understanding of the relative concerns of byproducts associated with each disinfecting agent. This will necessitate decisions based on the best information available at the time of evaluation, with flexibility to allow changes in disinfection approaches if developing scientific understanding dictates future changes.

In addition to formation of byproducts, another important consideration in evaluating alternative disinfecting agents is biodegradable organic carbon (BDOC) or assimilable organic carbon (AOC). Simply stated, BDOC or AOC levels can be significantly increased when strong oxidants change the characteristics of natural organic matter to a form that is more biodegradable. Added levels of BDOC or AOC can lead to undesirable microbial regrowth in distribution systems or intensify existing regrowth problems. While it is not often so labeled, in essence biodegradable organic matter is another form of byproduct. As discussed in Chapter 7, ozone may significantly increase BDOC or AOC levels depending on source water quality, but this effect occurs with other disinfectants as well. Where regrowth is a potential, formation of excess quantities of biodegradable organic matter may require a biodegradation process. Biodegradation is discussed in general in Chapter 2, and removal methods are discussed in Chapter 11. Costs for such processes will need to be considered, therefore, in any comparisons between disinfectants/oxidants.

Nondisinfection Objectives

Other areas that need to be thoroughly considered in evaluating alternative disinfectants relate to effects on treatment goals other than disinfection. These can include enhanced coagulation; oxidation of iron, manganese, and sulfide; in-plant control of nuisance biogrowths; removal of color; and control of tastes and odors. Each of these goals may be necessary for producing an acceptable finished water product and will need to be evaluated for each disinfection approach. Specific nondisinfection attributes of chlorine, chloramines, chlorine dioxide, and ozone are discussed in Chapters 4, 5, 6, and 7, respectively. Use of potassium permanaganate as an alternative oxidizing chemical for nondisinfection goals is discussed in Chapter 8. This type of application could be adopted to reduce the use of disinfecting chemicals for achieving nondisinfection goals. Although there is a need for understanding the byproducts formed by potassium permanganate as well, in some cases such application may help to reduce overall plant usage of disinfectants, thereby reducing overall byproduct formation.

Points of Disinfectant Application

With the growing need to develop alternative disinfection strategies to both control waterborne disease and limit the generation of byproducts, the point and the sequence of application of disinfectants has taken on more significance. In the past, disinfection concepts have not been as well defined and were often simply limited to the maintenance of a measurable residual at the plant and out in the distribution system. However, disinfection is now being considered in a much broader context, which requires considerable refinement in the planning of disinfection and the selection of the appropriate points of application.

The significance of the point or points of application of alternative disinfectants will vary with raw water quality, the particular baseline water treatment process, and the disinfecting agent under consideration. Initial design evaluation can consist of selection of alternative chemicals and points of application to achieve baseline treatment and the basic primary disinfection goal of pathogen kill. The effect of these alternatives on the formation of disinfection byproducts must then be considered. This evaluation is not entirely distinct from the evaluation of baseline processes, since there are usually interactions with baseline treatment systems that need to be considered. In fact, some of these interactions may ultimately cause a reevaluation of the baseline system to provide the approach or modification that better complements disinfection processes. An example would be selection of processes that are more effective in reducing oxidant demand or precursor content, thereby allowing for more effective use of disinfecting agents. As a part of these evaluations, in-plant tests or bench and pilot scale determinations may be needed to demonstrate which process combination best achieves the full range of objectives. Where necessary, modifications may be required in fine tuning the types of disinfectants used, the sequence of addition, and the location of chemical additions in the process train.

Except for ozone, all disinfectants may be added directly to the flow stream of the baseline treatment train to take advantage of the available mixing and detention in baseline plant structures. Use of ozone will require a separate, enclosed contact facility equipped to remove and destroy excess ozone. The separate facility would have to be inserted in the flow train at the desired point of ozone application, a condition that may be adversely affected by hydraulic limitations in existing plants if there is a shortage of head available.

Figure 13–4 shows typical addition points. Practically the only option available for slow sand filtration is postdisinfection in a contact chamber or in a clearwell that would provide the required detention. This is because most disinfectants provide a biocide action where predisinfection before the slow sand filter would tend to interfere with the biological character of the *schmutzdecke*, which is vital for effective slow sand filtration. An exception may occur in the case of ozone, which is highly reactive, can dissipate rapidly and can encourage *schmutzdecke* and other biological growth. As discussed in Chapter 11, preozonation can also improve the removal of color, TOC, and BDOC in slow sand filtration.

Conventional rapid rate filtration trains typically provide three possible points of disinfectant/oxidant application:

Pretreatment Location at the Head of the Plant

Disinfectant addition at this location can enhance flocculation; provide some advantages for primary disinfection as a result of detention through the remainder of the plant; achieve oxidative removal of undesired constituents such as color, tastes and odors, and iron and manganese; and achieve biocidal action to limit growths in downstream basins and in the filter media. A major advantage of this point of application is the opportunity for achieving combined pretreatment/disinfection goals along with the availability of greater contact time for achieving CT criteria. Some state agencies, however, are reluctant to grant CT credit prior to filtration. The major disadvantage of the pretreatment location is the higher level of disinfectant demand that can affect both disinfecting dosage re-

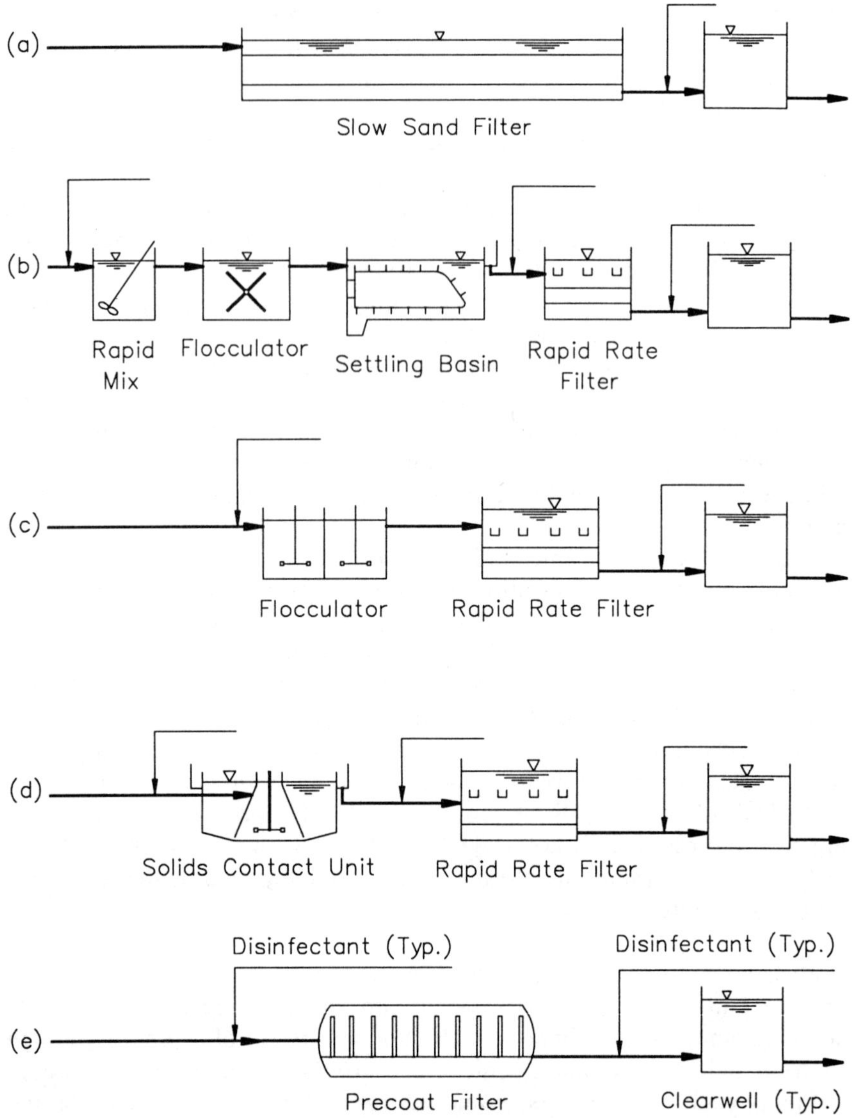

FIGURE 13–4. Typical water treatment process schematics: (a) slow sand filtration; (b) conventional rapid rate filtration; (c) direction filtration; (d) lime softening; (e) precoat fitration.

quirements and increase potential for byproduct formation, particularly where such demands are high. This is a consequence of both the higher disinfectant dose and the higher precursor levels in the raw water. Because of these adverse influences, addition at pretreatment locations will often be oriented more toward nondisinfection oxidation goals (i.e., iron, manganese, color, taste and odor removals, and enhanced coagulation) that might be accomplished at low to moderate disinfectant doses. In some situations, an alternative oxidant such as chlorine dioxide, ozone, or potassium permanganate might be used to partially or completely replace chlorine as an oxidant at this location. Where a disinfectant is added in pretreatment, some CT credit might also be gained, but a second downstream location, where conditions are more conducive to maintaining a reliable residual profile, may be more effective for achieving the bulk of the CT.

Prior to Filtration
This application point is available in two-stage rapid rate filtration systems that provide sedimentation or other first-stage solids removal processes ahead of filtration. Under these conditions, processes such as coagulation, flocculation, and first-stage solids removal can significantly reduce both disinfectant demand and the organic content associated with byproduct formation. This typically allows more efficient use of a disinfecting agent to achieve CT goals. Primary disinfection detention for this point of application is provided mainly by a contact chamber or clearwell storage, although some additional time can also be provided by filter influent structures and detention through the filters. Biocide action can be provided for the filter at this location along with an oxidized condition for maintaining an oxidized coating for manganese removal where this may be important. If these roles have been previously satisfied with chlorine, the need for alternative disinfectants to provide this capability should be confirmed prior to making any substitution.

After Filtration
At this location, detention is typically provided by the plant clearwell or by a separate contact chamber. Even where an upstream oxidant is added, this location may still be appropriate for achieving supplemental CT and for stabilizing disinfection residuals prior to introduction of flow into the distribution system.

Two points of application are available for the direct filtration process. Addition of a disinfectant in a pretreatment location (Figure 13–4) can be used both to enhance baseline treatment and to provide a biocide for the filter. Byproduct formation permitting, this application may provide primary disinfection, but a contact chamber or clearwell detention is likely to be required after the filters due to limited upstream tankage volume. Where concern for byproduct formation limits options, it may be possible to accomplish all or part of the treatment optimization and biocide goals with an oxidant like potassium permanganate; primary disinfection would then be accomplished with disinfectant addition and detention facilities after filtration using the second point of application shown on the flow diagram (Figure 13–4). Again, care must be exercised in assuring proper conditions for goals such as effective disinfection of pathogens and removal of manganese in cases where this is a concern.

Except for the implications of the relatively high pH levels generated within the process, application of disinfectants in the cold lime softening train may be considered to be similar to conventional treatment discussed above. Adjustments must be made for CT requirements as stipulated for pH variations in published criteria for free chlorine. Ozone residuals for complying with CT can also be difficult to maintain at elevated pH levels that frequently occur in softening; this effect on CT needs to be considered. In some locations pH adjustment may be appropriate to improve disinfectant performance. Requirements for a filter media biocide are often less common in cold lime softening, since the high pH can act to control growths. Adjustments of postsoftening pH may be required for effective ozonation.

In precoat filtration, disinfection is most often accomplished using a point of application and detention facilities after filtration. Under certain conditions, disinfectants might be used in a prefiltration location. One example is the use of ozone to condition particulates to improve filtration and color removal. In such cases, the primary purpose of the pretreatment additions would be to enhance the baseline process and not necessarily for achieving CT criteria for disinfection. Because of the provision of separate contacting facilities for ozone, however, it might also be possible to accomplish all or a part of the primary disinfection goals (CT) if sufficient detention time is provided in the ozone contact chamber. This decision will be influenced by the ozone demand at this location and its effect on the ozone dose required for meeting CT criteria.

Supplemental Precursor or DBP Removal Processes

Supplemental precursor removal strategies are those that achieve removals beyond that accomplished by normal baseline processes such as coagulation. Adsorption with activated carbon, for instance, is an example of a supplemental method for removal of organic precursors in water treatment. Where low-level removal of organics is sufficient, powdered activated carbon can sometimes accomplish such needed removals, but its effectiveness varies widely, so that specific testing would be required to confirm the removal capability. The tests would determine such parameters as quantity, mixing intensity, and contact time before or with flocculation that would be necessary. If greater removals are required, granular activated carbon might be considered, but the effectiveness and longevity of this process is also variable, and its applicability should be confirmed by testing as well. Initial tests can consist of determinations of equilibrium characteristics through GAC isotherms, which can then be followed with the RSSCT method for bench-scale evaluation of GAC column dynamics and, if warranted, by subsequent pilot testing. Care must be exercised to develop representative isotherm tests for use in these evaluations (2). In precoat filtration, some success has been experienced in reducing precursors by using synthetic resins (in powdered form) or PAC to supplement the precoat.

Preoxidants also can be considered for supplemental precursor removal. Under some conditions, ozone, chlorine dioxide, and potassium permanganate can achieve precursor reductions. These oxidants can also reduce the demand for chlorine and other downstream disinfectants, which allows for less byproduct formation and improved conditions for maintaining disinfecting residuals in meeting secondary disinfection goals.

The applicability of preoxidants for supplementary precursor removal is extremely variable, and care must be exercised to avoid an increase in precursor content when conditions or dosages are inappropriate (see Chapters 7 and 8). As a result, these alternatives require site-specific testing to ensure that the process is a reliable as well as cost-effective treatment.

Biodegradation processes can reduce precursor content as well as disinfectant demands. One previously mentioned process enhancement for this type of approach is the use of ozone prior to a biodegradation step to increase susceptibility to biodegradation, thereby increasing the overall removal capability of biodegradation processes.

Distribution System Evaluation

Distribution system evaluations primarily rely on existing distribution system data. Typically, these data can provide information on parameters such as coliforms, heterotrophic plate counts, and disinfectant residual. Past data can be compiled according to location in the distribution system to identify the points of highest bacteriological levels (not necessarily greater than applicable standards) or areas subject to low disinfectant residual. In many cases, these spots can then be compared with distribution system attributes using existing maps and hydraulic network models to help identify areas of low flow and the extremities within the system. Note that while dead ends can be easily identified as areas of concern, problems can occur at other locations where flow converges from opposite directions and at storage tanks. Low flow conditions occur at points of convergence due to lack of outflow.

More refined distribution system water quality models may be employed in some situations. These approaches can be relatively expensive and can involve a major effort to calibrate and maintain the model. Even where use of these models is contemplated, it would be helpful to prescreen data by the above approach in order to identify the important features to be modeled.

Laboratory methods also are available for comparative in-pipe evaluations of alternative secondary disinfection agents. These methods can include flow through pipe segments and rotating pipeline reactors, which are intended to simulate a variety of effects on in-pipe phenomena. The actual experience with and assessment of applicability of these methods is presently somewhat limited.

Resolution of microbial problems can be multifaceted and can require some of the following disinfection approaches:

- Rechlorination stations to maintain disinfecting residuals in areas where residual depletion is a problem
- Use of disinfectant with decreased reactivity to allow longer residual and improved disinfectant penetration of biofilm locations (e.g., increase pH when using free chlorine or conversion to chloramines in finished water)
- Improved corrosion control to minimize tuberculation and deposits that can shield microbes from disinfecting agents
- Improved hydraulic patterns in distribution system to reduce detention time
- Use of biodegradation processes to remove biodegradable organic material that can encourage microbial growth in the distribution system

Resolving Conflicting Disinfection Goals and Problems

Many of the conflicting issues have already been discussed in this chapter, such as creating new byproducts by changing disinfectants; reducing the concentration of iron, manganese, tastes and odors by deferring the disinfectant feed point; and increased formation of BDOC. Adjusting pH within water treatment plants also can have some important and sometimes conflicting effects that relate to meeting both disinfection and baseline treatment goals. These effects need careful consideration when evaluating conflicting goals as illustrated by the pH phenomena below.

Disinfection

The CT criteria for chlorine disinfection are affected by pH. Higher CT levels are required at higher pH. These considerations may have an effect on the selected pH through clearwells and other tankage being used for CT. In the case of ozone, pH levels that are too high result in rapid degradation and difficulty in maintaining sufficient residual for the time, *T*.

Coagulation

Coagulation processes are significantly affected by pH. For alum, an optimum region for turbidity removal is frequently in the pH range of 6 to 7, whereas an optimum pH of 5 to 6 is frequently better for removal of organic constituents such as color and disinfection byproduct precursors. Sometimes a compromise pH near 6 is best for coagulation to achieve both goals. As long as adequate turbidity removals can be achieved, a lower pH might be selected if disinfection byproduct precursor removal is critical.

Aluminum Residual

The need for control of aluminum residual is a result of the concerns over the possible adverse effects of excess residuals. Excessive levels of aluminum in filter effluent may be an indicator of partial dissolution of floc and associated deterioration in the filtration process. Optimum pH to minimize aluminum solubilization in the coagulation and filtration processes is in the range of 6 to 7. Emphasizing this need in treatment could conflict with the use of a very low pH for disinfection byproduct precursor removal.

Manganese Removal

In many plants, a critical location for manganese removal is within the filters. By maintaining an oxidant residual, an oxidized coating can be developed in the media that initially adsorbs and subsequently oxidizes any residual manganese that remains at this point in the process. Although not widely appreciated, this removal process can provide an extremely important polishing step for achieving low manganese levels in finished water. The key factor in this process is the maintenance of an oxidized residual across the filters using chlorine (or some other oxidant). While a slightly alkaline pH would also be desired to enhance this phenomenon, it may conflict with goals for minimizing aluminum residuals and obtaining effective turbidity removal. Therefore, some compromise to a lower-than-desired pH level for manganese removal may need to be considered. The outcome of these several adjustments may require careful consideration in some cases. However, effective removal of manganese by these oxidized coatings has been reported to still occur at slightly acidic pH levels of 6.1 to 6.2 as long as an oxidant is applied (8).

Corrosion Control

pH can have a significant effect on most corrosion control strategies where corrosion approaches can require a pH greater than 7.0 and sometimes higher than 8.0 in finished water. This higher pH frequently conflicts with the pH desired across filtration processes both for achieving turbidity removal and minimizing aluminum residuals and also reduces the primary disinfection effectiveness of free chlorine, which results in a higher CT requirement. As a consequence, adjustment to a higher pH for corrosion control might best be deferred to a point downstream of filtration. The optimum pH for some corrosion control agents, such as zinc orthophosphate, can be lower than for other approaches so each case must be considered on its own merits.

Disinfection Byproduct Formation

Formation of disinfection byproducts is significantly affected by pH. THM levels are increased as pH is raised, a factor that has caused some utilities to keep pH levels as low as possible. While this strategy may be appropriate for controlling THMs, it may not be helpful in controlling the larger range of halogenated byproducts where formation is increased as pH is reduced. These effects may need to be reviewed with the development of new standards for disinfection byproducts.

INITIAL TESTING

Development of a disinfection test program is somewhat site and situation specific, but there are general features applicable to most situations. These are summarized in Figure 13–5. Most programs begin with a compilation of existing data and a review of plant treatment objectives and operating experiences. This typically involves significant input from the plant staff. Many aspects of water treatment are site specific, and the personal observations of plant operations staff can be an important starting point for determining the background on cause and effect of treatment features. Additional analysis can then be undertaken to further characterize the treatment system with respect to specific areas of interest.

Initial testing typically involves screening tests to determine demands for alternative disinfectants and levels of byproduct formation as indi-

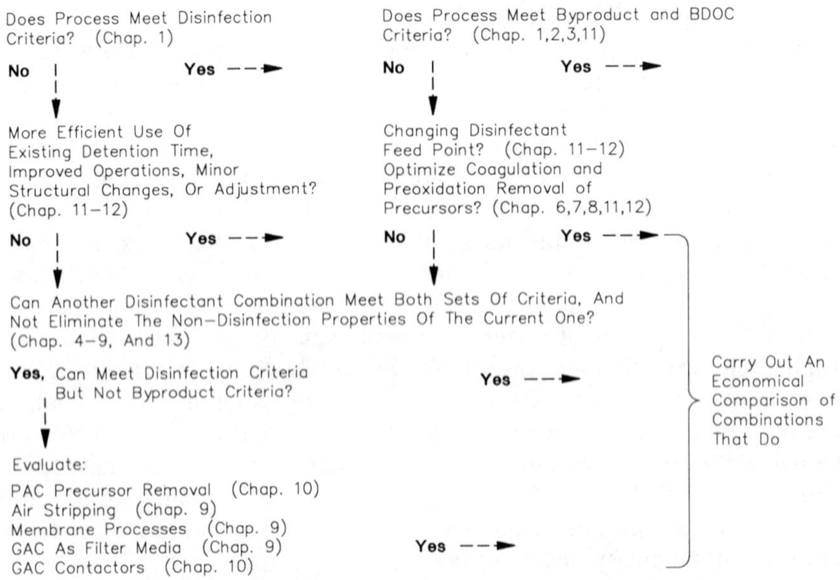

FIGURE 13–5. Typical disinfection strategy decision process.

cated by THM and TOX results. Analyses of additional byproducts may be indicated depending on future regulations. Where applicable, the relative effectiveness as oxidants for constituents such as iron, manganese, color, and tastes and odor should be determined. This testing phase may also involve evaluation of organic precursor removal in existing baseline processes. In many plants, evaluation of alternative coagulants and coagulant conditions such as pH and dosage may also be included. The particular parameters of interest in this type of testing are reduction in the THM formation potential and other measures of precursor content. Because of the time and labor required for obtaining results for the formation potential of specific byproducts such as THM, surrogate parameters such as UV absorbance at 254 μm should be considered for some of the initial screening assessments. These screening assessments can be used to select priority chemical dosage ranges and conditions for more detailed testing (see Figure 11–4 for an example of the use of UV absorbance at 254 μm for selecting a priority dosage condition). Choice of other areas of testing may become more site specific. These will depend on specific water quality conditions and treatment goals.

Many initial testing programs rely on bench scale testing. These methods require minimal support equipment and have considerable flexibility for examining a wide range of process options at a relatively low cost compared to requirements for more equipment and work-intensive procedures in continuous pilot testing. Initial bench scale testing can also provide details that will allow for more informed planning of a subsequent and more costly pilot study phase.

The primary purpose of a test program is to determine the relative effectiveness of applicable disinfection and baseline treatment alternatives for achieving the full range of water quality objectives, including control of pathogens and disinfection byproducts. In essence, bench scale testing involves the simulation of dynamic processes using a batch-type approach. In the actual water treatment plant or even in a pilot scale simulation, a continuous water flow at a fixed rate is subjected to a succession of process steps. In the bench scale or batch approach, each of the pertinent process steps must be simulated in individual vessels using chemical feed and mixing in proportion to that used in the full-scale application. While these tests frequently require some manipulation to more closely simulate process sequences, considerable advantage is provided in terms of simplicity and flexibility.

Time between steps sometimes is an important factor in disinfection bench tests, especially where more than one disinfectant or oxidizing chemical is to be employed. Some reactions are almost instantaneous; others take more time. Unless the timing between batch tests is reasonably correct, the initial reaction of a first-stage disinfectant may proceed so far that the byproducts or byproduct ratios produced by the addition of a second oxidant may not indicate true process conditions. These features should be considered in establishing test protocols.

Not all process steps can be reasonably simulated on a bench scale, but some simulations are more important than others so that this limitation may not present an insurmountable obstacle. For instance, although it would not be possible to exactly simulate precoat or rapid rate filtration on a bench scale for testing of alternative applications of disinfectants, it is possible for the bench procedure to produce a general simulation. Data for removals of constituents such as precursors, color, iron, and manganese can be reasonably indicated, and a general indication of tendencies for turbidity removal can be obtained. However, simulation of precise levels of turbidity and particle removal is not possible using these approaches. Larger-scale alternative methods must be employed where these questions can be specifically addressed.

Meaningful bench scale simulations of certain phenomena are more difficult to achieve. An example would be a test situation where preparation of the disinfectant itself involves a dynamic process such as the generation of small quantities of chlorine dioxide for bench scale use. The generation of ozone is also a dynamic process, but in this case flow through ozone pilot testing should be considered in place of bench scale for initial testing. Pilot facilities will require a pump and connecting piping or hose to deliver flow to a pilot contacting column that can be made portable for repeated use.

In general, bench tests of disinfectants may be divided into two categories:

1. *Chemical addition following initial treatment by baseline processes.* Samples are subjected to alternative baseline process simulations such as coagulation and sedimentation. The primary objective of this testing is to evaluate benefits of baseline processes on subsequent disinfection processes. Typical of the beneficial effects afforded by baseline processes are reduced disinfectant demand and removal of a portion of the disinfection byproduct precursors.
2. *Predisinfection (and/or oxidation) prior to or in conjunction with baseline processes.* A typical objective of these evaluations is to evaluate the effects of disinfectant/oxidant alternatives for enhancing baseline process goals. Possible nondisinfection benefits that can be achieved by this approach are improved coagulation; oxidation of iron, manganese, and sulfides; removal of tastes and odors; removal of color; and enhanced removal of disinfection byproduct precursors.

Baseline Process Tests

Benchtop procedures such as jar testing are part of accepted water treatment practice. This text, therefore, concentrates on specific procedures that relate more specifically to disinfection practice. Where possible, components of an existing baseline process train can provide samples to be used for disinfection tests, thereby avoiding the need for simulations of baseline processes. This approach should be used as much as possible to avoid problems with scale-up and also simplify test procedures.

A readily available tool used to prepare and analyze baseline process samples is the standard jar test assembly with variable speed mixers. Where chemical addition alternatives may precede filtration, the filter sample would be prepared in the jar test assembly. A Buchner funnel apparatus (as shown in Figure 13–6) for large samples or filter funnels can be used to simulate filtration. Note that the intent of this approach is to provide a general simulation of filtration effects as a basis for initial testing of a baseline system to compare relative effects of alternative disinfection

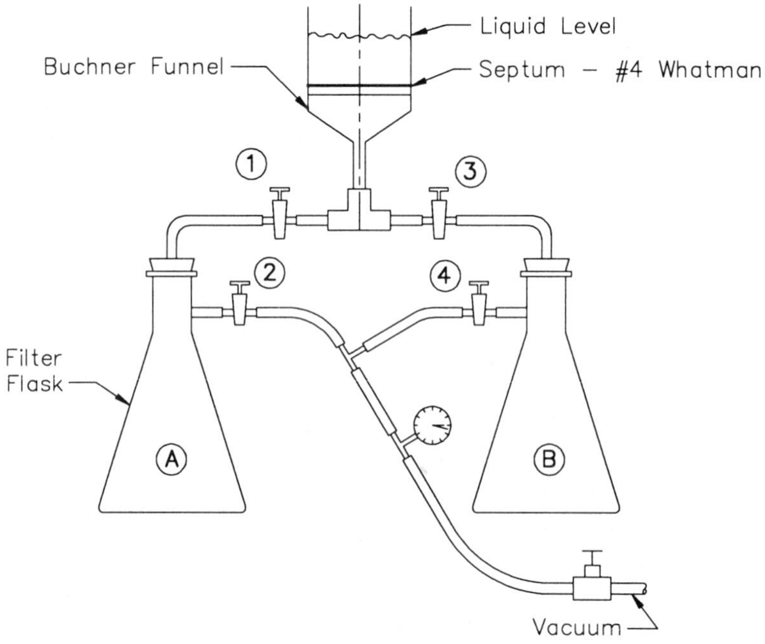

FIGURE 13–6. Buchner funnel filter arrangement.

approaches. As previously discussed, other larger-scale methods may be required for more definitive simulation of the actual filtration process for specific turbidity- and particle-removal characteristics. Test procedures will vary with the type filtration process described below.

Precoat (DE) Filtration

The principal variable in bench scale precoat filter tests is the grade or size of media. The sequential steps for the precoat filter sample preparation are shown in Table 13–2. As indicated, a media such as the Johns-Manville Hyflow grade, a common gradation in drinking water treatment, would be used first. The filtrate (Step 10) then would be checked for turbidity. If the turbidity is higher than a desired target level, the test sample preparation should be repeated using the next finer grade DE until a sample with less than target level of turbidity is achieved. That sample is then used for subsequent disinfection tests. While a reasonably achieved target level in precoat filtration of many waters is 0.2 NTU, some variations in target levels may be necessary for differing water quality characteristics. For the most part, most DE filter applications can achieve target

TABLE 13–2. Buchner Funnel Test Procedure—Precoat Filtration Sample Preparation[a,b,c]

Procedure (see Figure 13–6)

1. In a separate beaker, stir the diatomaceous earth admixture (Hyflow Grade or equivalent, about 4 to 8 g/l) into liquid to be filtered in 4-inch diameter-funnel.
2. Close all valves.
3. Turn on vacuum.
4. Open valves 1 and 2.
5. Pour slurry into funnel.
6. Adjust vacuum to desired flow (slow and steady to maintain liquid depth over septum).
7. When enough slurry is filtered to form a precoat on the septum, open valves 3 and 4.
8. Close valves 1 and 2.
9. Remove filter flask A and pour contents into Buchner funnel.
10. Use filtrate in flask B for subsequent disinfection tests.

[a] The liquid level in the Buchner funnel must be kept as high as possible at all times to avoid disturbing the precoat as new slurry is added.
[b] If the filter cake is allowed to become dry, cracking will occur and filtrate quality may not be acceptable.
[c] A glass fiber filter should be used in place of the Whatman #4 paper filter where disinfection byproduct formation testing is to be performed. Otherwise, some organic material may be eluted from the paper filter.

levels much lower than the EPA criteria for precoat filters, set at 1.0 NTU for 95 percent of samples (4). Some states, however, may stipulate more stringent criteria, so regulatory and other site-specific factors will need to be considered to determine a reasonable target turbidity for each case.

For some source waters it is advantageous to use preozonation for achieving certain oxidation related benefits. Ozone can be effective in conditioning colloidal particulates for more effective precoat filter removal. Ozone in this application also may achieve primary disinfection goals. Either bench scale or short term pilot scale methods of ozone addition can be used in a test sequence to both condition the particulates for filtering and provide a sample that will be useful to determine byproduct generated by a secondary disinfectant, such as chlorine or chloramines. Such tests may also be used to determine ozone demand.

Additives or amendments to the precoat are sometimes used to remove source water organic matter. The more common additives are PAC and ground synthetic adsorbing resins. The ratio of such additives is generally on the order of 50 percent and more of the precoat used. In the precoat filter sample preparation, PAC or resin would be added to the admixture in Step 1 (Table 13–3) in varying proportions for the subsequent disinfection tests. The objective here would be to reduce organics sufficiently to achieve acceptable byproduct levels for the selected disin-

TABLE 13–3. Buchner Funnel Test Procedure—Granular Filtration Sample Preparation[a,b,c]

Procedure (see Figure 13–6)

1. In a separate beaker, stir the diatomaceous earth admixture (Hyflow Grade, about 4 to 8 g/l), pour into 1-liter coagulated sample (from jar test) and mix slowly.
2. Close all valves.
3. Turn on vacuum.
4. Open valves 1 and 2.
5. Pour slurry into funnel.
6. Adjust vacuum to desired flow (slow and steady to maintain liquid depth over septum).
7. When enough slurry is filtered to form a precoat on the septum, open valves 3 and 4.
8. Close valves 1 and 2.
9. Remove filter flask A and pour contents into Buchner funnel.
10. Use filtrate in flask B for subsequent disinfection tests.

[a] The liquid level in the Buchner funnel must be kept as high as possible at all times to avoid disturbing the precoat as new slurry is added.
[b] If the filter cake is allowed to become dry, cracking will occur and filtrate quality may not be acceptable.
[c] A glass fiber filter should be used in place of the Whatman #4 paper filter where disinfection byproduct formation tests are being performed. Otherwise, some organic material may be eluted from the paper filter.

fectants. It should be noted that the bench scale resin tests will yield only general qualitative results. The effectiveness of resin in removing organics over a prolonged filter run can be determined only in pilot testing.

Rapid Rate Filters

The basic jar test procedure can be used to simulate many features of the rapid rate filter process. Under this procedure, coagulants and other chemicals are added to a sample, then mixed and settled. Supernatant is withdrawn as the finished product for analysis. In general, this approach yields a relatively well-clarified supernatant that can yield reasonable approximations of most phenomena. The approach and assembly shown in Figure 13–6 for the precoat filter can often be used to simulate filtration where large quantities of filtered water are desired. Alternatively, use of a paper filter that has been rinsed with distilled water such as a Whatman #40, can effectively simulate the effects of filtration where small quantities of filtered water are needed for subsequent testing. Where THM or other DEP formation analyses are to be performed, a 1 μm glass fiber should be used to avoid leaching of organics from the filter paper. Sand/granular media approaches also are viable (9).

In the case of the Buchner funnel filtration approach for simulating rapid rate filtration, the coagulated sample would be prepared using jar test equipment as shown in Table 13–3. Alternative coagulants or alternative amounts of coagulants would be prepared and would serve as the base for the admixture in Step 1. The DE additive simply helps to improve the porosity of the coagulated admixture, thereby permitting a reasonable rate of filtration.

If it proves difficult to attain the desired target turbidity with the Buchner funnel test (typically 0.10 to 0.20 NTU), a finer grade of DE may be used. Care must be exercised in this test, however, to be sure that the use of finer DE does not permit the addition of less coagulant than would normally be required for actual rapid rate filtration. Its role in this test is primarily to facilitate filtration to prepare samples for subsequent testing of alternative disinfectants for treatment of filtered water.

The rapid rate filter sample would be prepared in the same manner described regardless of whether the direct filtration or the conventional two-stage solids removal mode was employed in actual treatment.

Cold Lime Softening

Except for the precipitation of hardness, the cold lime softening baseline process tests would be the same as those for the rapid rate filter described above. In this case the jar tests involve the addition of lime to precipitate hardness. If solids contact systems are to be used, solids levels are allowed to build up in full scale units by internal recycle that enhances the softening reaction. This recycle can be simulated in jar testing by running a series of tests in which the supernatant is poured off, saving the sludge from each test step, thereby allowing sludge buildup in the jar. This can be repeated over three to four test steps before a supernatant sample is finally collected for analysis and further testing.

If coagulants, such as ferric chloride, are to be used to enhance the settling of the precipitates, the coagulants should be added to the test jar to simulate the sequence of additions in the process as closely as possible. For instance, if hardness is to be removed in a solids contact type unit, lime might be added to the process flow before it enters the unit or directly to the internal mixing zone of the unit itself. A coagulant aid also might be added directly to the same mixing zone, or it might be added in an in-line coagulation mode to the settled effluent entering the filter. The first test step can simulate the sequence of chemical additions and levels of mixing and settling provided in actual process. If a coagulant is to be added to the filter influent, a 2.0-liter settled sample might be drained from the initial test jar for transfer to a second jar for coagulant addition and mixing. This second sample could then be filtered by one of the methods described for rapid rate filtration. Note that in all cases, only the supernatant should be added to the filter, since precipitated lime tends to clog the filters.

Disinfectant Evaluations

The essential features of the disinfection tests include mixing the disinfectant at the desired concentration and then holding the mixture for the detention time that would be afforded in actual treatment. Table 13–4 lists some common combinations of disinfectants that might be tested. Combinations selected for testing may be reduced by considering some of the effects of the characteristics listed in Table 13–1.

For many of the basic disinfection simulations, a jar test apparatus will suffice, although other mixing arrangements can be used as well. Two-liter square beakers available for use with this equipment generally provide sufficient volume for a full range of testing. This equipment has versatility for evaluating a number of phenomena that require the addition and mixing of chemical disinfecting agents in a source water. In this type

TABLE 13–4. Typical Disinfection Combinations That Can Be Tested During Bench Tests[a,b,c]

Run	Pretreatment Addition	Intermediate Addition	Posttreatment Addition
A	None	None	Chlorine or chloramine
B	None	Chlorine	Chlorine, chloramine, or none
C	Chlorine	None	Chlorine, chloramine, or none
D	Potassium permanganate	Chlorine	Chlorine, chloramine, or none
E	Ozone	None	Chlorine or chloramine
F	Ozone	Ozone	Chlorine or chloramine
G	None	Ozone	Chlorine or chloramine
H	Ozone/PAC	Chlorine or none	Chlorine, chloramine, or none
I	PAC	Chlorine	Chlorine, chloramine, or none
J	Chlorine dioxide	None	Chlorine or chloramine
K	Chlorine dioxide/PAC	Chlorine or none	Chlorine, chloramine, or none

[a] Various disinfection combinations can be tested during a jar test. These illustrate some general combinations that can be considered.

[b] Typical addition sequences would consist of the following:

Pretreatment addition. Chemicals added either prior to or in conjunction with the coagulants. Some chemicals, such as potassium permanganate or PAC, may include a prescribed contacting time prior to coagulant addition.

Intermediate addition. Chemicals added to supernatant collected following the settling period.

Posttreatment addition. Chemicals added following intermediate addition. These additions may follow a filtration simulation.

[c] For postchloramination, add ammonia after proper contact with free chlorine. Different prechlorine contact times and alternative sequences of chlorine and ammonia addition can be evaluated for effects on disinfection byproduct formation (see Chapter 5).

of testing, different dosages of either a single disinfectant or several disinfectants can be tested in parallel. Typically, tests should start by determining the demand. A measured amount of disinfectant should be added, followed by rapid stirring for about 1 minute. After the stirring is halted, a sample can be removed and tested for an initial residual. The holding period should simulate actual detention, although additional samples can be obtained as desired to assess the residual profile over time.

Samples also can be withdrawn for analysis of disinfection byproduct formation. However, care must be exercised in the mixing and storage of these samples, since some of these byproducts are volatile and can be displaced from open vessels into the air. Air space–free bottles should be used for storage of these samples over any period. In addition, care should be exercised in the mixing and transfer of samples. Where these samples are in contact with a disinfecting residual to determine the effect of an ongoing reaction, storage should be in the dark since light accelerates the dissipation of many disinfectants. Analyses can consist of initial byproduct formation as well as samples incubated over time to determine formation potential. A final disinfectant residual should be measured to ensure that the sample is exposed to the test disinfectant for the specified incubation period. It is also important to specify and control the pH and temperature at which a reaction is taking place.

Jar test equipment can be effectively used for all disinfectants except ozone. For ozone tests, bench scale testing can be achieved by bubbling ozone through a column of water. After an amount of ozone is bubbled to achieve the desired dosage simulation, the cylinder can be allowed to stand for the time that approximates detention in process. Samples may then be withdrawn for analysis. An excess of ozone often occurs in benchtop application. As a consequence, analysis of the ozonated/filtered sample for ozone byproducts would be more useful for qualitative rather than quantitative determinations. An alternative to this bench scale approach would be short-term pilot testing with continuous flow systems (1 to 10 gpm) that yield better approximations of the dosing conditions in a full-scale ozone system.

Where simulations require two or three successive bench scale operations conducted in sequence, it is important to observe or approximate the time that is expected to be provided for each step. This is especially important for the sequence of chlorine and ammonia additions to form chloramines. Time of contact also can be important for byproduct formation with other disinfecting agents and for oxidation reactions with constituents such as iron and manganese.

Analyses conducted to determine the byproducts generated by each disinfection step and by the total process train will depend on the disinfectant/oxidant combinations used. Byproducts that will be associated with the use of the different disinfectants have been discussed before. These are summarized in Table 13–1, along with several other nondisinfecting capabilities.

Surrogates

Many of the chemical analyses required for DBPs and their precursors are costly and require significant time for results to develop. As a result, it is often desirable to adopt surrogates for these contaminant determinations for screening tests and as a guide for day-to-day test programs. There are a number of surrogates available, discussed in detail in Chapter 3. These include TOC, DOC, TOX, UV absorbance at 254 nm, and color. Of these, both DOC and UV absorbance at 254 nm appear to be useful general indicators of organic precursor content, with UV absorbance at 254 nm being more practical for rapid results. UV absorbance at 254 nm also tends to yield better correlation for many situations. TOX can be a useful surrogate for halogenated disinfection byproducts not identified by selected specific analyses. The presence of certain nitrogen species (nonammonia components of total Kjeldahl nitrogen) can also be of interest for assessing variations in disinfectant demands and the potential for formation of byproducts such as organic chloramines. Other surrogates might be considered based on site-specific concerns.

Evaluation of Biodegradable Material

Increasing concerns for biogrowth in distribution systems are leading to a need to evaluate the biodegradable material that is associated with alternative treatment protocols. Most of the chemical disinfecting agents are capable of partially oxidizing naturally occurring organic matter to make it more biodegradable. This effect varies, with some disinfecting agents creating more of a problem than others. Ozone, in particular, has been observed to greatly increase the levels of biodegradable organic matter, so evaluations of these phenomena would be especially important for this disinfectant.

Two types of general testing methods have been developed, as discussed in Chapter 2. Original methods were based on level of growth of selected bacteria that are applied to the sample. Results were then converted to an equivalent level of growth for a defined organic food source. These original test methods were termed assimilable organic carbon (AOC), and results were expressed in terms of bacterial growth levels that corresponded to a given level of acetate as a food source, yielding AOC values in units of micrograms of acetate equivalents per liter.

More recently methods based on measured change in dissolved organic carbon (DOC) content have been developed. These methods involve the measurement of the change in DOC content that results from exposure of a sample to bacterial degradation. The quantity removed is termed biodegradable organic carbon (BDOC) and is expressed in terms of mg/l of DOC removed in the test. Several other measures of biodegradable organic material are available, including a coliform growth response procedure that has been developed by the U.S. EPA.

A variety of technique variations are available within each of the two general method categories. It is difficult to draw firm conclusions on the best technique to use, since these methods are still being developed. However, general conclusions can be reached with both AOC and BDOC methods as long as they are being performed by a competent laboratory. Trends of biodegradability can then be established for comparing the effects of different alternatives.

Stock Solutions

One critical feature of testing for both baseline and disinfection processes is the accuracy of chemical addition. Because such small volumes of chemicals are often used, an apparent slight error can have significant impact on the test results. It is important, therefore, to prepare stock solutions of the chemicals at appropriate dilutions that provide measurable volumes for addition. A wide range of chemicals might be used in the tests. Preparation of a few of the more common solutions is discussed below. Accuracy in measuring the chemicals added to solution is the most important feature in each preparation. It is also important to prepare fresh stock solutions to avoid inconsistencies and deterioration associated with aged solutions.

Alum Solution

The standard liquid alum solution is approximately 36° Baume providing 5.34 lb of filter alum in a gallon weighing 8.34 lb/gal × sp.gr. of 1.33 = 11.1 lb/gal of liquid or 49 percent. To make a 2 percent solution, add 15.8 ml to make 0.5 l. One ml of stock yields 10 mg/l when added to a 2 liter jar test beaker. It is important to note that alum in solutions of 1.0 percent or less will not provide accurate results, since the alum will usually preflocculate in the solution. This constraint should be recognized when these solutions are prepared.

Polymer Solution

Most liquid polymers have a concentration of approximately 1 g/ml or 10^6 mg/l. Both concentrated and diluted polymer solutions are viscous liquids that are most conveniently measured by use of disposable syringes. Adding 1 ml to 1 liter of water will produce a solution with a concentration of approximately 0.1 percent. This is a convenient dilution for many testing situations since 2 ml of this solution added to a standard 2 liter jar test beaker will produce a dosage of approximately 1.0 mg/l. For precision, adjustment to actual polymer dose can be achieved by multiplying this approximate dose by the specific gravity of the polymer.

While the above level of dilution is convenient for many liquid polymer compositions, some emulsion polymers are extremely viscous and need to be further diluted for proper handling. Dry polymers must be weighed and carefully added to an intensively stirred solution to ensure proper mixing. Additional details on polymer preparation are available in Ref. 9.

Chlorine Solution

Assume commercial bleach is 5 to 5.15 percent free chlorine. Dilute 1:100 to yield a solution of approximately 500 mg/l. Because some variation in bleach and stock solution contents can occur, the stock solution chlorine content should be specifically measured on each day of testing.

Ammonia Solution

Ammonium sulfate or ammonium chloride, both available as a salt, can be used to prepare ammonia stock solutions. Compute the ammonia concentration based on the nitrogen content of the salt.

Chlorine Dioxide Solution

Chlorine dioxide will need to be generated at the test site. It will irritate the mucous membrane and has a noxious effect similar to that of chlorine. Breathing chlorine dioxide vapor should be avoided, and the following procedures should be carried out in a well-ventilated area.

One method for generating chlorine dioxide in the laboratory is described in *Standard Methods* (10). An alternative method calls for the preparation of three dilute solutions of specified concentration. When these solutions are mixed in designated proportions, a dilute concentration of 1,000 ppm of chlorine dioxide is obtained. It is recommended that the three solutions be initially mixed to produce no more than 400 ml total and that the operation be carried out in a chemical hood. As experience and confidence in handling is obtained, the quantity can be increased.

The three solutions to be prepared are as follows:

- *Solution A, acid.* Add 5.0 g of 37 percent hydrochloric acid to demineralized water to make 1,000 ml.

- *Solution B, hypochlorite.* Add 31.4 g of 5.25 percent sodium hypochlorite solution diluted to 1,000 ml with demineralized water. As an alternate, 11.0 g of 15 percent sodium hypochlorite can be used.
- *Solution C, anthium dioxide.* Add 60 ml of 5 percent anthium dioxide (International Dioxide, Inc., Kingston, RI) to demineralized water to give 1,000 ml of solution.

Mix 200 ml of Solution A with 100 ml of Solution B. Stir well for 2 minutes. Add 100 ml of Solution C and continue stirring. Check the pH and be sure it is below 4.0. If it is not, add more Solution A.

The resulting mixture will turn yellow and will contain approximately 1,000 ppm of chlorine dioxide with little free chlorine. The solution should be stored in a brown glass bottle and kept at 40°F. The solution should be standardized on preparation and restandardized before each use since shelf life is short.

SUPPLEMENTAL TESTING AND EVALUATION

While bench scale test procedures can provide invaluable data for the planning and design of disinfection improvements, it is essential that the limitations of these tests be understood. The nature of these limitations will vary according to the particular source water and treatment features of each situation. Two basic limitations of bench scale testing are (1) capability to simulate dynamic treatment processes and (2) capability to evaluate long-term variations and future trends in source water quality.

Specific decisions are sometimes required to separate issues to be examined at bench scale from those to be explored in pilot studies. For example, bench scale isotherm tests to determine the effectiveness of GAC in removing source water organics will indicate removal possibilities, but will not provide specific criteria regarding system dynamics that can be important in the design and operation of prototype facilities. Determining such criteria will require flow through testing. Similarly, bench tests may be useful to indicate how ozonation may benefit a particular process train. However, because it is almost impossible to accurately control low rates of ozone feed, bench tests only give general indications of the required ozone dosage rates to achieve the desired results. Better indications can be achieved in short-term pilot tests, which can be considered as an alternative to bench test methods. In another area of evaluation, biodegradation methods for removal of BDOC require that a biogrowth be established in a test system. This is not well suited to batch systems and will require a continuous flow type of system with adequate time to establish biogrowth equilibrium.

The principal difficulties with disinfection studies in pilot plant operation are associated with maintaining continuous, steady flow of disinfectant addition. At the low rate of disinfectant addition, chemical pumps typically operate on a pulse feed mode. This slug-type chemical addition may give erratic results unless a process mixing or detention element is located downstream of the chemical feed point. Individual pilot plant situations must be reviewed to determine the most meaningful method of integrating the disinfection components of the overall process. To the extent possible, existing baseline treatment effluents should be used in order to avoid complexities of simulating baseline processes at a pilot testing scale. However, this may not be possible where alternative processes are to be tested in combination with disinfection processes.

No matter which scale of the testing is used, source water quality variations and trends are always a concern when developing design data. It is not unusual for test programs, even those of a year or more in duration, to take place at a time when source water quality is better than historical worst-case conditions. Many factors combine to affect source water quality. For example, annual variations in rainfall as well as inflow and outflow patterns can affect reservoir cycles in ways that affect algal growth patterns and chemical and biological cycles. Because worst-case conditions may not occur during a test period, some judgment may be required in evaluating data.

Source water quality during the period of a test program should serve as the benchmark to compare with past water quality extremes and anticipated future trends. Where seasonal influence on source water quality is significant, the benchmark data should include either a full 12-month period that encompasses the test period or testing that focuses on representative periods during the year. Anticipated future trends also might be estimated. For reservoir sources where a potential for increased eutrophication may exist, it may prove helpful to compare the benchmark water quality data with those of nearby watercourses where eutrophication may be more advanced than in the subject water source. Where limnological comparisons indicate a reasonable relationship, water samples from the nearby watercourse can be used in the disinfection test program to illustrate possible future treatment conditions. However, some care must be exercised in making these comparisons since internal reservoir dynamics can significantly influence water quality at the point of withdrawal. For example, reservoir outlet designs frequently allow multiple withdrawal levels. Water quality found in the surface of an eutrophic lake may not characterize conditions found at a lower level where withdrawal might be contemplated, so that effects at different depths may also have to be considered.

The general intent of the source water quality data review and comparison is to determine the relative effectiveness of alternative disinfection regimes in producing water with acceptable byproduct levels under extreme water quality conditions that have either occurred before or are expected to exist in the future. Where test data for extreme source water quality conditions are not available, more general methods will be necessary to estimate trends. Changes in byproduct levels must be estimated or extrapolated using available test data and predicted source quality trends. In the end, it may not prove practical to develop definitive estimates of future trends. In these situations, process flexibility features should be considered to allow flexibility in design to accommodate possible changes in treatment conditions. To the extent possible, watershed management and protection should be undertaken in order to limit adverse effects.

LONG-TERM PLANNING FOR DISINFECTION

Planning for disinfection involves both short- and long-term components. Short-term planning components generally involve specific criteria associated with existing or imminent regulations. These criteria provide specific targets for testing and evaluation as discussed throughout the preceding portion of this chapter. However, a broader long-term focus is also important in planning disinfection strategies; scientific understanding of many aspects of disinfection is still developing with no clear end point in sight. Critical areas of growing understanding include characterization of new waterborne diseases that continue to be discovered (Chapter 2), emerging understanding of microbial regrowth in distribution systems (Chapter 2), improving capability to identify increasing numbers of disinfection byproducts (Chapter 3), and ongoing development of methodologies for evaluating health effects (Chapter 3). It is likely that future regulations will develop over a long period as understanding improves in each of these areas. As a result, a long-term planning posture needs to be incorporated along with the more specific short-term steps being undertaken to meet identified regulatory criteria.

A critical element in long-term planning is *flexibility*. This often involves general planning concepts in plant design that frequently do not require major commitment in capital, such as the following:

1. Availability of additional site area to accommodate future treatment methodologies along with layout flexibility to accommodate appurtenant chemical storage and feed facilities.
2. Hydraulic concepts to allow the insertion of new processes in the treatment train in the future. This may require providing piping stubs,

additional head at critical points, and hydraulic structures that will allow flows to converge at convenient tee locations at which to insert or connect a new process. In this regard, many existing plants do not offer convenient connection locations between sedimentation basins and filters, which can make future insertion of a new process difficult. Complex piping arrangements in other portions of treatment plants can also create difficulties.

3. Deeper filter boxes to allow eventual conversion to deep bed GAC filter adsorber systems for achieving biodegradation. For example, an empty contact time of approximately 10 minutes might be desirable for this type of approach. If a filter is designed for a hydraulic loading of 4 gpm/sf, a media depth of 5.3 ft would yield a 10-minute empty bed contact. Additional media depth might be considered for a sand layer at the bottom of a filter to remove fine particles that are released from the GAC bed above and which may contain bacteria that are difficult to remove by disinfectants. (When GAC is used for biodegradation, GAC regeneration is not an issue and sand mixing with the GAC is not a problem.) Even if the initial media is installed to a lesser depth than that required by these criteria, the filter box can be designed for the ultimate media depth.

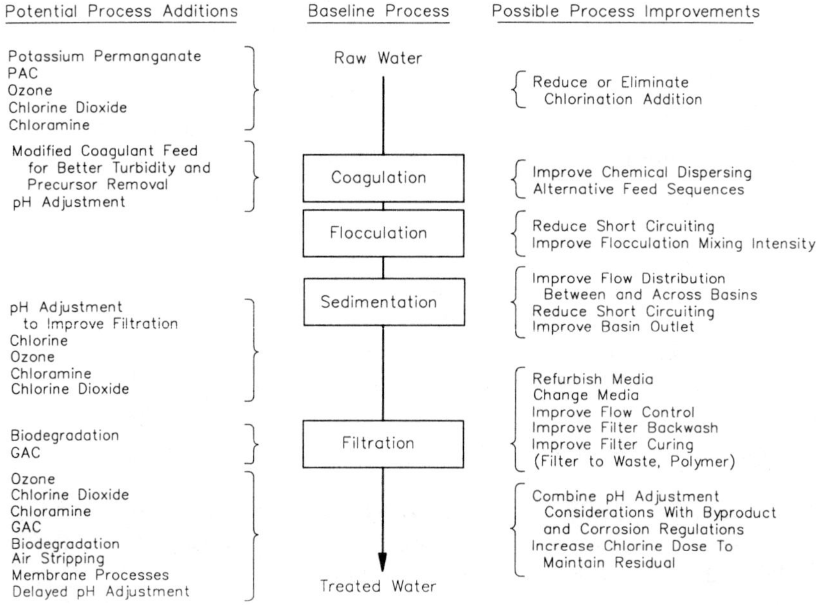

FIGURE 13–7. Potential adjustments and future process additions to baseline treatment.

4. Flexibility in electrical systems for simple modification to accommodate additional loads for possible power-intensive treatment technologies, such as ozone, ultraviolet radiation, and membrane processes.

Development of flexibility concepts involves an assessment of critical points for process incorporation. This is illustrated for a conventional rapid rate filtration system in Figure 13–7. In most cases, space and allowance for future incorporation of processes can be provided without specifically delineating which process combination might ultimately be selected.

References

1. Hudson, H. E., Jr. 1981. *Water clarification processes*. New York: Van Nostrand Reinhold.
2. Randtke, S. J., and V. L. Snoeyink. 1983. Evaluating GAC adsorptive capacity. *JAWWA* 75: 406–13.
3. McGuire, M. J., et al. 1989. *Optimization and economic evaluation of granular activated carbon removal*. Report for AWWA Research Foundation, Denver, CO.
4. U.S. EPA. 1989. *Guidance manual for compliance with the filtration and disinfection requirements for public water systems using surface water sources*. EPA 68-01-6989. Washington, DC: U.S. Environmental Protection Agency, Office of Drinking Water.
5. ASCE/AWWA. 1990. *Water treatment plant design*, 2nd ed. New York: McGraw-Hill.
6. White, G. C. 1986. *Handbook of chlorination*, 2nd ed. New York: Van Nostrand Reinhold.
7. Richard P. Arber Associates. 1986. City of Thornton pilot plant project: Treatment alternatives for controlling chlorinated organic contaminants in drinking water. Report under U.S. EPA Agreement CR-809333-01, September 1986.
8. Knocke, W. R., et al., 1990. Alternative oxidants for the removal of soluble iron and manganese. Report for AWWA Research Foundation, Denver, CO, March 1990.
9. Dentel, S. K., et al., 1989. *Polymer selection in water treatment plants*. Guidance manual prepared for AWWA Research Foundation, Denver, CO.
10. APHA, AWWA, WPCF. 1989. *Standard methods for the examination of water and wastewater*, 17th ed. Clesceri, et al., eds. Washington, DC: American Public Health Association.
11. Klerks, P. L., and P. C. Fraleigh. 1991. Controlling adult zebra mussels with oxidants. *JAWWA* 83(12): 92–100.
12. Cameron, G. N., J. M. Symons, S. R. Spencer, and J. Y. Ma. 1989. Minimizing THM formation during control of the Asiatic clan: A comparison of biocides. *JAWWA* 81(10): 53–62.

Index